THE FACTS
of LIFE

D1403945

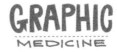

GRAPHIC
MEDICINE

Susan Merrill Squier and Ian Williams, General Editors

Editorial Collective
MK Czerwiec (Northwestern University)
Michael J. Green (Penn State University College of Medicine)
Kimberly R. Myers (Penn State University College of Medicine)
Scott T. Smith (Penn State University)

Books in the Graphic Medicine series are inspired by a growing awareness of the value of comics as an important resource for communicating about a range of issues broadly termed "medical." For healthcare practitioners, patients, families, and caregivers dealing with illness and disability, graphic narrative enlightens complicated or difficult experience. For scholars in literary, cultural, and comics studies, the genre articulates a complex and powerful analysis of illness, medicine, and disability and a rethinking of the boundaries of "health." The series includes original comics from artists and non-artists alike, such as self-reflective "graphic pathographies" or comics used in medical training and education, as well as monographic studies and edited collections from scholars, practitioners, and medical educators.

Other titles in the series:

MK Czerwiec, Ian Williams, Susan Merrill Squier, Michael J. Green, Kimberly R. Myers, and Scott T. Smith, *Graphic Medicine Manifesto*

Ian Williams, *The Bad Doctor: The Troubled Life and Times of Dr. Iwan James*

Peter Dunlap-Shohl, *My Degeneration: A Journey Through Parkinson's*

Aneurin Wright, *Things to Do in a Retirement Home Trailer Park: . . . When You're 29 and Unemployed*

Dana Walrath, *Aliceheimers: Alzheimer's Through the Looking Glass*

Lorenzo Servitje and Sherryl Vint, eds., *The Walking Med: Zombies and the Medical Image*

Henny Beaumont, *Hole in the Heart: Bringing Up Beth*

The FACTS of LIFE

Paula Knight

The Pennsylvania State University Press | University Park, Pennsylvania

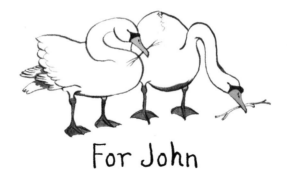

For John

Library of Congress Cataloging-in-Publication Data

Names: Knight, Paula, author, illustrator.
Title: Facts of life / Paula Knight.
Other titles: Graphic medicine.
Description: University Park, Pennsylvania : The Pennsylvania State University Press, 2016. | Series: Graphic medicine
Summary: "A graphic memoir and visual exploration of the stigma-inducing healthissues of miscarriage, childlessness, and chronic medical conditions" –Provided by publisher.
Identifiers: LCCN 2016051423 | ISBN 9780271078465 (pbk. : alk. paper)
Subjects: | MESH: Infertility, Female–psychology | Abortion, Habitual–psychology | Chronic Disease–psychology | Mothers--psychology | Social Stigma | Health Knowledge, Attitudes, Practice | Graphic Novels | Autobiography
Classification: LCC RG201 | NLM WP 17 | DDC 618.1/78--dc23
LC record available at https://lccn.loc.gov/2016051423

Printed in Latvia
Published by The Pennsylvania State University Press,
University Park, PA 16802-1003

First published by Myriad Editions,
www.myriadeditions.com

The Pennsylvania State University Press is a member of the Association of American University Presses.

It is the policy of The Pennsylvania State University Press to use acid-free paper. Publications on uncoated stock satisfy the minimum requirements of American National Standard for Information Sciences—Permanence of Paper for Printed Library Material, ANSI Z39.48–1992.

PROLOGUE

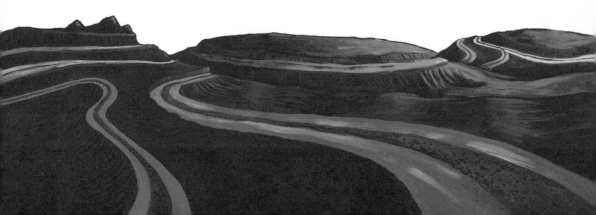

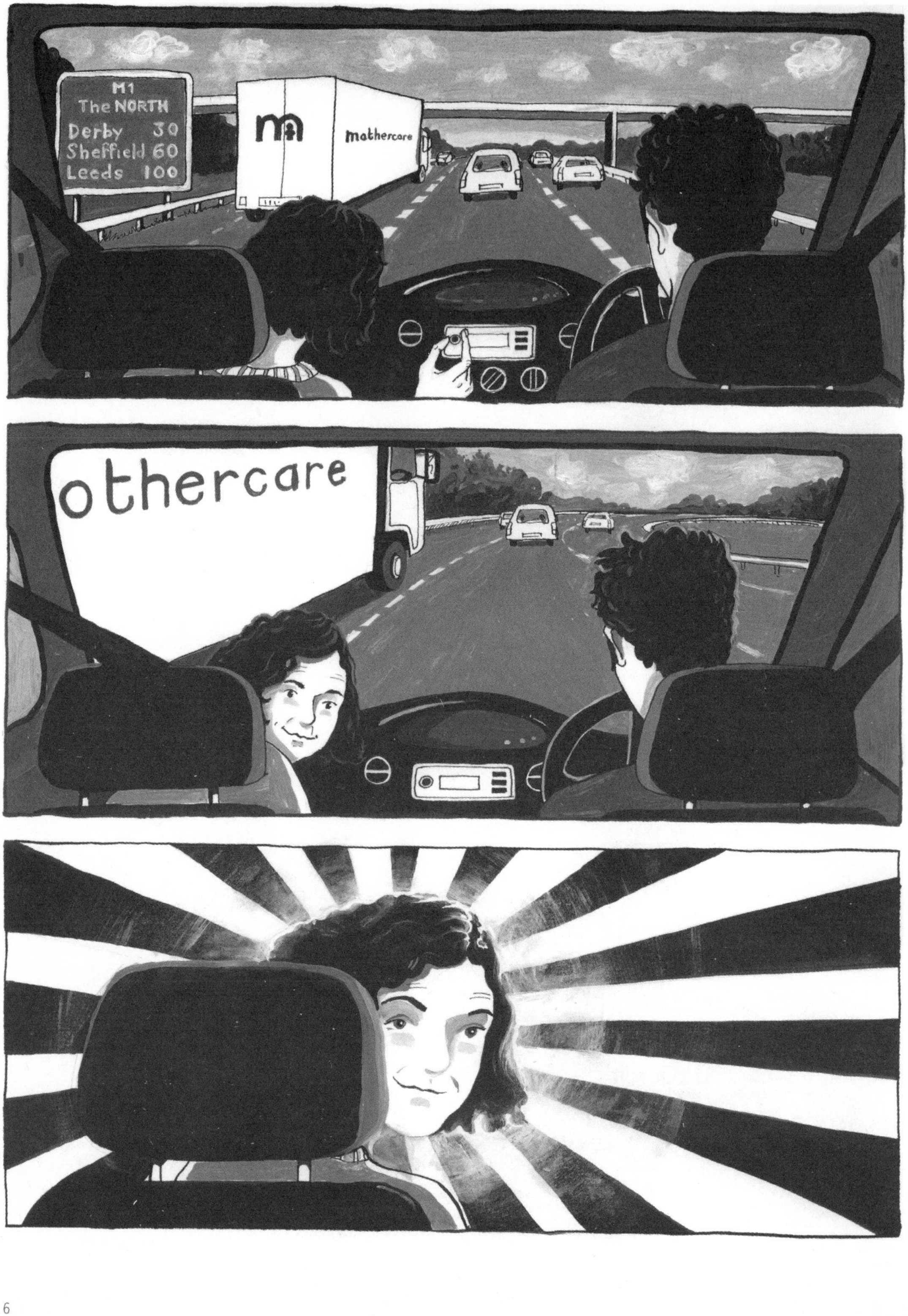

M1
The NORTH
Derby 30
Sheffield 60
Leeds 100
mothercare
othercare

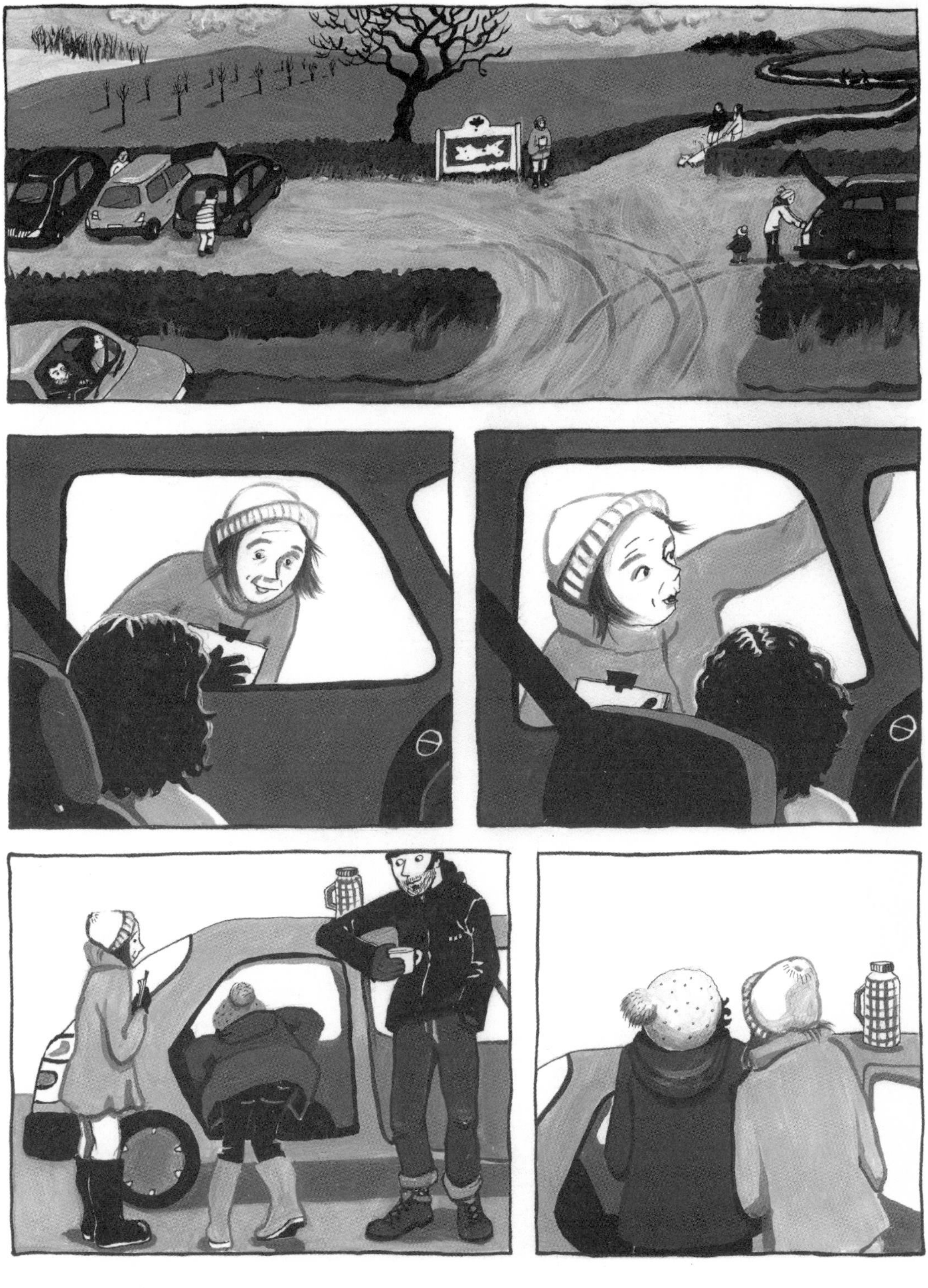

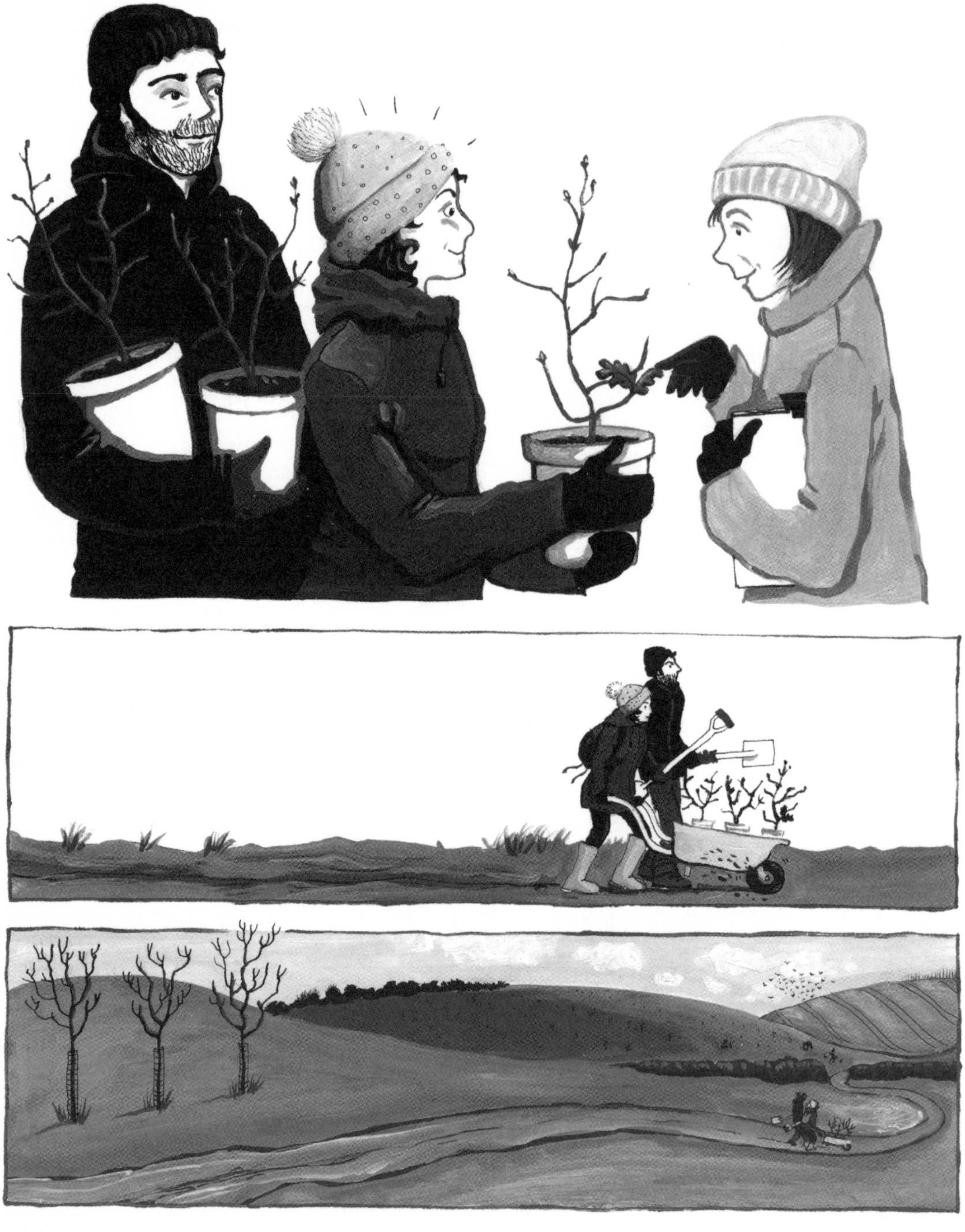

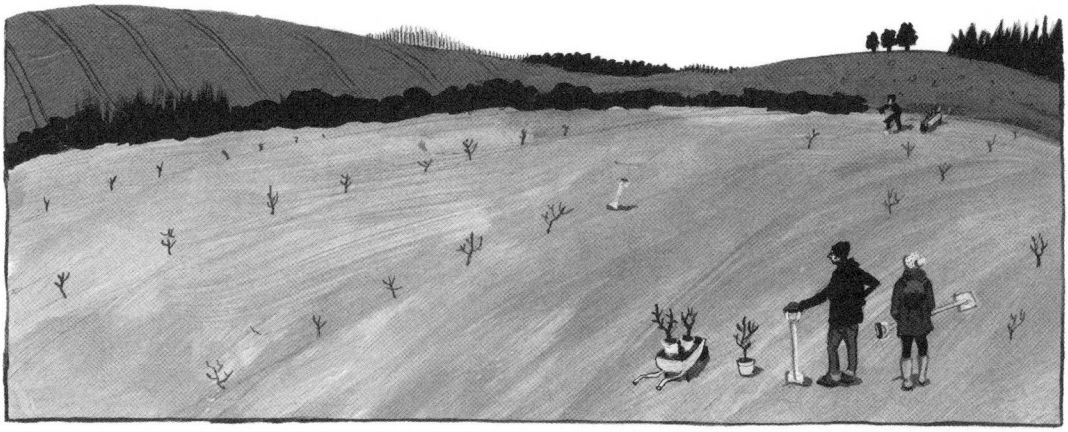

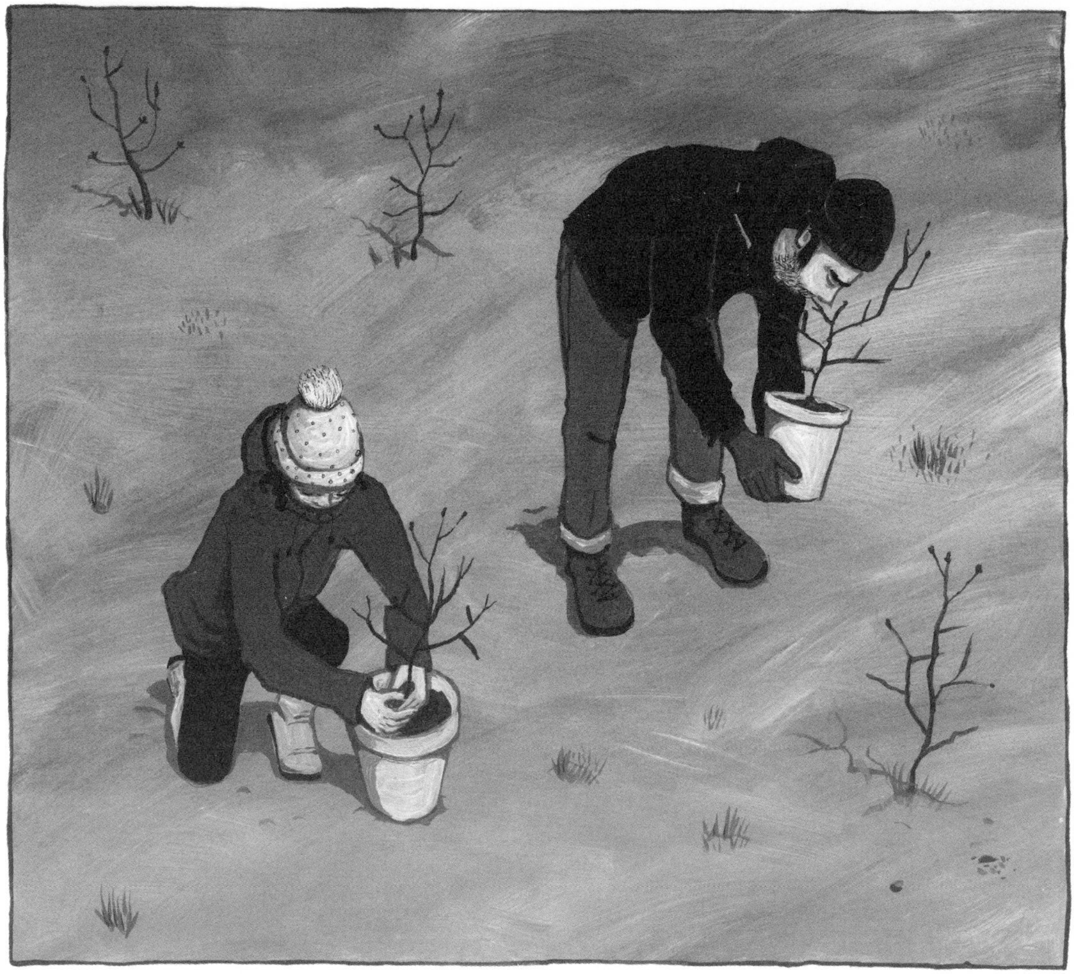

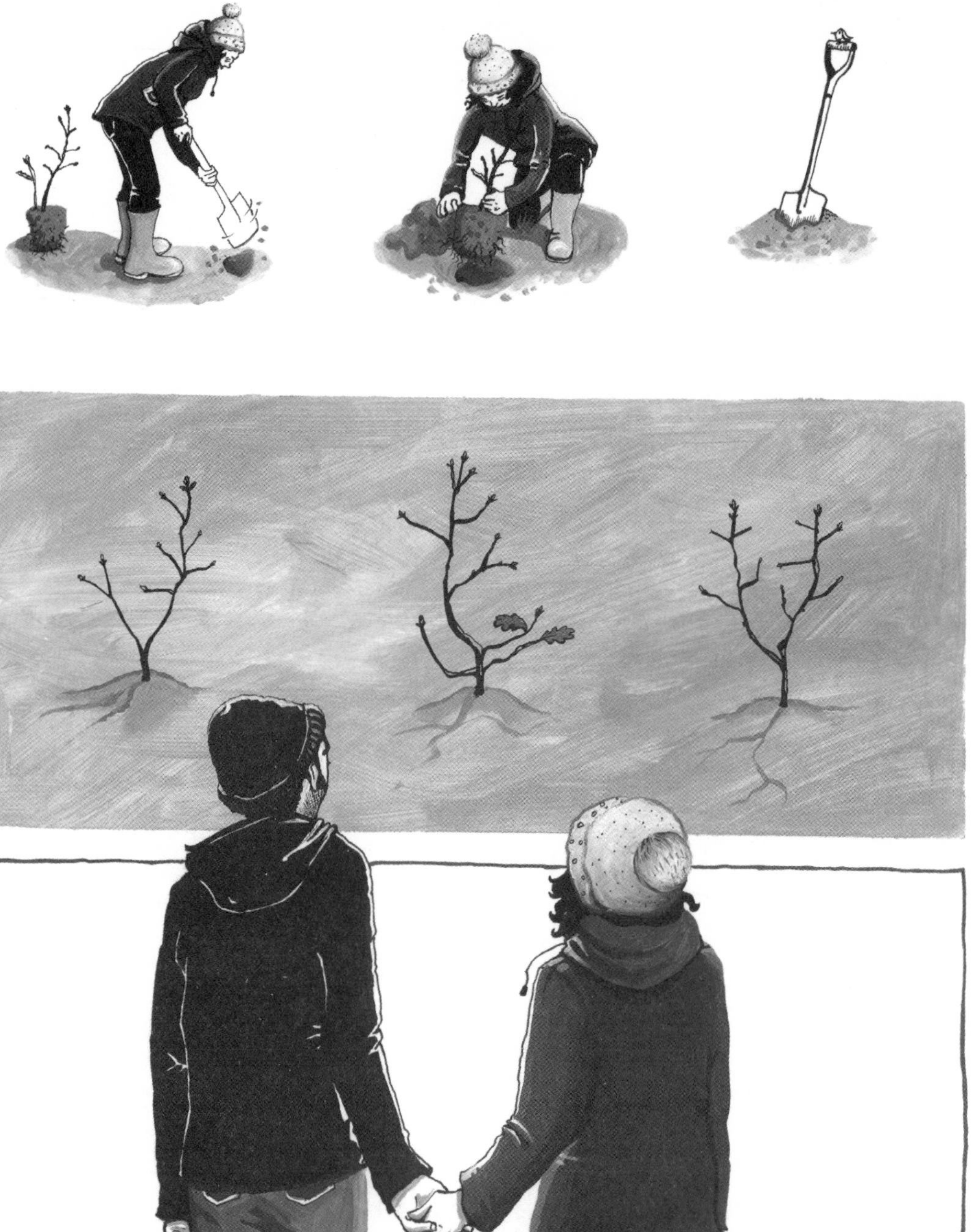

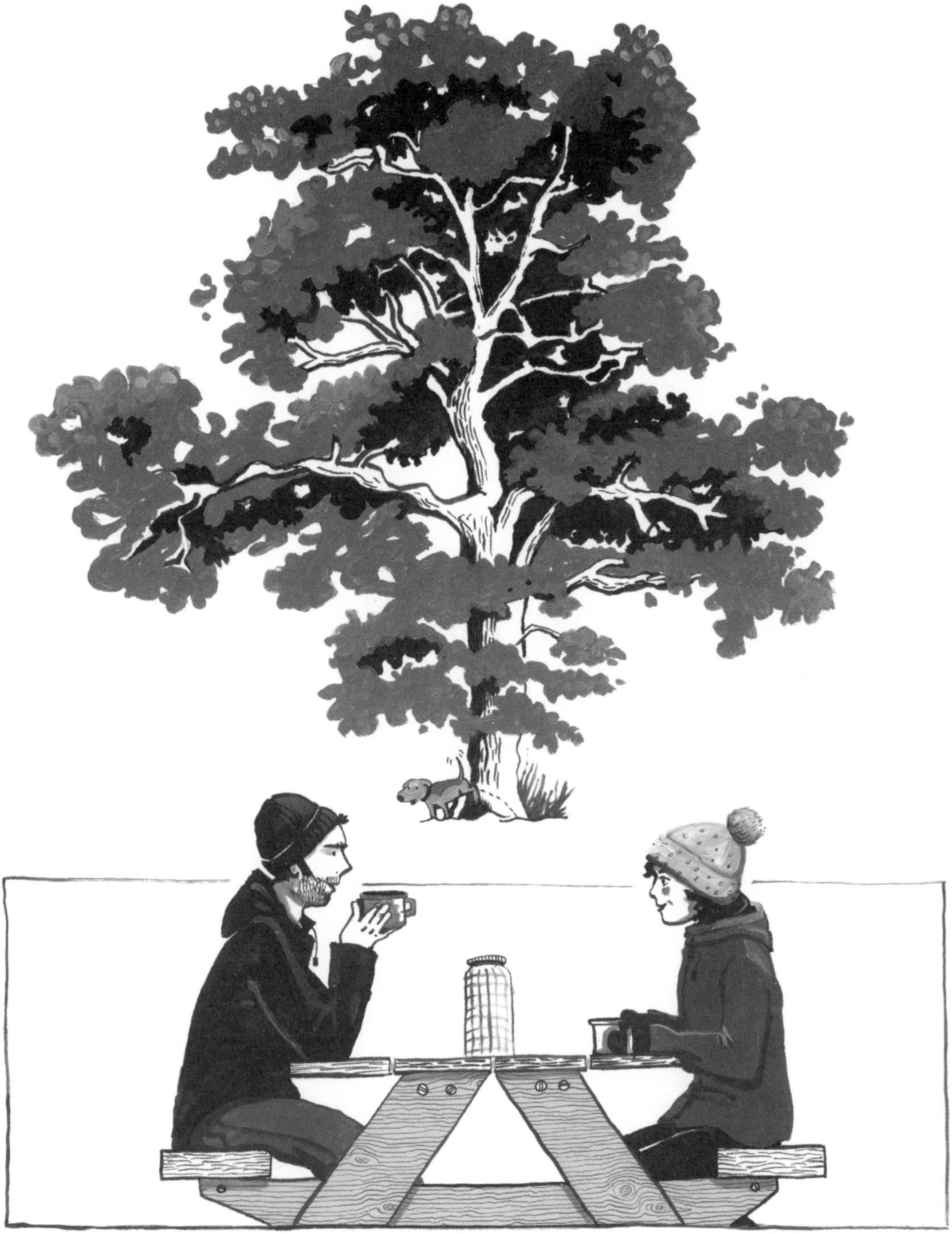

ONE

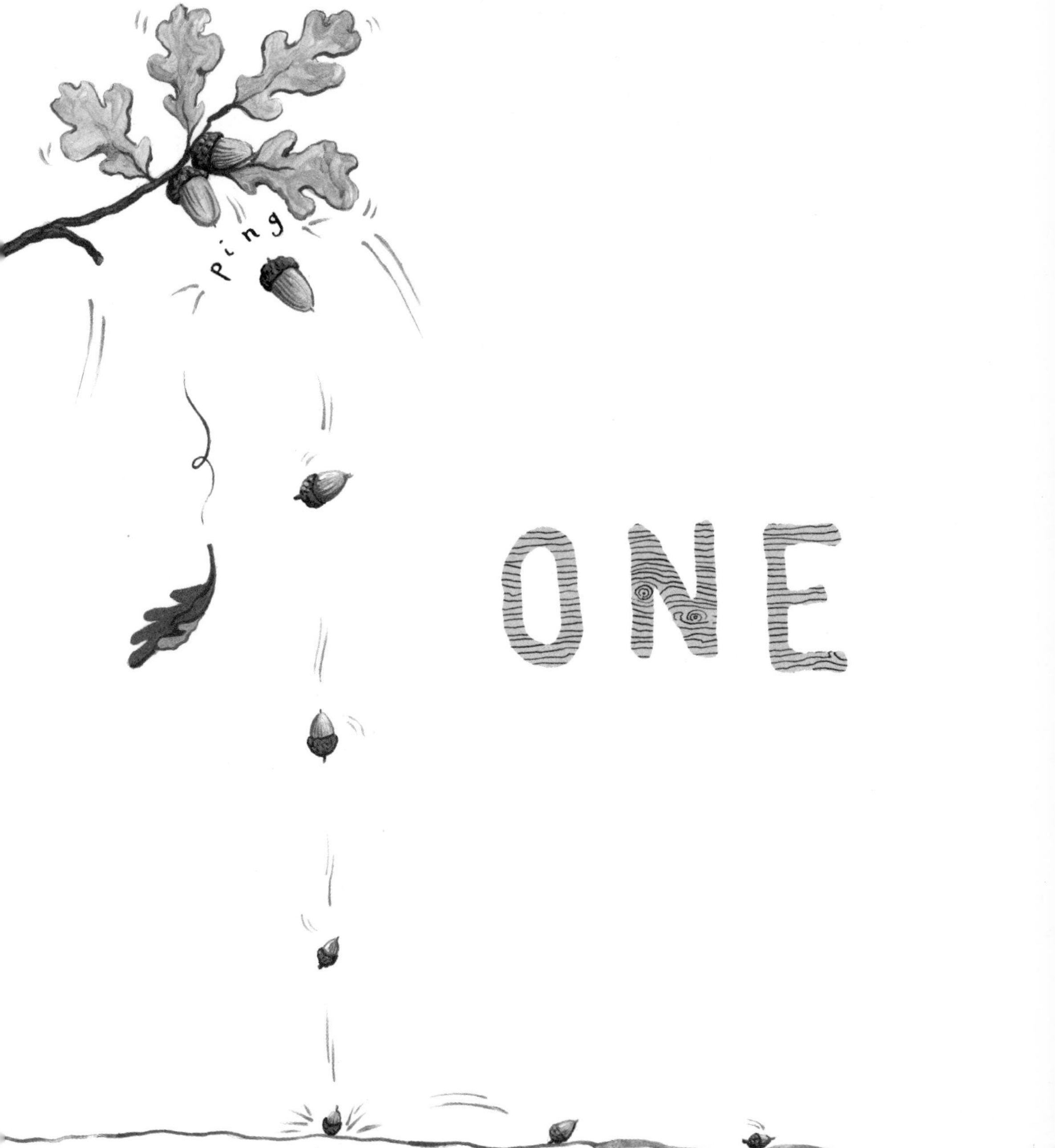
ping
plop

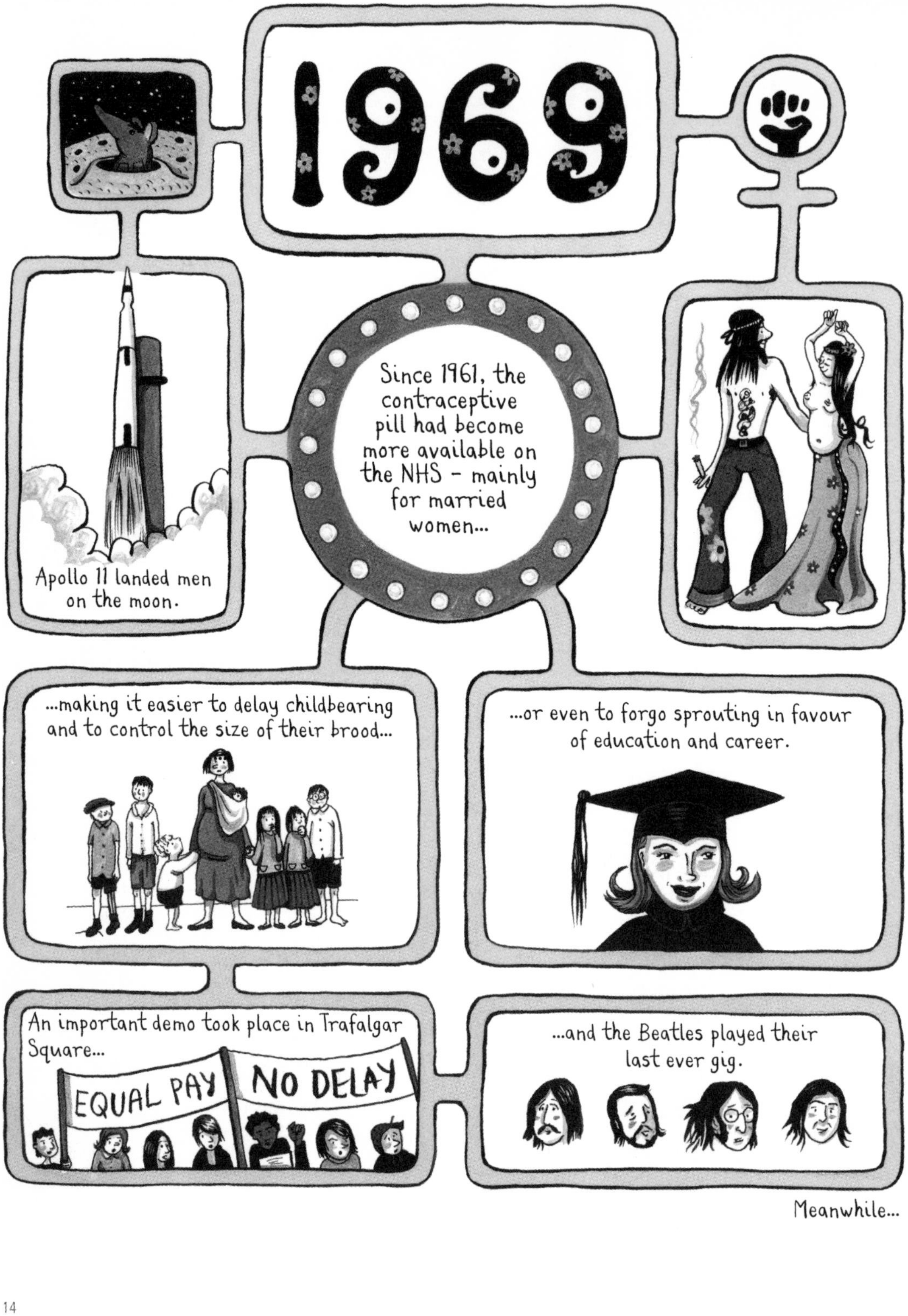
1969
Apollo 11 landed men on the moon.
Since 1961, the contraceptive pill had become more available on the NHS - mainly for married women...
...making it easier to delay childbearing and to control the size of their brood...
...or even to forgo sprouting in favour of education and career.
An important demo took place in Trafalgar Square...
EQUAL PAY
NO DELAY
...and the Beatles played their last ever gig.
Meanwhile...

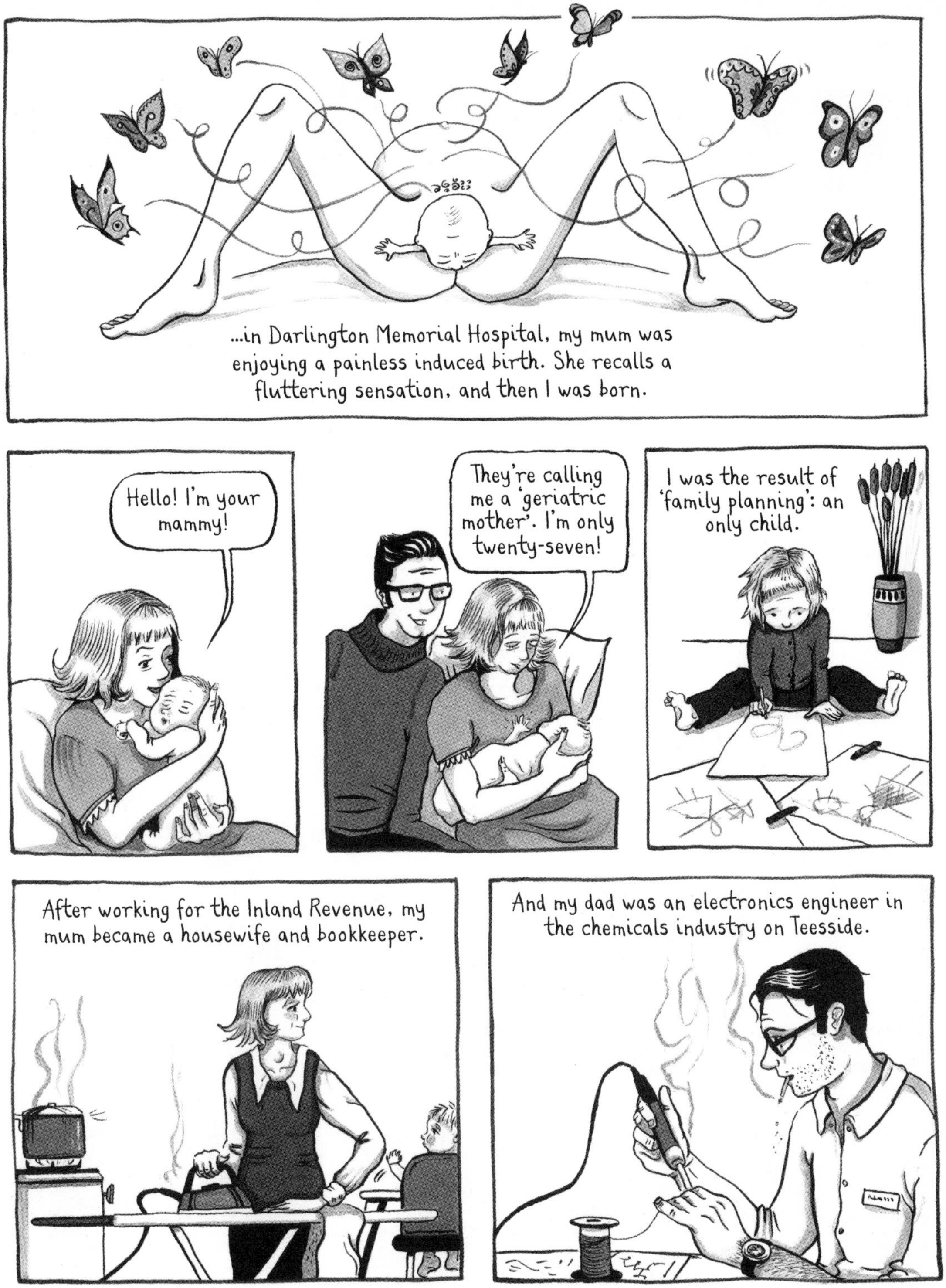
...in Darlington Memorial Hospital, my mum was enjoying a painless induced birth. She recalls a fluttering sensation, and then I was born.
Hello! I'm your mammy!
They're calling me a 'geriatric mother'. I'm only twenty-seven!
I was the result of 'family planning': an only child.
After working for the Inland Revenue, my mum became a housewife and bookkeeper.
And my dad was an electronics engineer in the chemicals industry on Teesside.

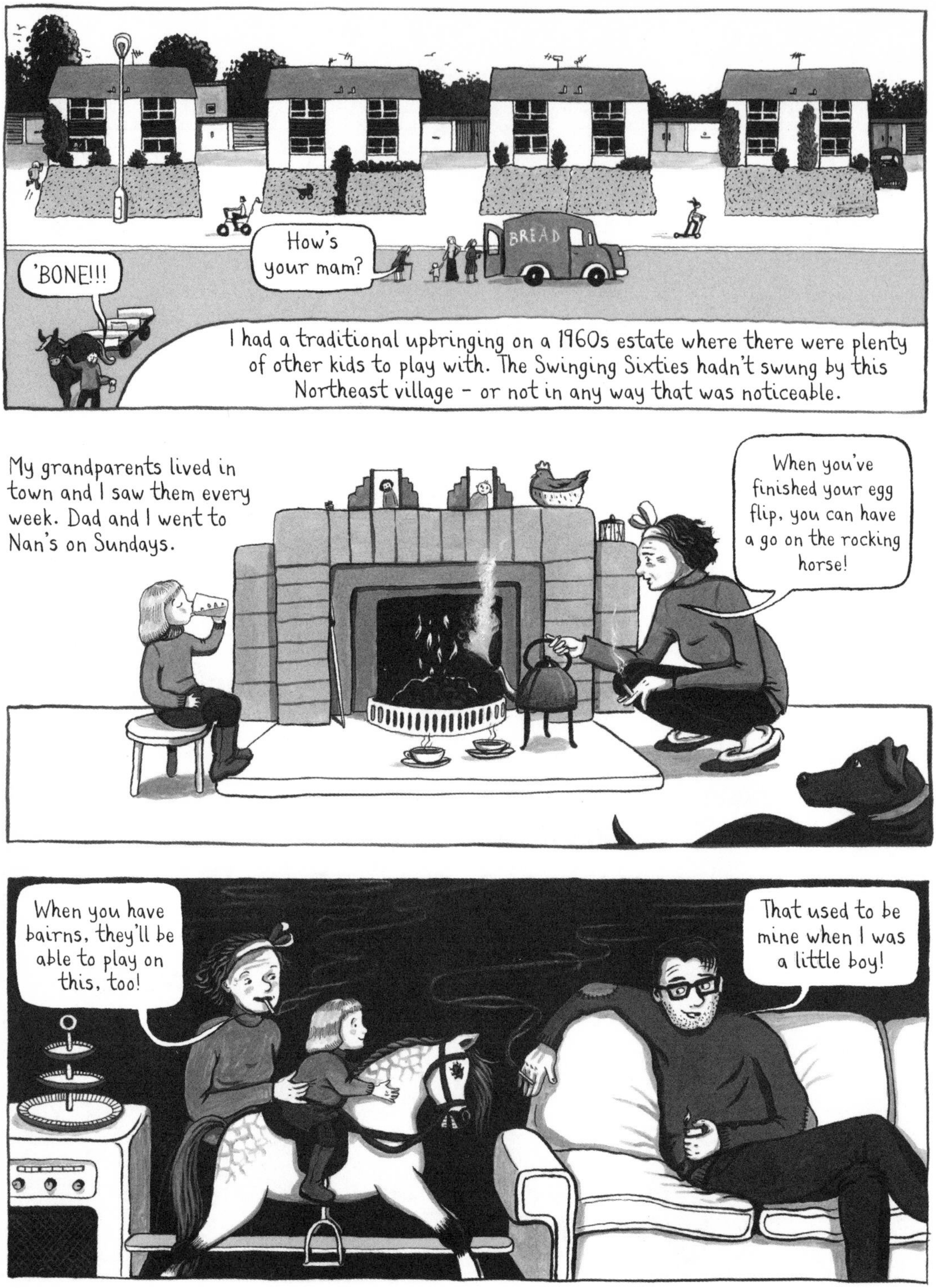
How's your mam?
'BONE!!!
BREAD
I had a traditional upbringing on a 1960s estate where there were plenty of other kids to play with. The Swinging Sixties hadn't swung by this Northeast village - or not in any way that was noticeable.
My grandparents lived in town and I saw them every week. Dad and I went to Nan's on Sundays.
When you've finished your egg flip, you can have a go on the rocking horse!
When you have bairns, they'll be able to play on this, too!
That used to be mine when I was a little boy!

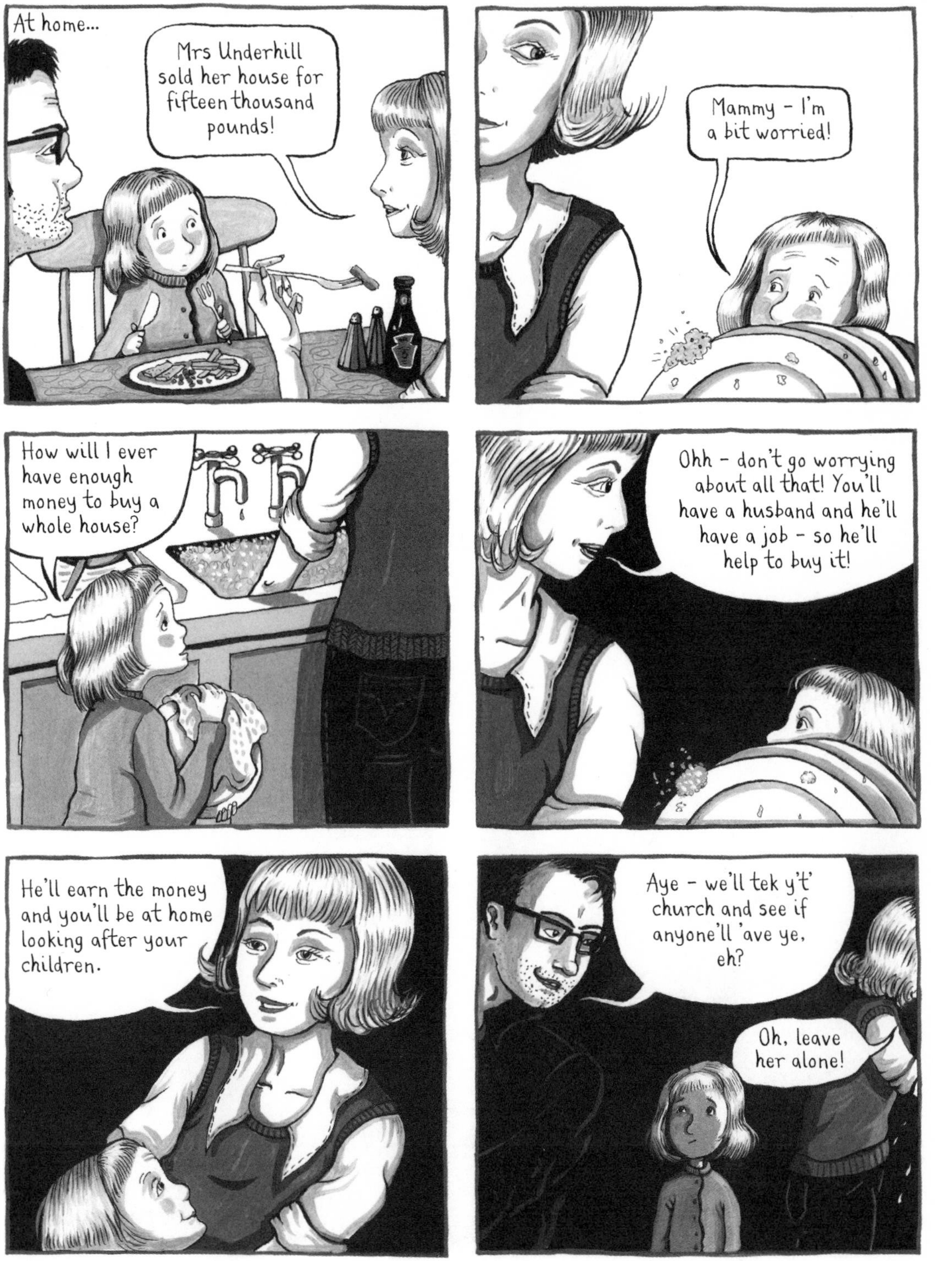
At home...
Mrs Underhill sold her house for fifteen thousand pounds!
Mammy - I'm a bit worried!
How will I ever have enough money to buy a whole house?
Ohh - don't go worrying about all that! You'll have a husband and he'll have a job - so he'll help to buy it!
He'll earn the money and you'll be at home looking after your children.
Aye - we'll tek y't' church and see if anyone'll 'ave ye, eh?
Oh, leave her alone!

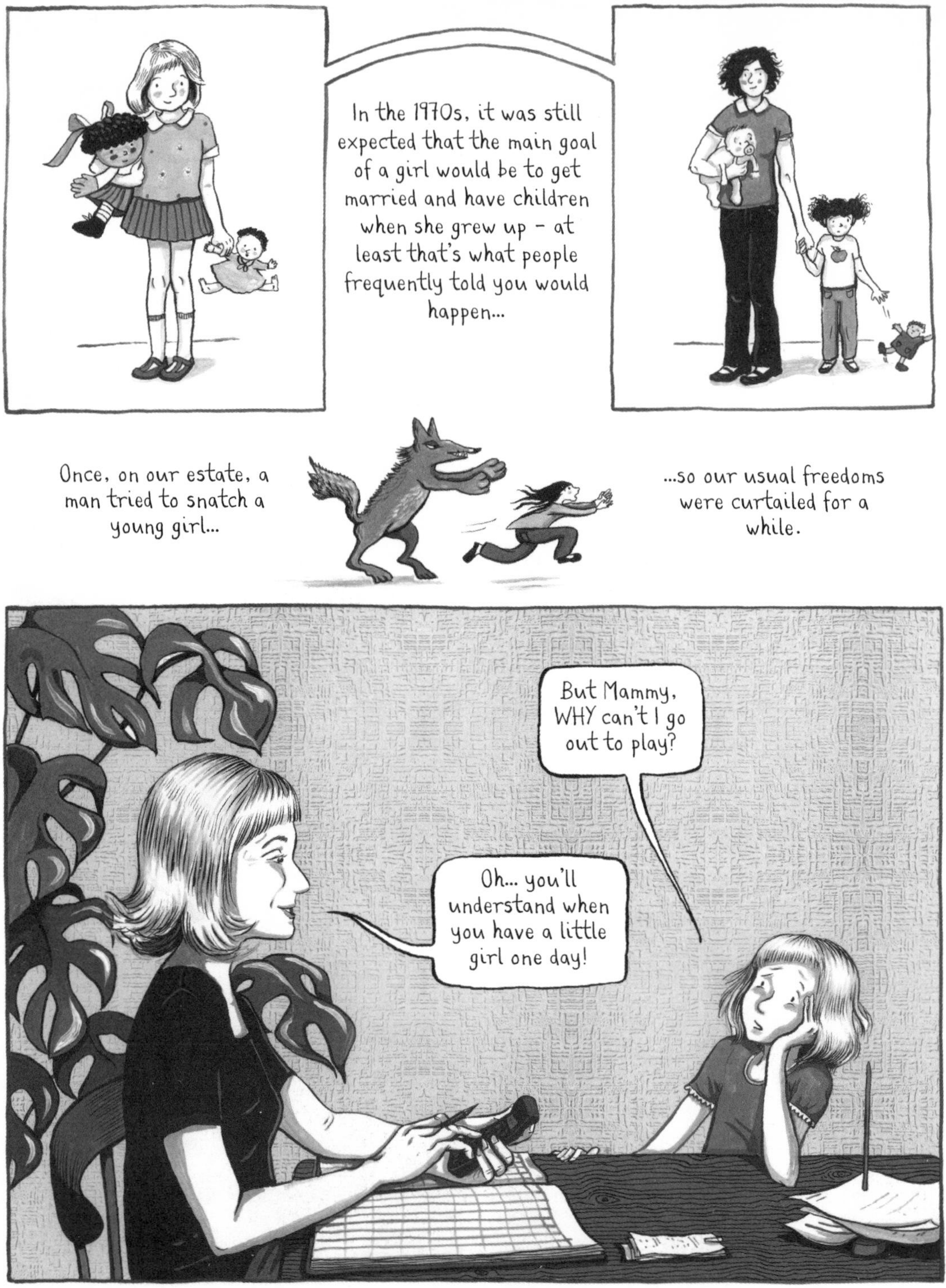
In the 1970s, it was still expected that the main goal of a girl would be to get married and have children when she grew up - at least that's what people frequently told you would happen...
Once, on our estate, a man tried to snatch a young girl...
...so our usual freedoms were curtailed for a while.
But Mammy, WHY can't I go out to play?
Oh... you'll understand when you have a little girl one day!

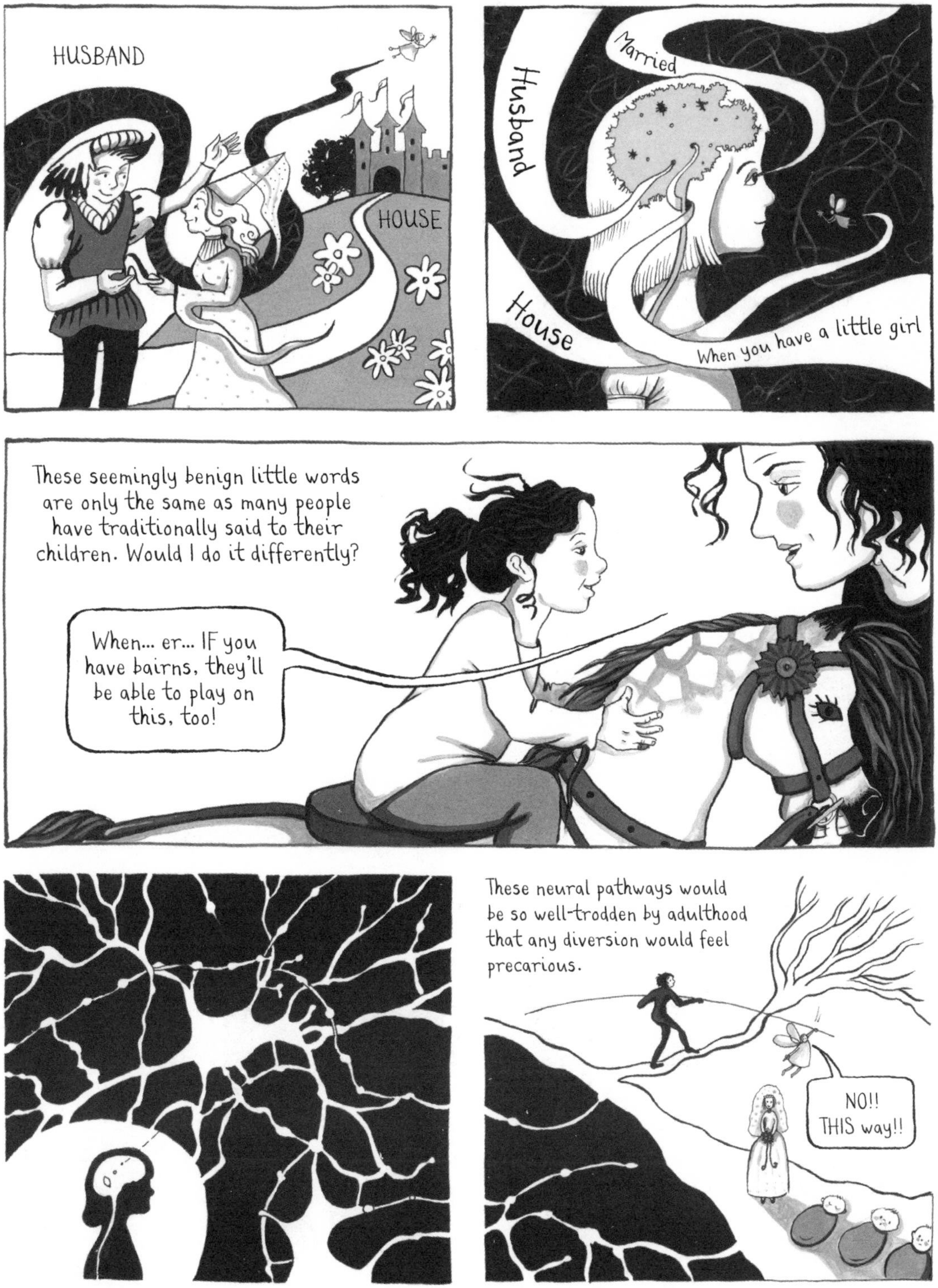
HUSBAND
HOUSE
Married
Husband
House
When you have a little girl
These seemingly benign little words are only the same as many people have traditionally said to their children. Would I do it differently?
When... er... IF you have bairns, they'll be able to play on this, too!
These neural pathways would be so well-trodden by adulthood that any diversion would feel precarious.
NO!! THIS way!!

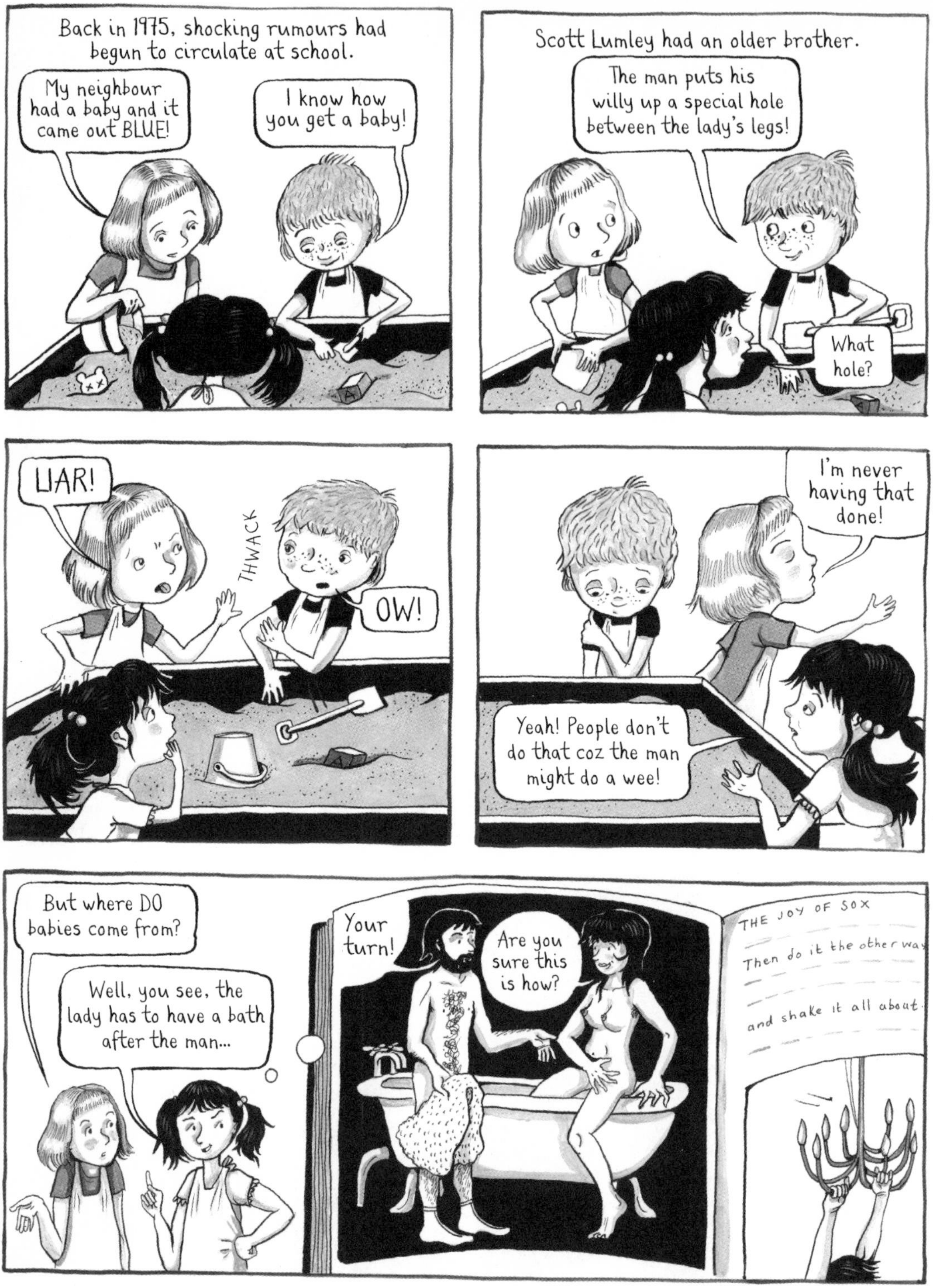

Back in 1975, shocking rumours had begun to circulate at school.
My neighbour had a baby and it came out BLUE!
I know how you get a baby!
Scott Lumley had an older brother.
The man puts his willy up a special hole between the lady's legs!
What hole?
LIAR!
THWACK
OW!
I'm never having that done!
Yeah! People don't do that coz the man might do a wee!
But where DO babies come from?
Well, you see, the lady has to have a bath after the man...
Your turn!
Are you sure this is how?
THE JOY OF SOX
Then do it the other wa
and shake it all about.

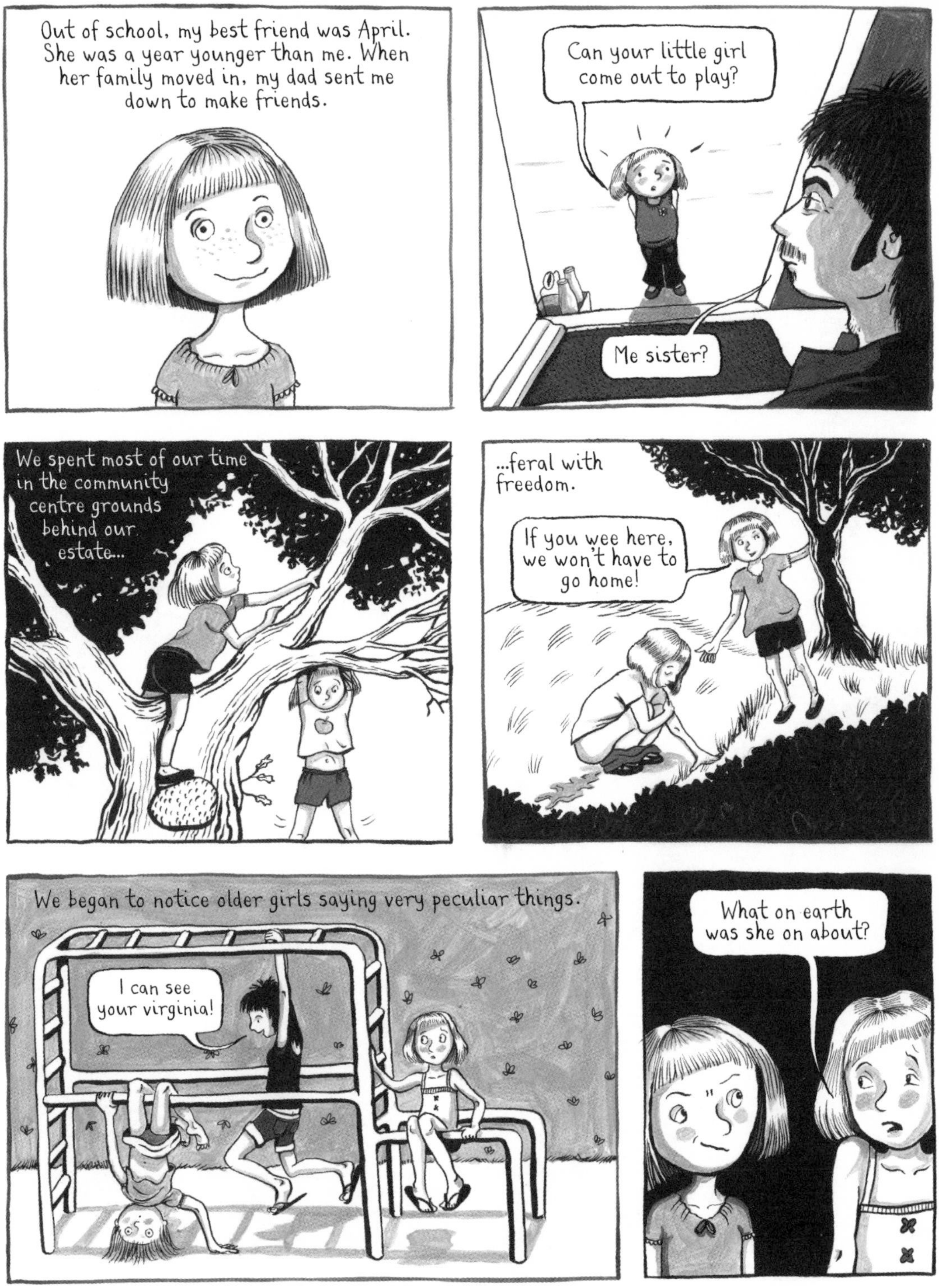

Out of school, my best friend was April. She was a year younger than me. When her family moved in, my dad sent me down to make friends.
Can your little girl come out to play?
Me sister?
We spent most of our time in the community centre grounds behind our estate...
...feral with freedom.
If you wee here, we won't have to go home!
We began to notice older girls saying very peculiar things.
I can see your virginia!
What on earth was she on about?

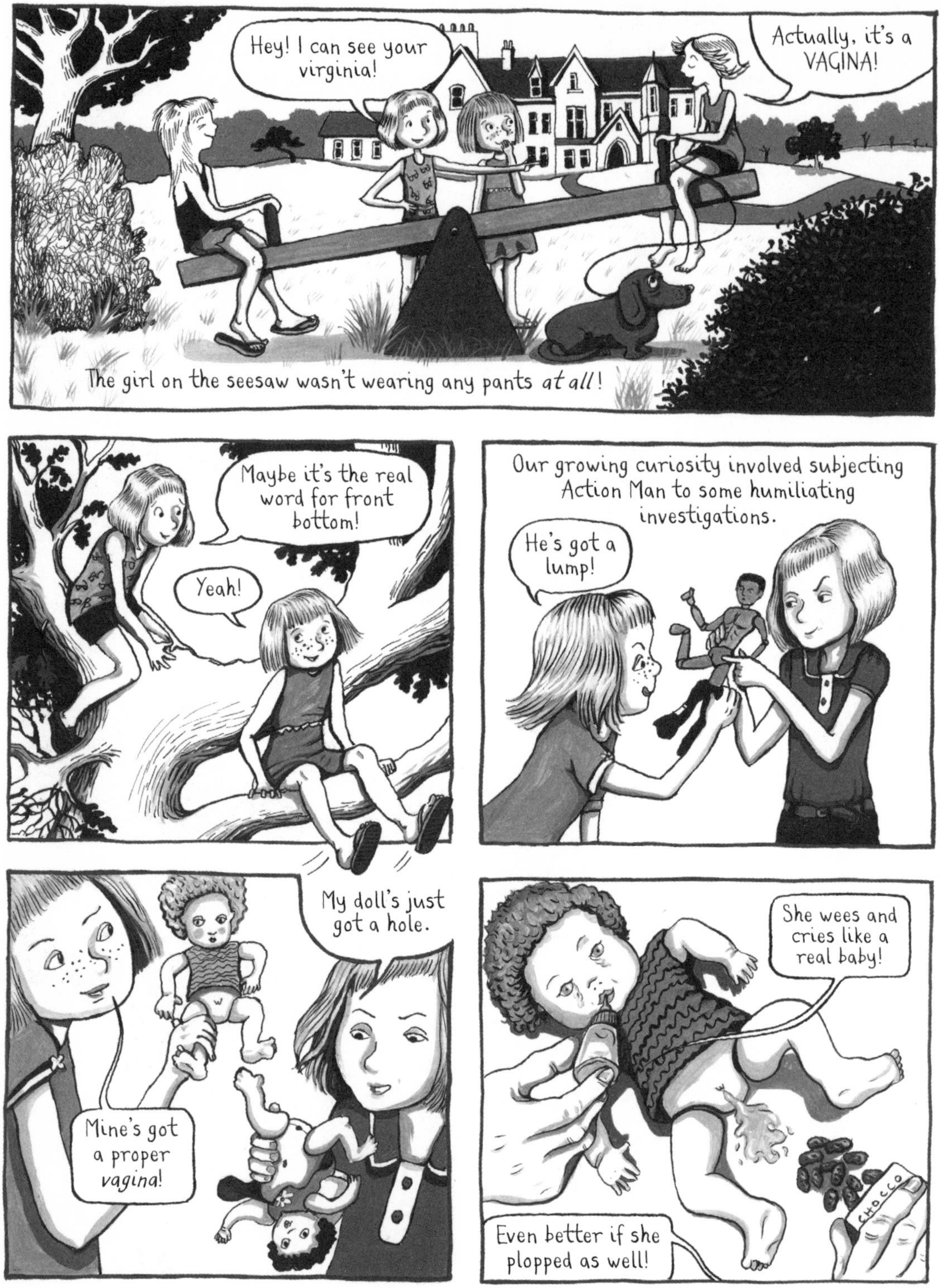
Hey! I can see your virginia!
Actually, it's a VAGINA!
The girl on the seesaw wasn't wearing any pants *at all*!
Maybe it's the real word for front bottom!
Yeah!
Our growing curiosity involved subjecting Action Man to some humiliating investigations.
He's got a lump!
My doll's just got a hole.
Mine's got a proper *vagina*!
She wees and cries like a real baby!
Even better if she plopped as well!

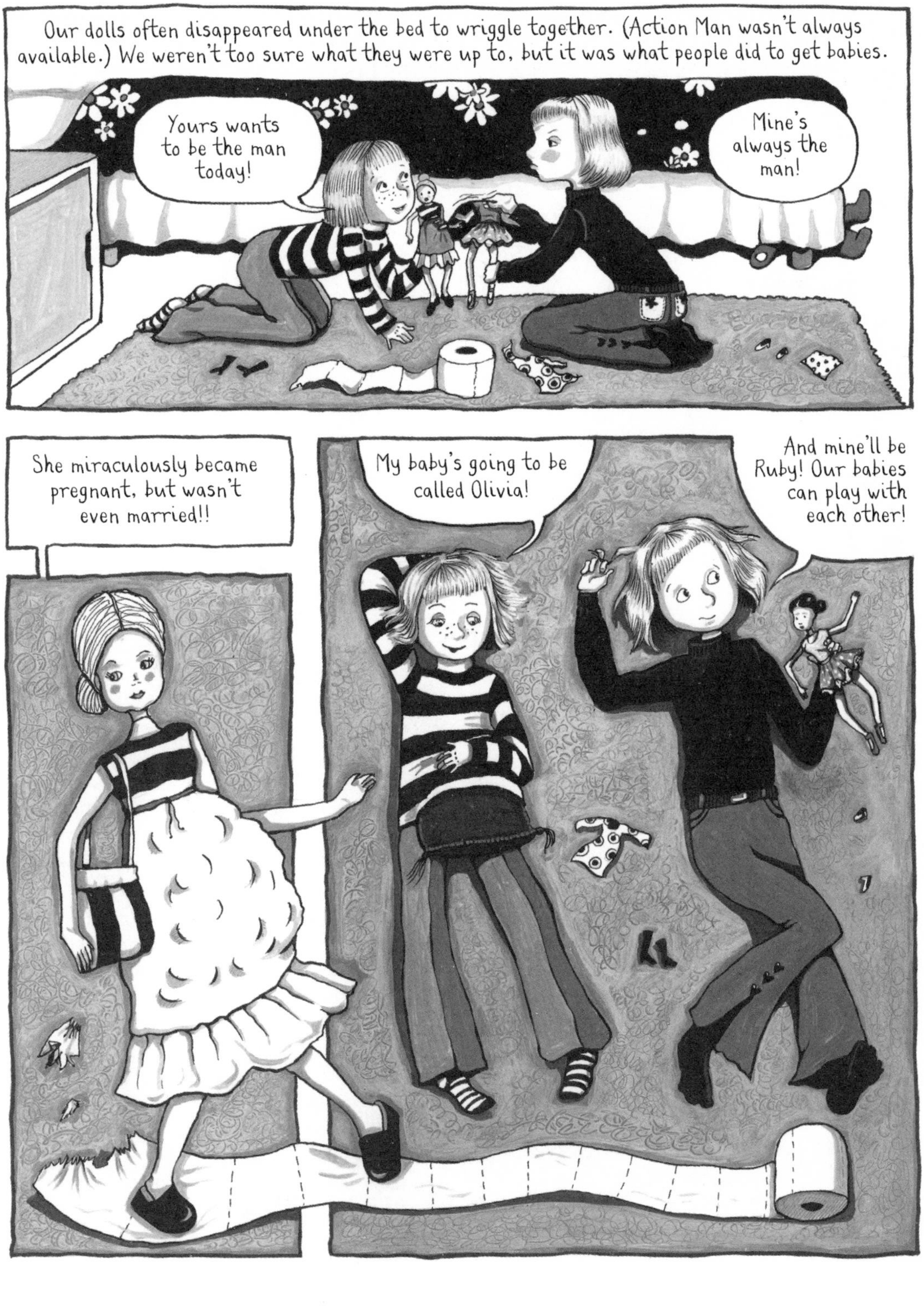
Our dolls often disappeared under the bed to wriggle together. (Action Man wasn't always available.) We weren't too sure what they were up to, but it was what people did to get babies.
Yours wants to be the man today!
Mine's always the man!
She miraculously became pregnant, but wasn't even married!!
My baby's going to be called Olivia!
And mine'll be Ruby! Our babies can play with each other!

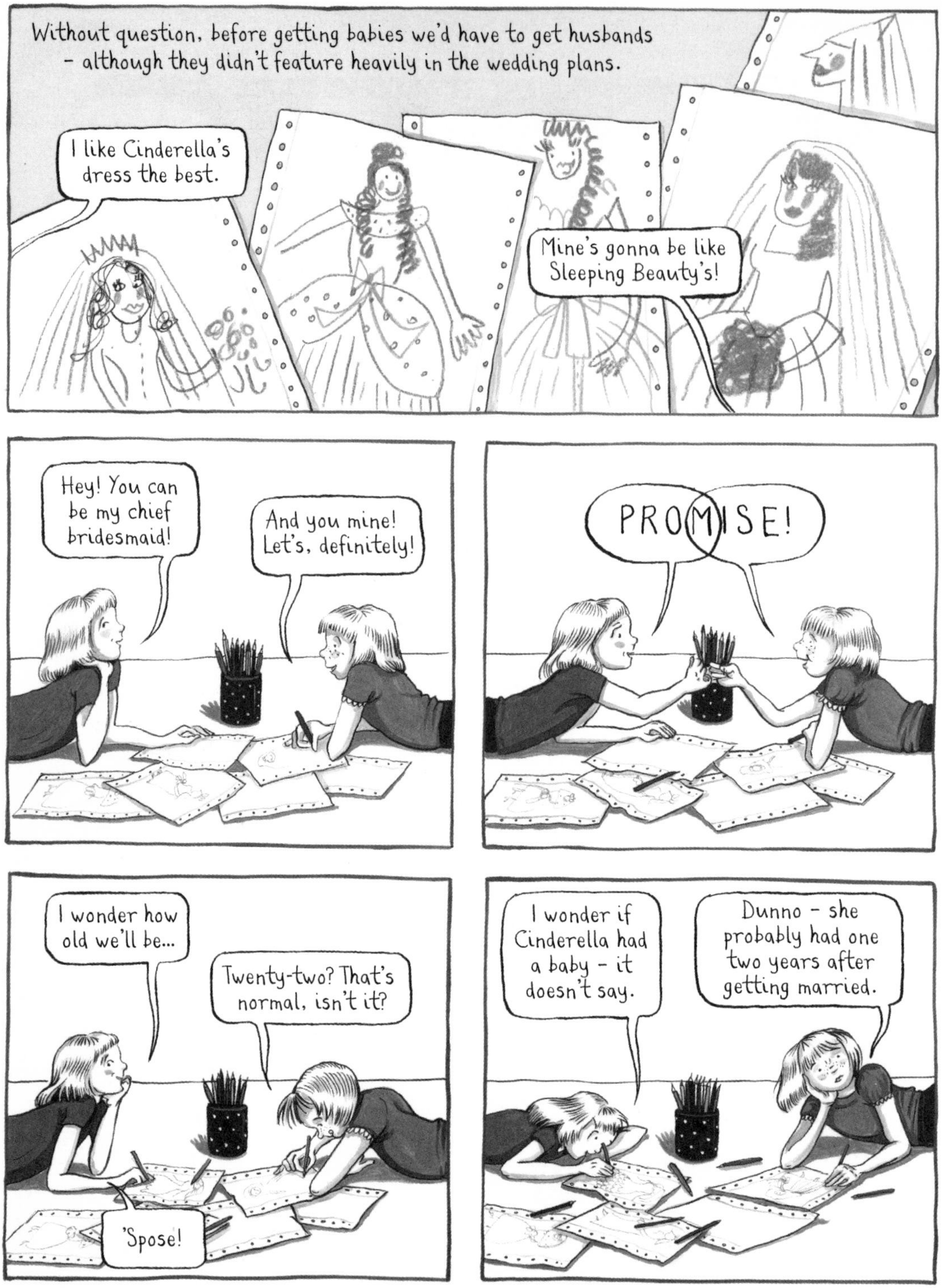
Without question, before getting babies we'd have to get husbands – although they didn't feature heavily in the wedding plans.
I like Cinderella's dress the best.
Mine's gonna be like Sleeping Beauty's!
Hey! You can be my chief bridesmaid!
And you mine! Let's, definitely!
PROMISE!
I wonder how old we'll be...
Twenty-two? That's normal, isn't it?
'Spose!
I wonder if Cinderella had a baby – it doesn't say.
Dunno – she probably had one two years after getting married.

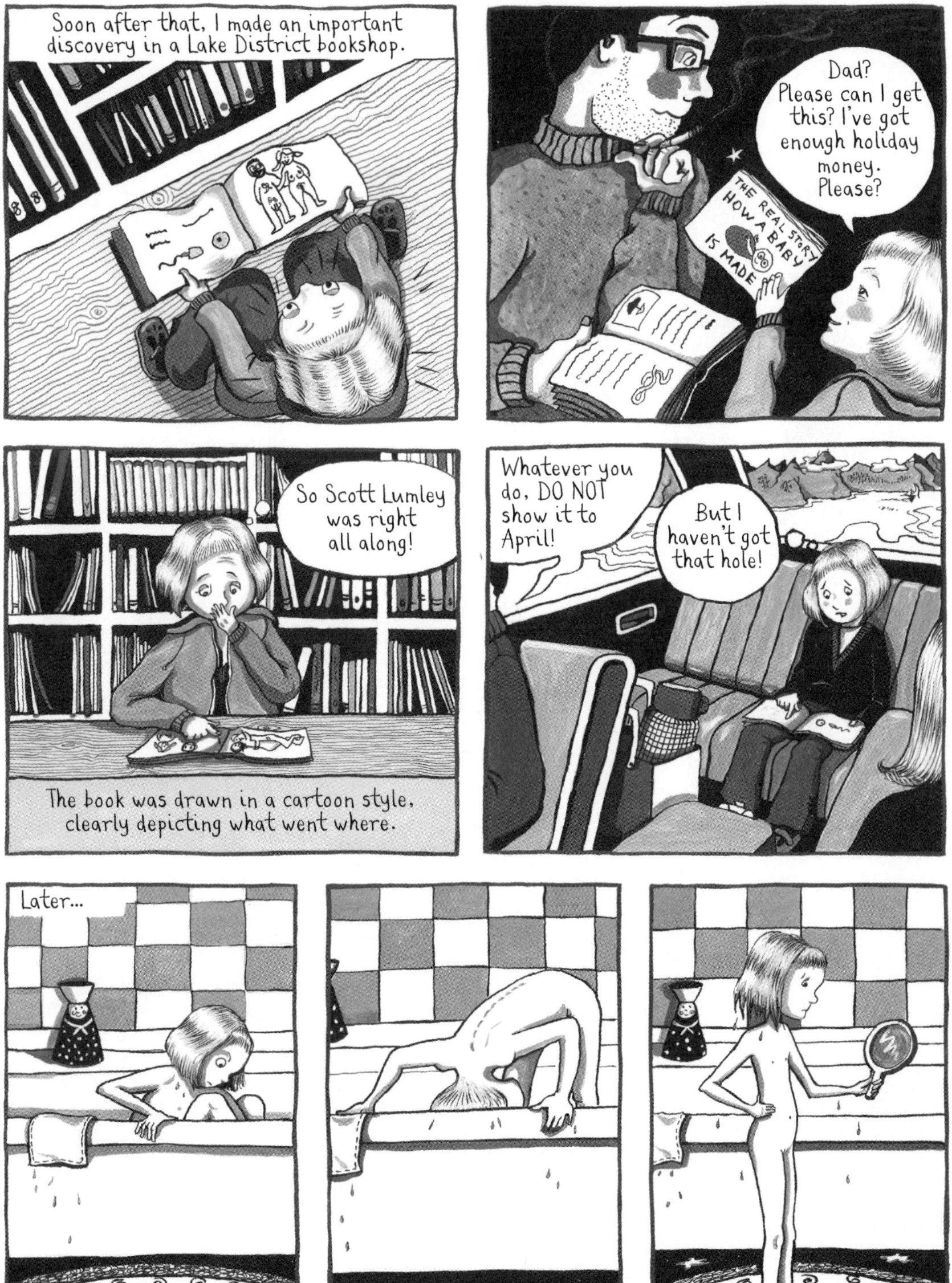
Soon after that, I made an important discovery in a Lake District bookshop.
Dad? Please can I get this? I've got enough holiday money. Please?
THE REAL STORY HOW A BABY IS MADE
So Scott Lumley was right all along!
The book was drawn in a cartoon style, clearly depicting what went where.
Whatever you do, DO NOT show it to April!
But I haven't got that hole!
Later...

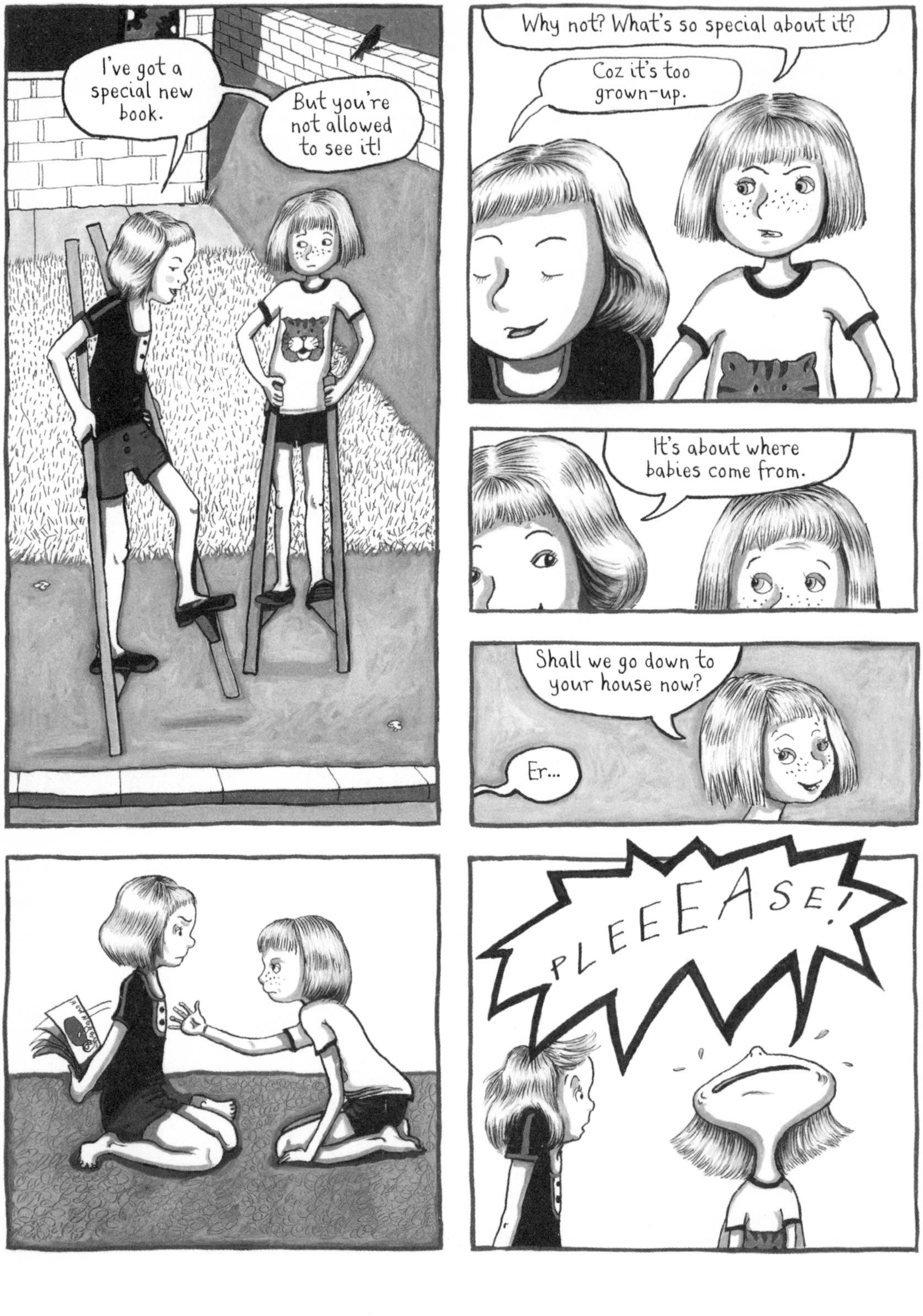
I've got a special new book.
But you're not allowed to see it!
Why not? What's so special about it?
Coz it's too grown-up.
It's about where babies come from.
Shall we go down to your house now?
Er...
PLEEEEASE!

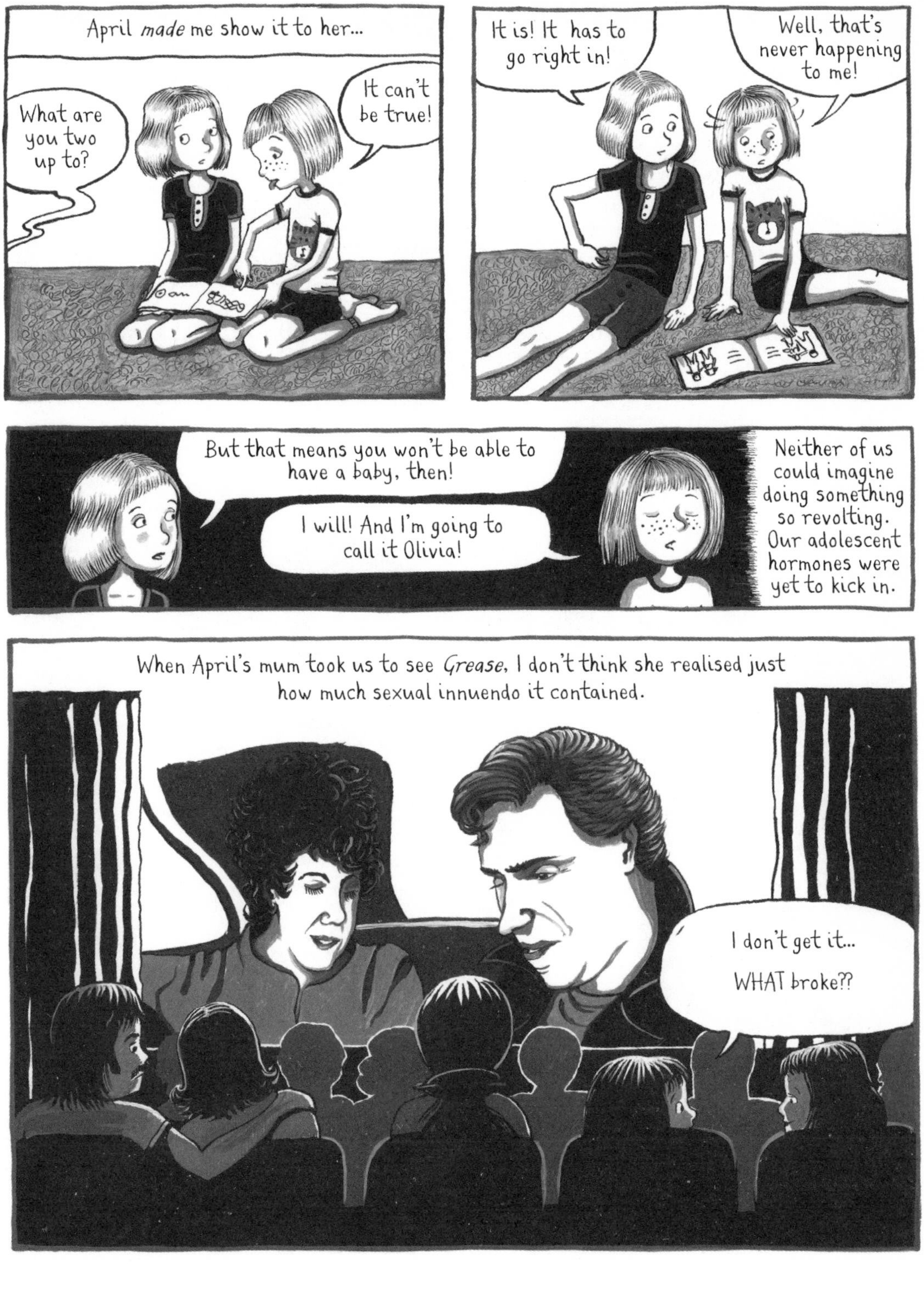
April *made* me show it to her...
What are you two up to?
It can't be true!
It is! It has to go right in!
Well, that's never happening to me!
But that means you won't be able to have a baby, then!
I will! And I'm going to call it Olivia!
Neither of us could imagine doing something so revolting. Our adolescent hormones were yet to kick in.
When April's mum took us to see *Grease*, I don't think she realised just how much sexual innuendo it contained.
I don't get it...
WHAT broke??

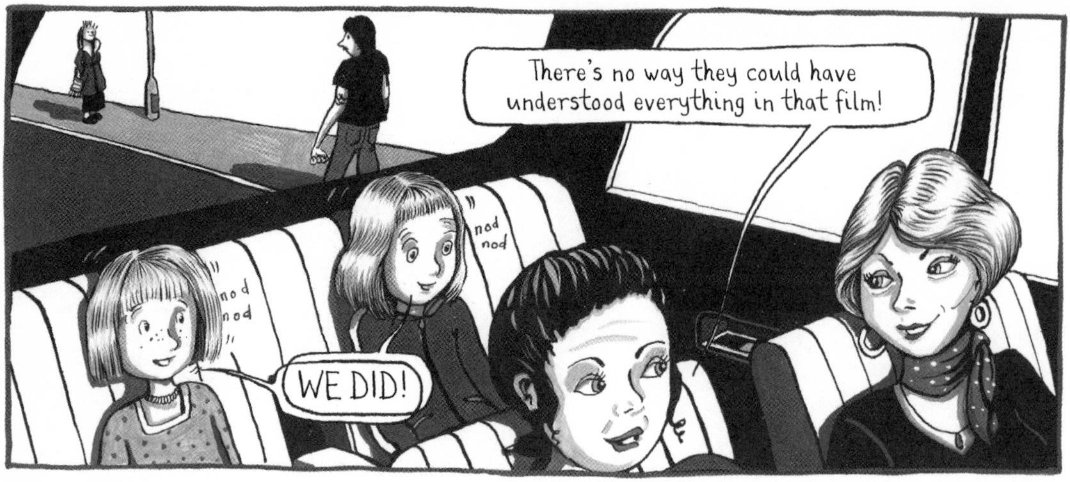
There's no way they could have understood everything in that film!
nod nod
nod nod
WE DID!

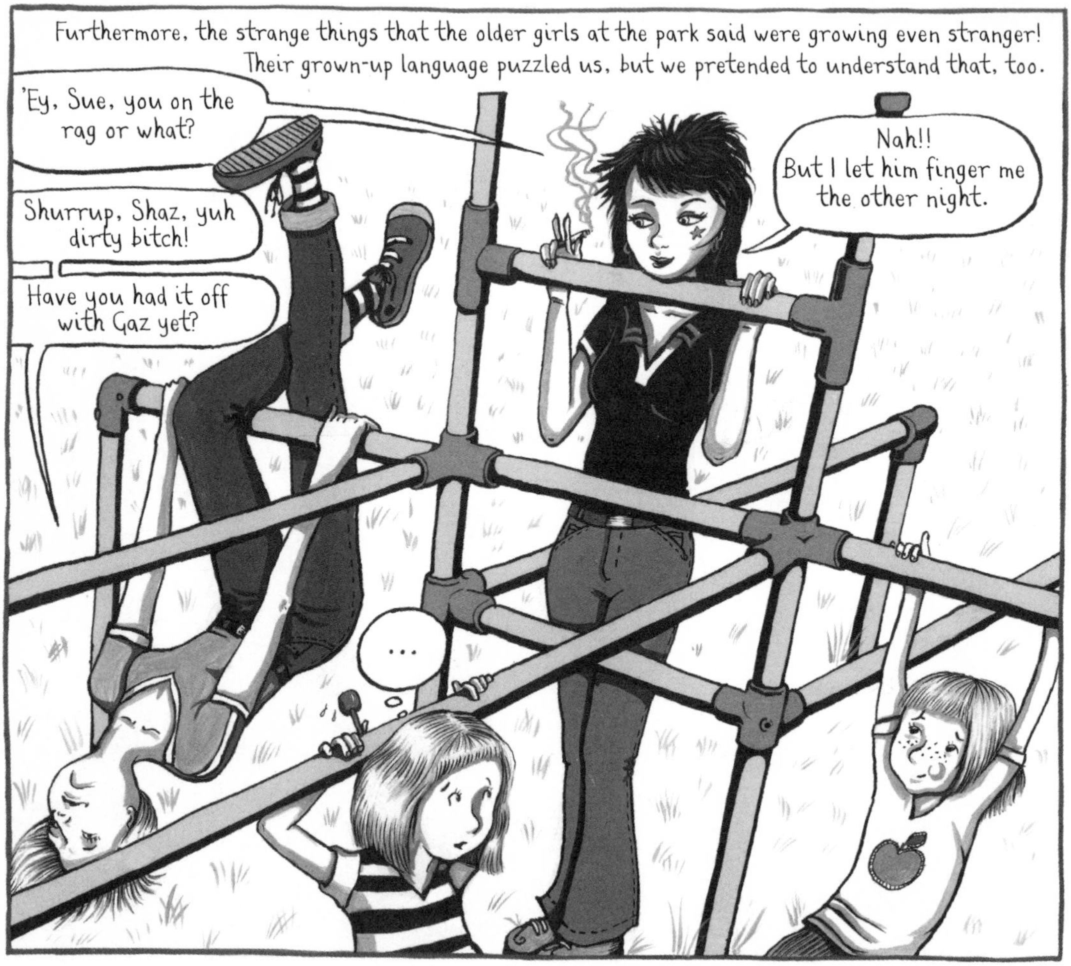
Furthermore, the strange things that the older girls at the park said were growing even stranger! Their grown-up language puzzled us, but we pretended to understand that, too.
'Ey, Sue, you on the rag or what?
Nah!! But I let him finger me the other night.
Shurrup, Shaz, yuh dirty bitch!
Have you had it off with Gaz yet?
...

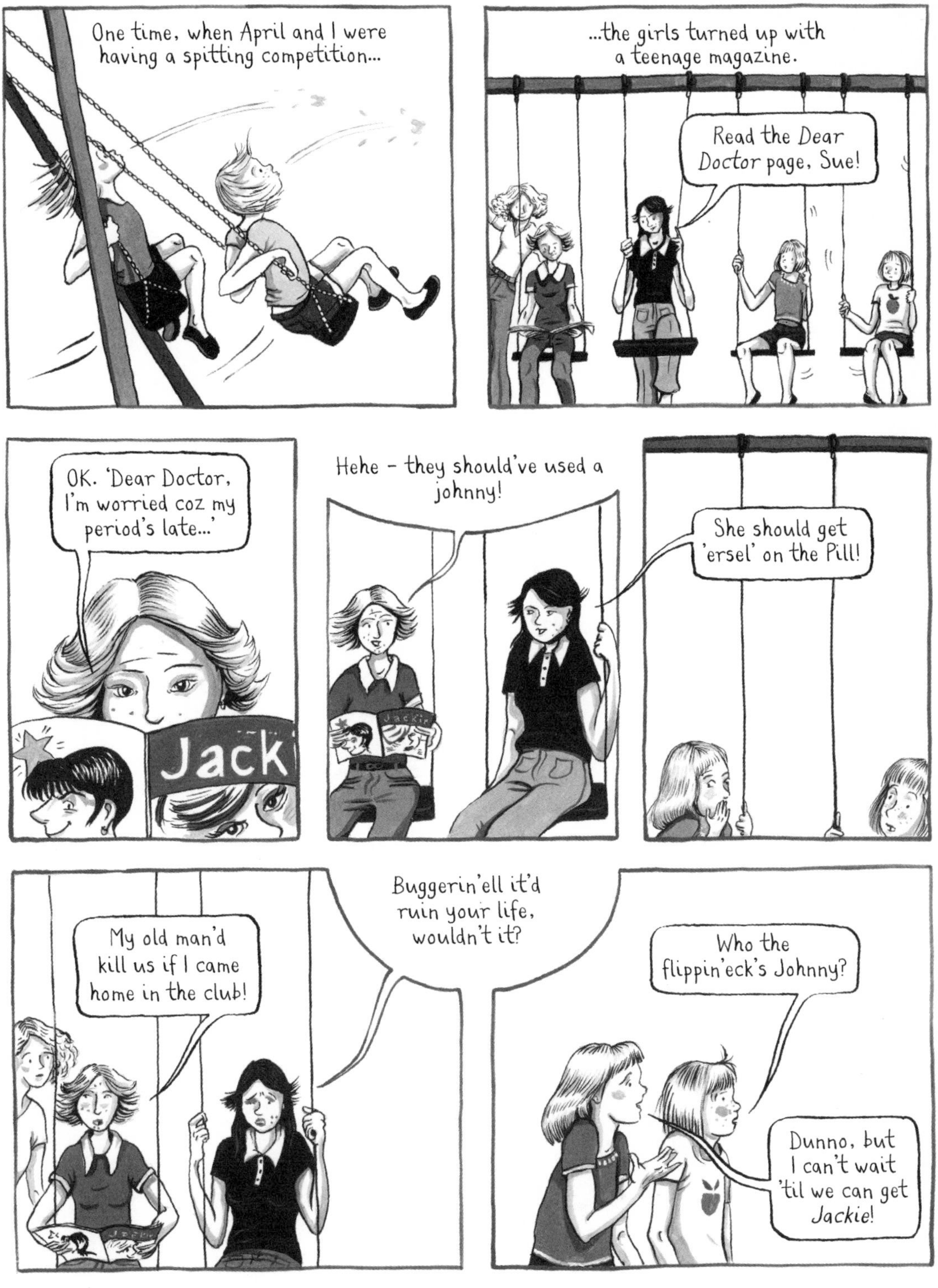
One time, when April and I were having a spitting competition...
...the girls turned up with a teenage magazine.
Read the *Dear Doctor* page, Sue!
OK. 'Dear Doctor, I'm worried coz my period's late...'
Jack
Hehe – they should've used a johnny!
She should get 'ersel' on the Pill!
My old man'd kill us if I came home in the club!
Buggerin'ell it'd ruin your life, wouldn't it?
Who the flippin'eck's Johnny?
Dunno, but I can't wait 'til we can get *Jackie*!

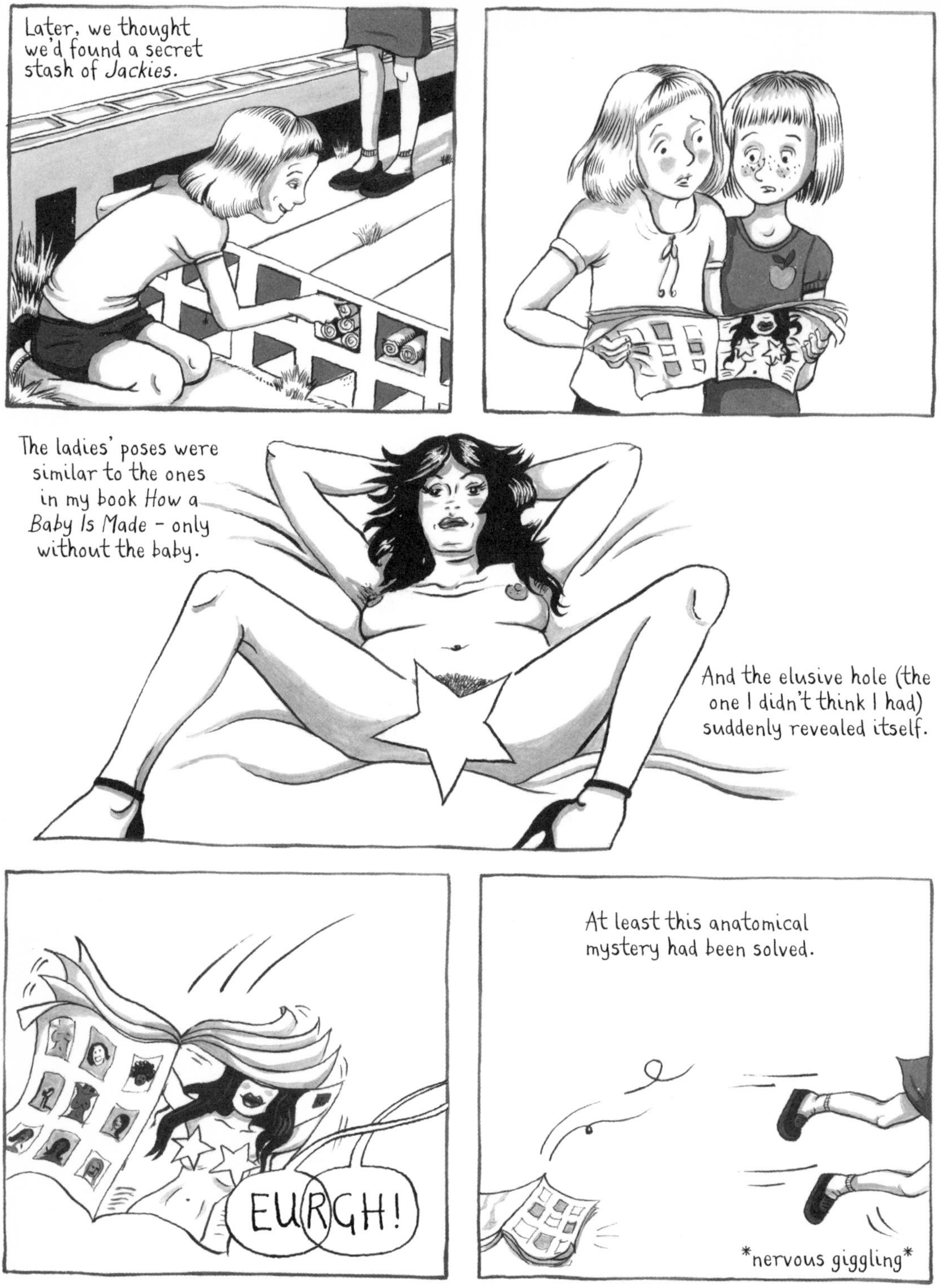
Later, we thought we'd found a secret stash of *Jackies*.
The ladies' poses were similar to the ones in my book *How a Baby Is Made* – only without the baby.
And the elusive hole (the one I didn't think I had) suddenly revealed itself.
EURGH!
At least this anatomical mystery had been solved.
nervous giggling

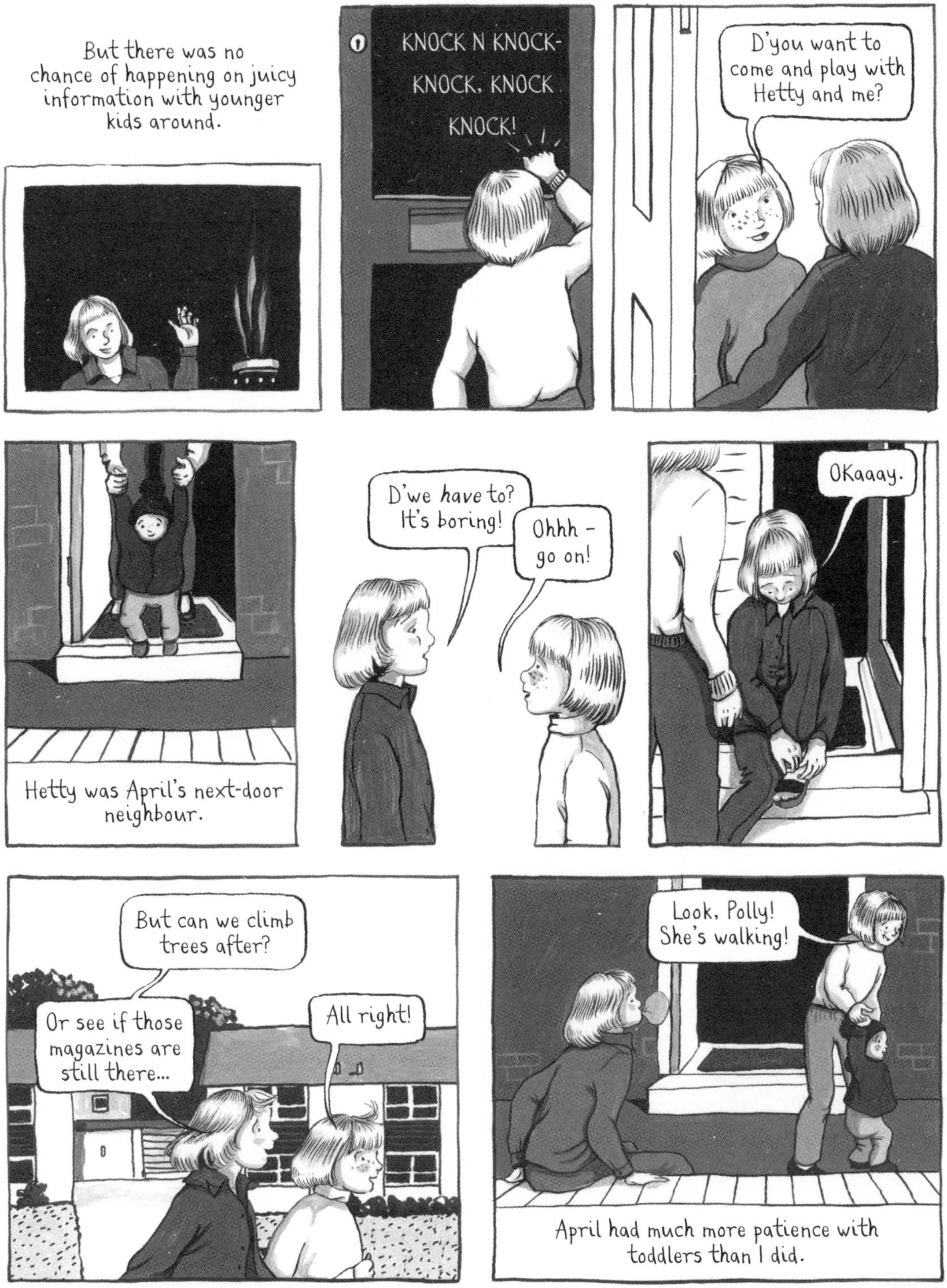

But there was no chance of happening on juicy information with younger kids around.
KNOCK N KNOCK-KNOCK, KNOCK KNOCK KNOCK!
D'you want to come and play with Hetty and me?
Hetty was April's next-door neighbour.
D'we *have* to? It's boring!
Ohhh - go on!
OKaaay.
But can we climb trees after?
Or see if those magazines are still there...
All right!
Look, Polly! She's walking!
April had much more patience with toddlers than I did.

I preferred seeing if we could get all the way down Hetty's driveway on one rollerskate without putting the other foot down.

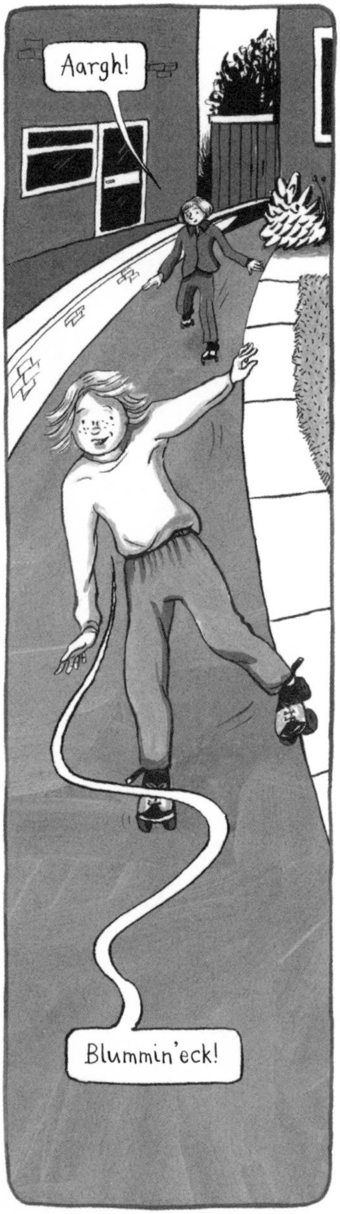
Aargh!
Blummin'eck!

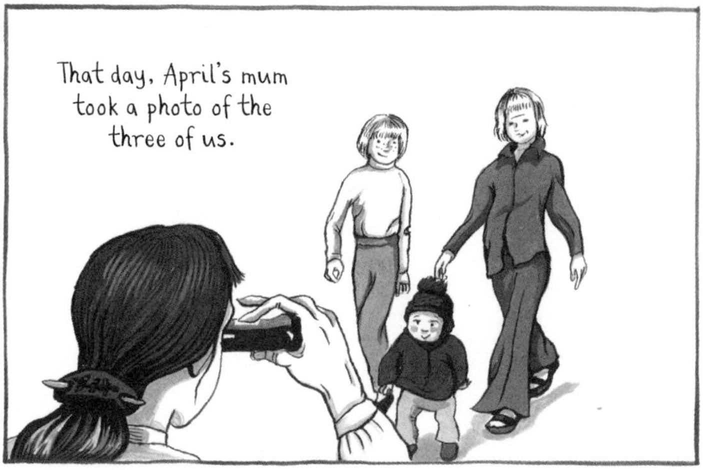
That day, April's mum took a photo of the three of us.

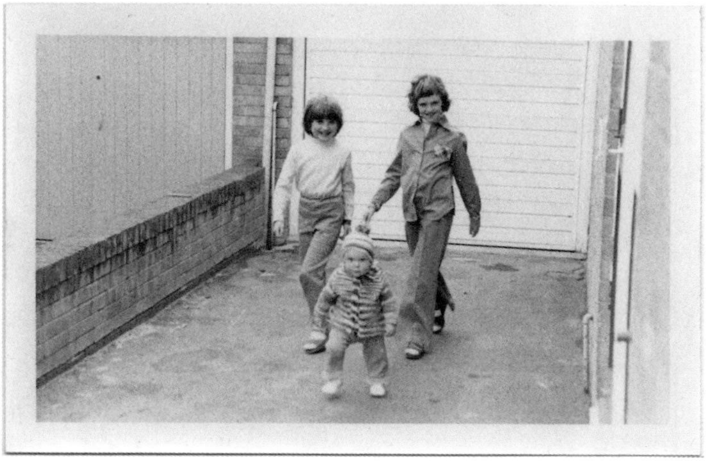

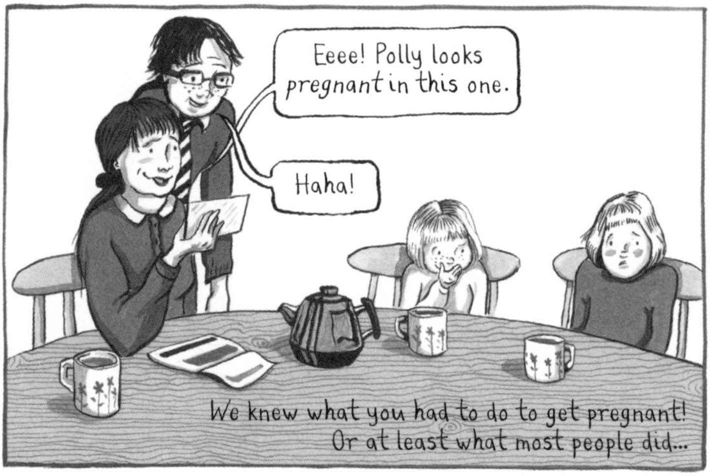
Eeee! Polly looks pregnant in this one.
Haha!
We knew what you had to do to get pregnant! Or at least what most people did...

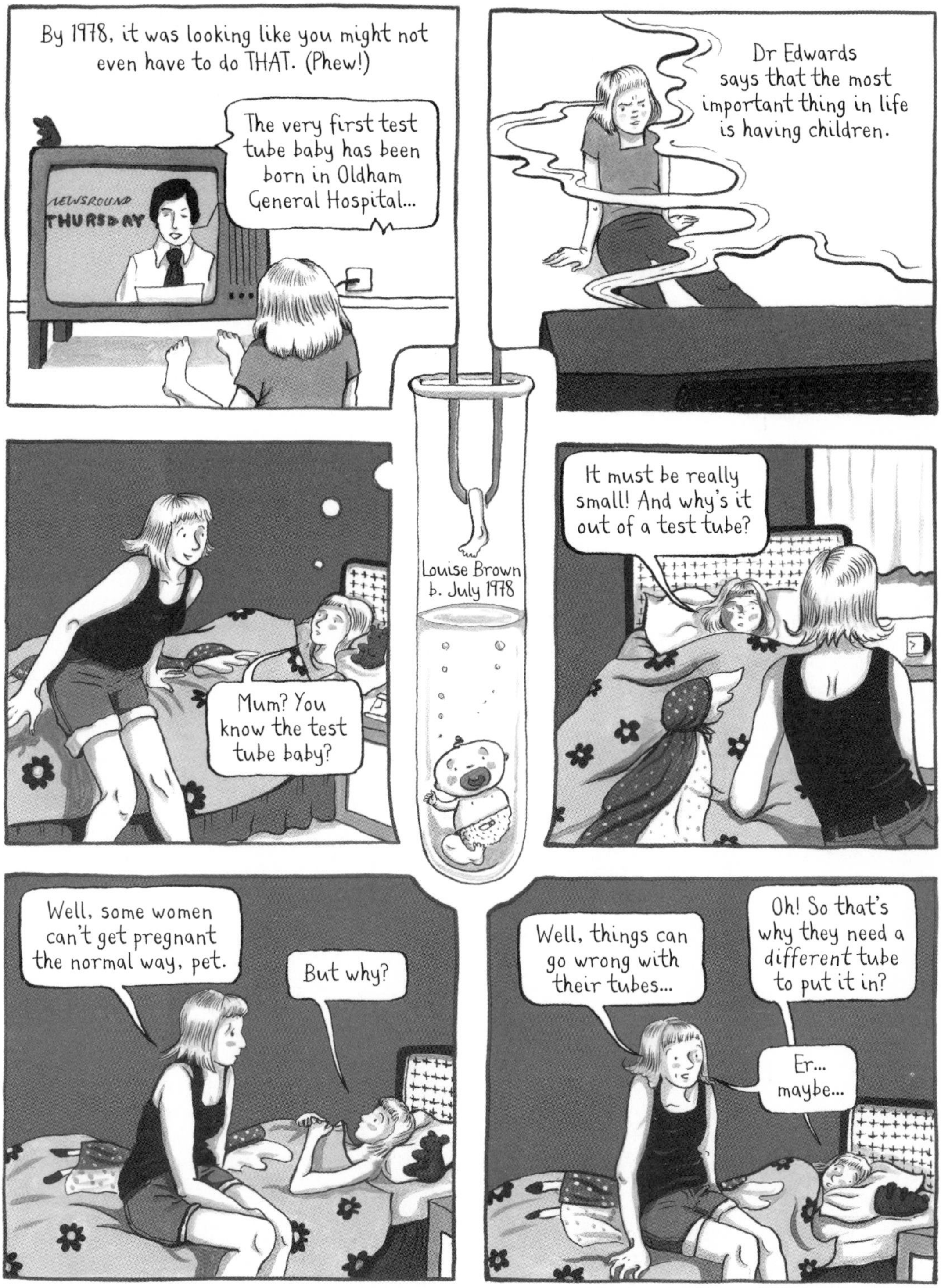
By 1978, it was looking like you might not even have to do THAT. (Phew!)
NEWSROUND
THURSDAY
The very first test tube baby has been born in Oldham General Hospital...
Dr Edwards says that the most important thing in life is having children.
Louise Brown b. July 1978
Mum? You know the test tube baby?
It must be really small! And why's it out of a test tube?
Well, some women can't get pregnant the normal way, pet.
But why?
Well, things can go wrong with their tubes...
Oh! So that's why they need a different tube to put it in?
Er... maybe...

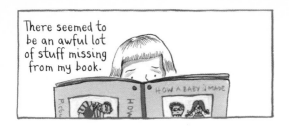

There seemed to be an awful lot of stuff missing from my book.

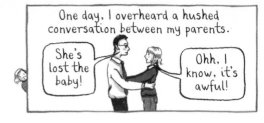

One day, I overheard a hushed conversation between my parents.

She's lost the baby!

Ohh, I know, it's awful!

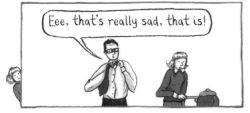

Eee, that's really sad, that is!

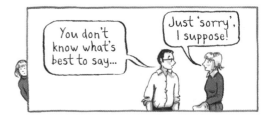

You don't know what's best to say...

Just 'sorry', I suppose!

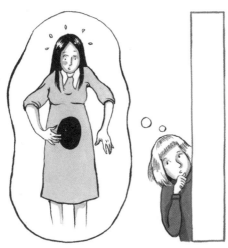

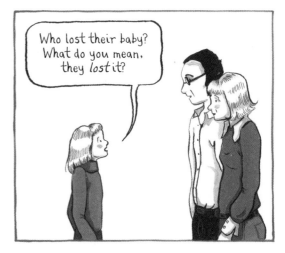

Who lost their baby? What do you mean, they *lost* it?

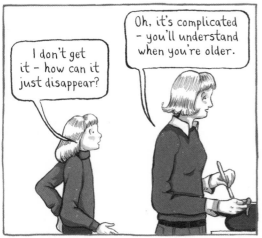

I don't get it - how can it just disappear?

Oh, it's complicated - you'll understand when you're older.

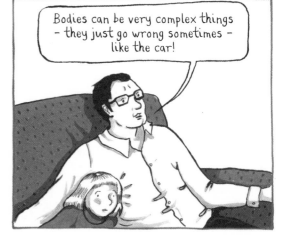

Bodies can be very complex things - they just go wrong sometimes - like the car!

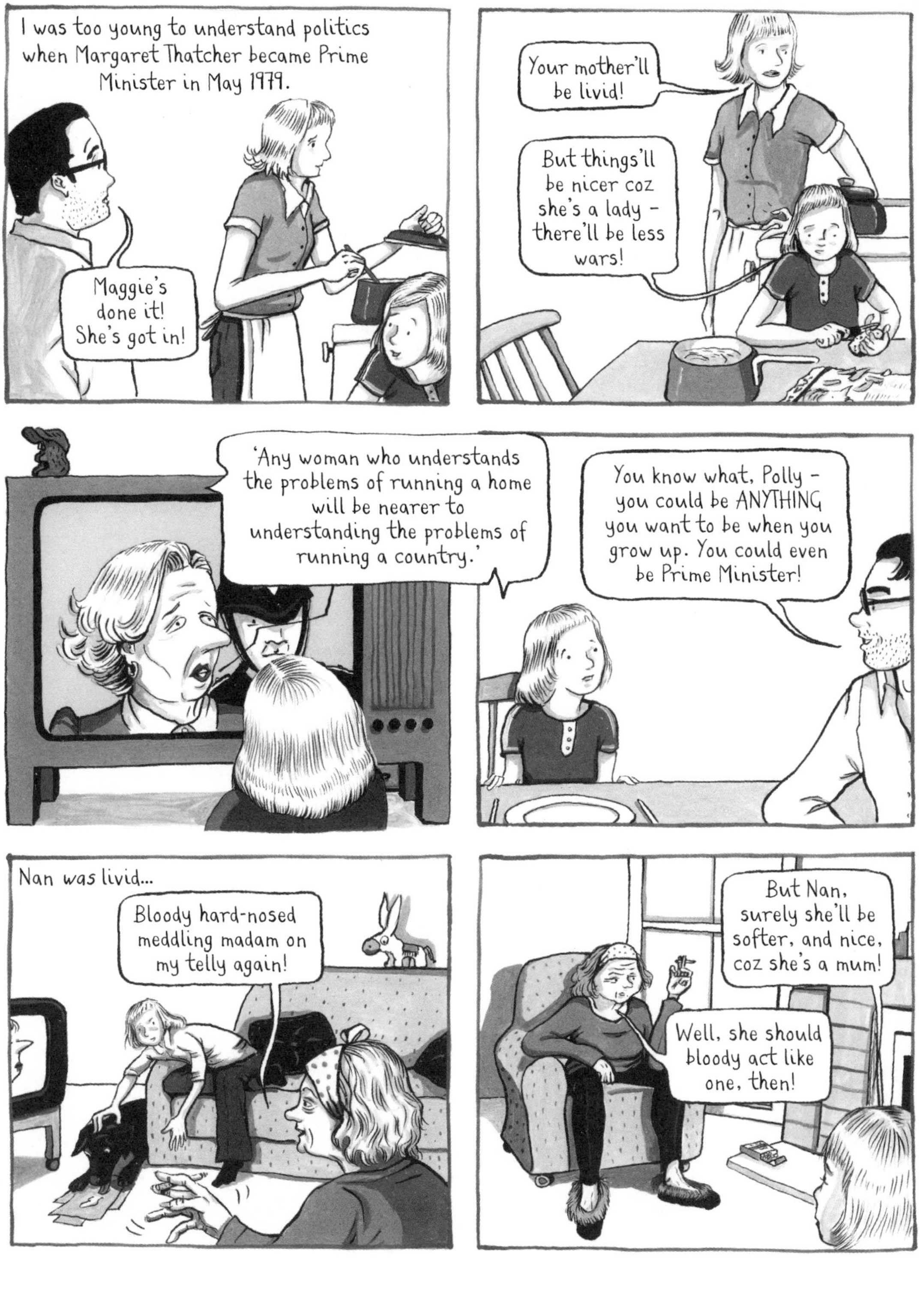
I was too young to understand politics when Margaret Thatcher became Prime Minister in May 1979.
Maggie's done it! She's got in!
Your mother'll be livid!
But things'll be nicer coz she's a lady - there'll be less wars!
'Any woman who understands the problems of running a home will be nearer to understanding the problems of running a country.'
You know what, Polly - you could be ANYTHING you want to be when you grow up. You could even be Prime Minister!
Nan was livid...
Bloody hard-nosed meddling madam on my telly again!
But Nan, surely she'll be softer, and nice, coz she's a mum!
Well, she should bloody act like one, then!

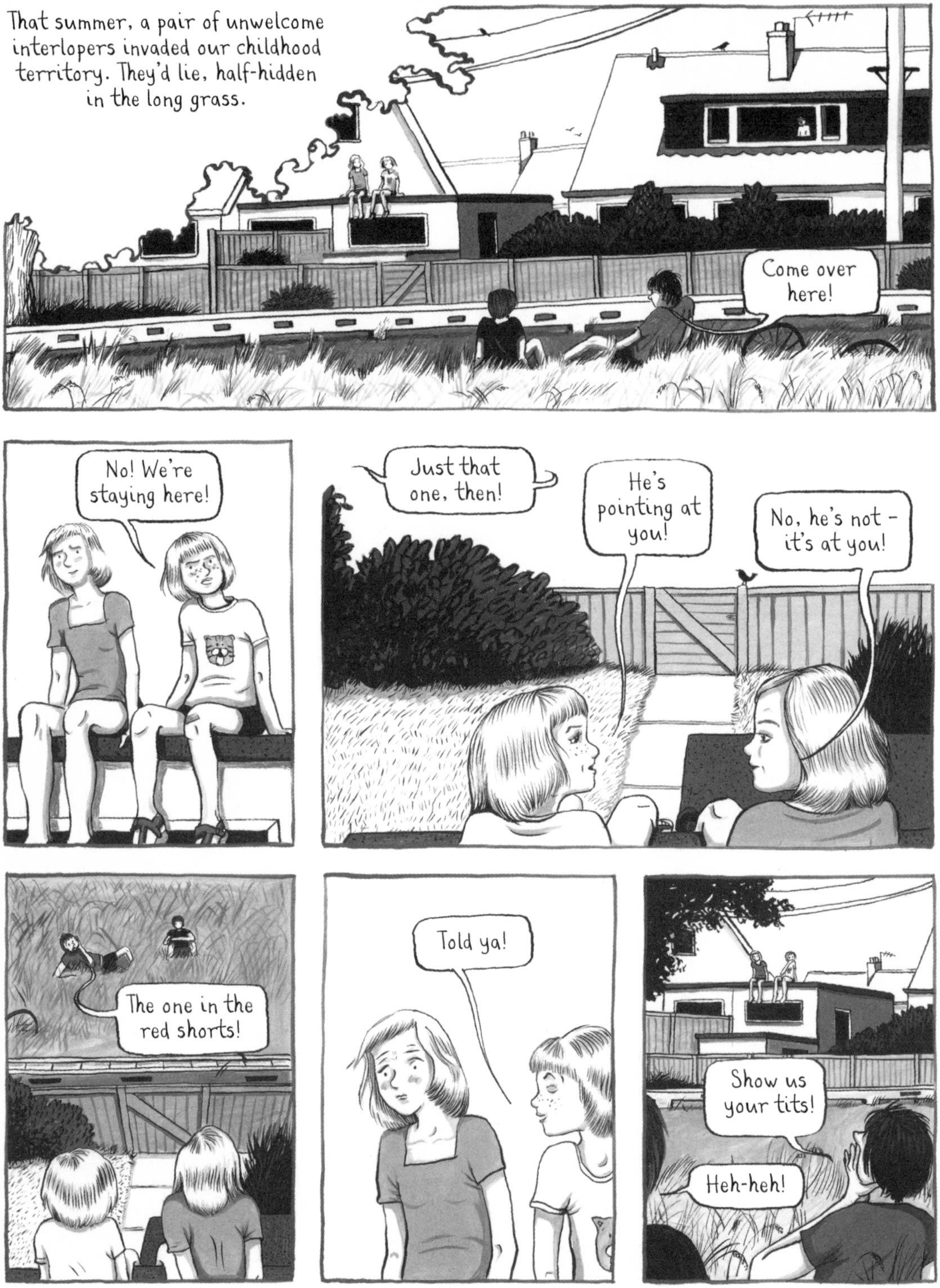
That summer, a pair of unwelcome interlopers invaded our childhood territory. They'd lie, half-hidden in the long grass.
Come over here!
No! We're staying here!
Just that one, then!
He's pointing at you!
No, he's not - it's at you!
The one in the red shorts!
Told ya!
Show us your tits!
Heh-heh!

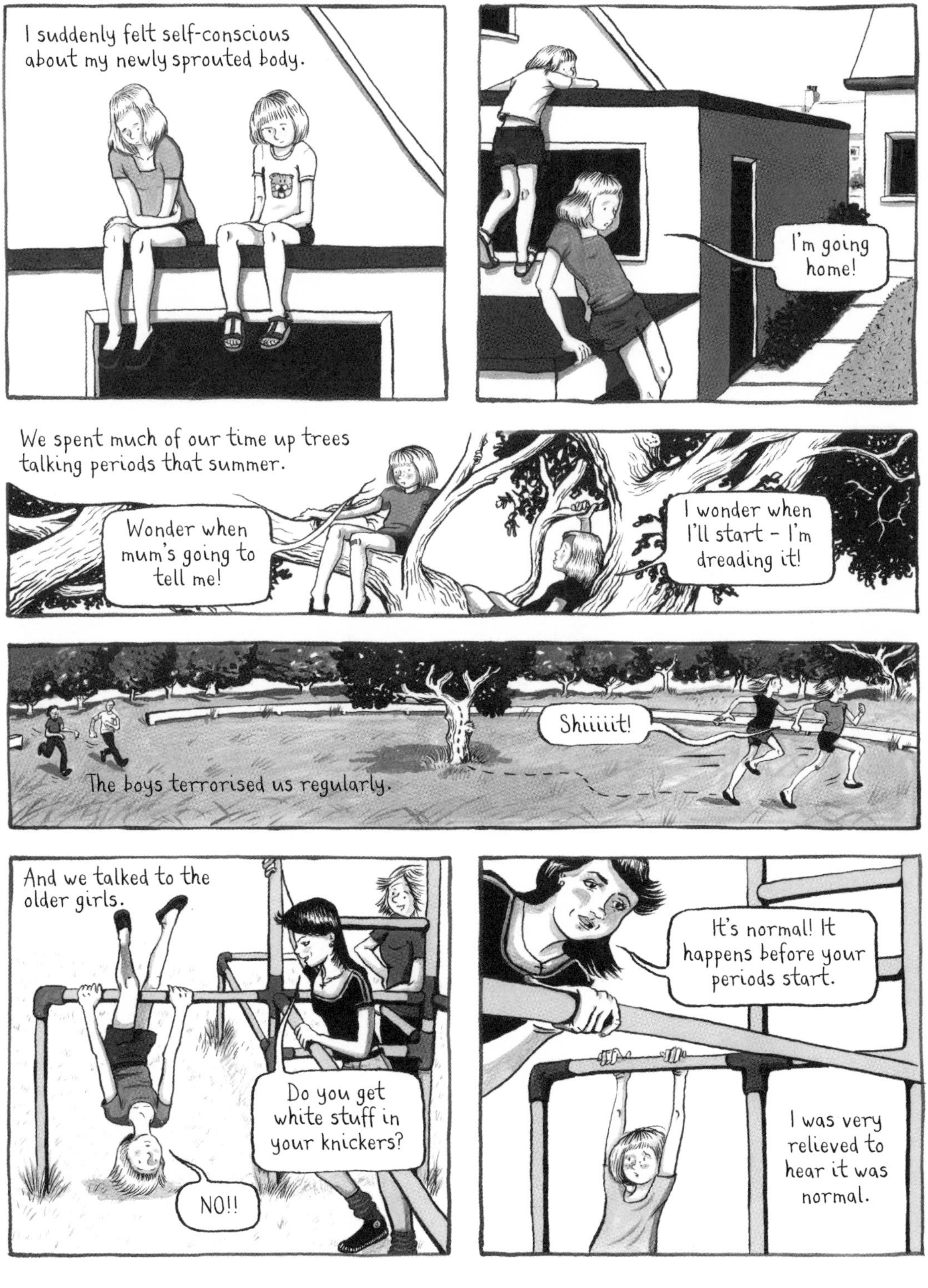
I suddenly felt self-conscious about my newly sprouted body.
I'm going home!
We spent much of our time up trees talking periods that summer.
Wonder when mum's going to tell me!
I wonder when I'll start - I'm dreading it!
Shiiiiit!
The boys terrorised us regularly.
And we talked to the older girls.
Do you get white stuff in your knickers?
NO!!
It's normal! It happens before your periods start.
I was very relieved to hear it was normal.

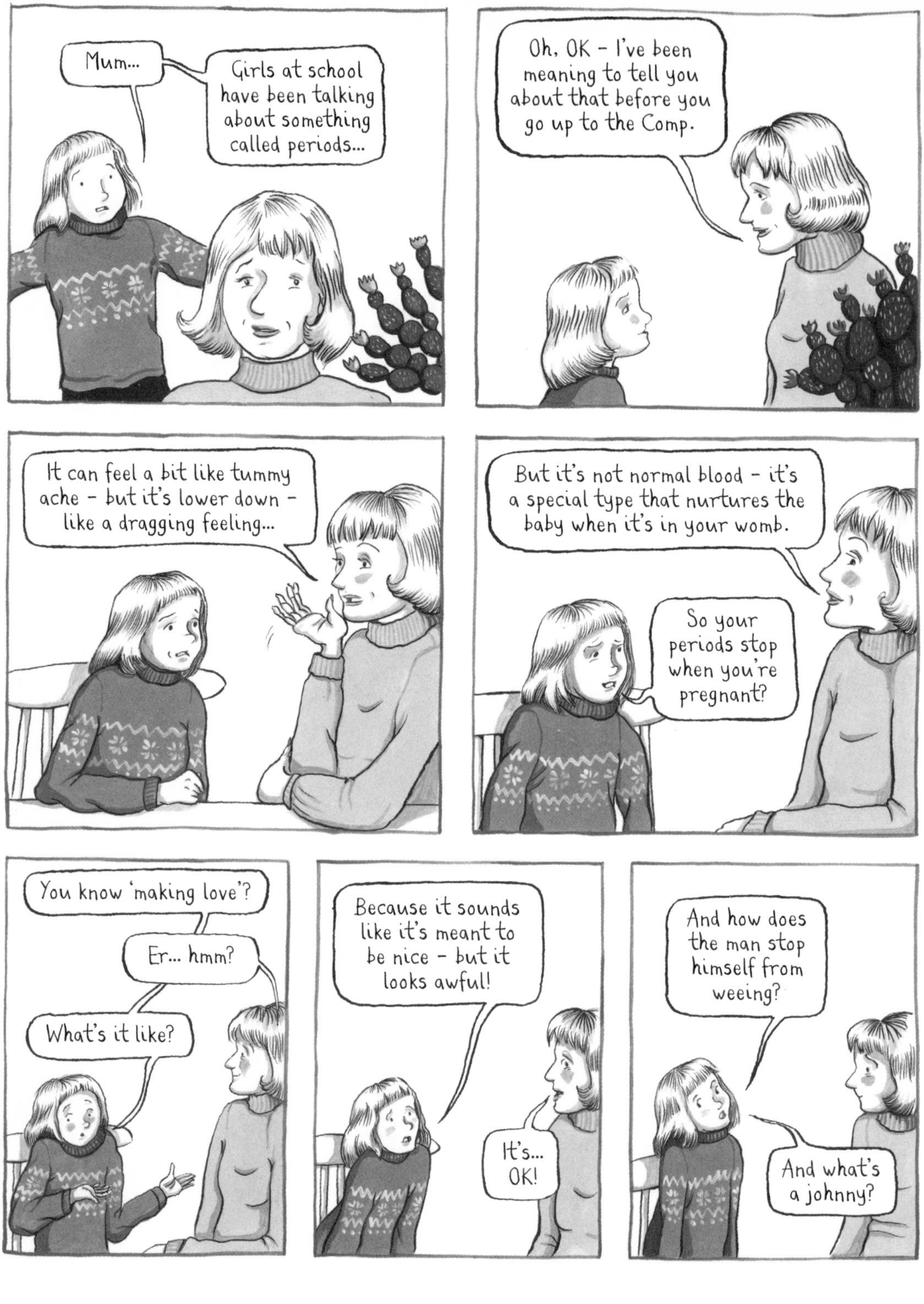
Mum...
Girls at school have been talking about something called periods...
Oh, OK – I've been meaning to tell you about that before you go up to the Comp.
It can feel a bit like tummy ache – but it's lower down – like a dragging feeling...
But it's not normal blood – it's a special type that nurtures the baby when it's in your womb.
So your periods stop when you're pregnant?
You know 'making love'?
Er... hmm?
What's it like?
Because it sounds like it's meant to be nice – but it looks awful!
It's... OK!
And how does the man stop himself from weeing?
And what's a johnny?

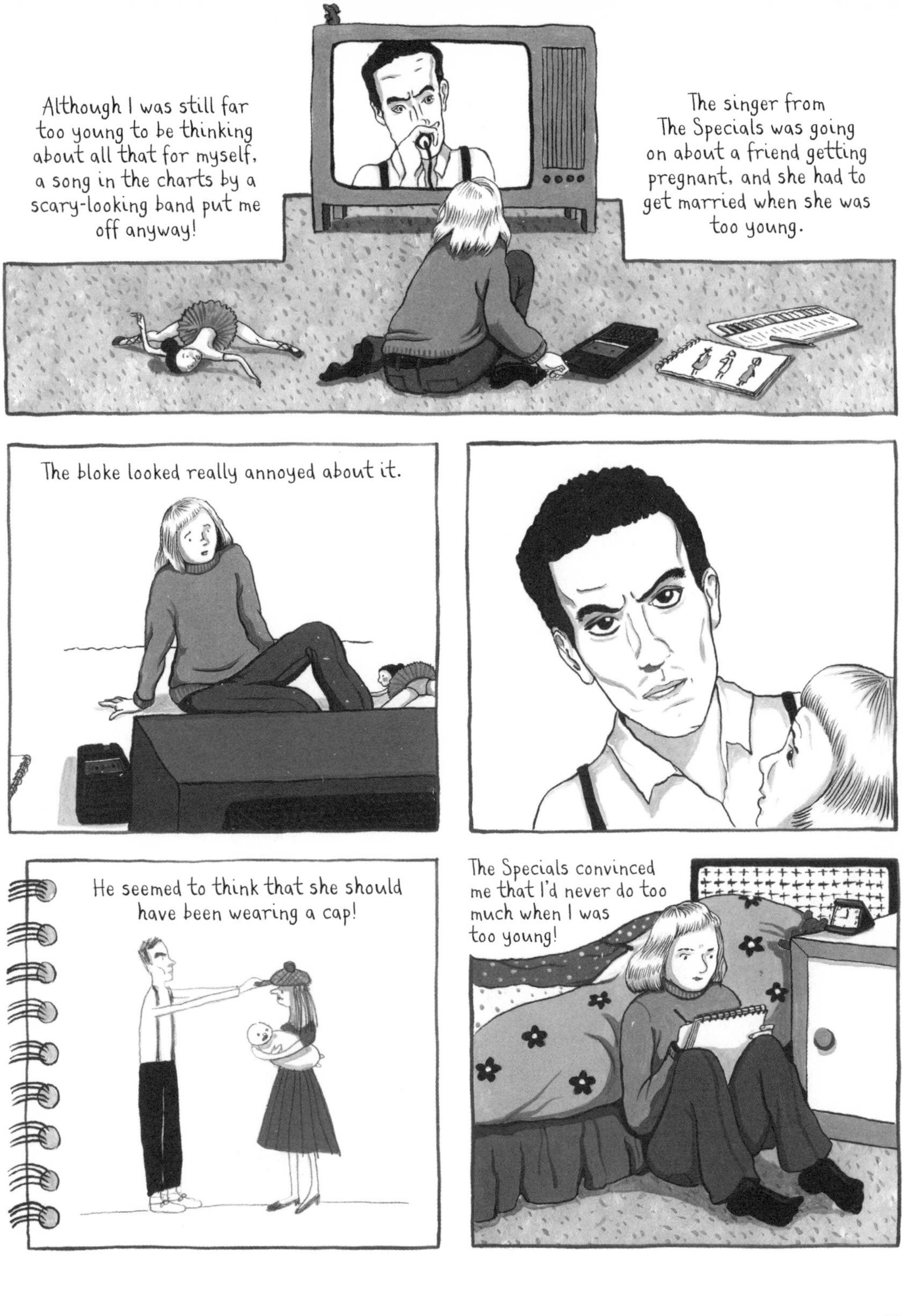
Although I was still far too young to be thinking about all that for myself, a song in the charts by a scary-looking band put me off anyway!
The singer from The Specials was going on about a friend getting pregnant, and she had to get married when she was too young.
The bloke looked really annoyed about it.
He seemed to think that she should have been wearing a cap!
The Specials convinced me that I'd never do too much when I was too young!

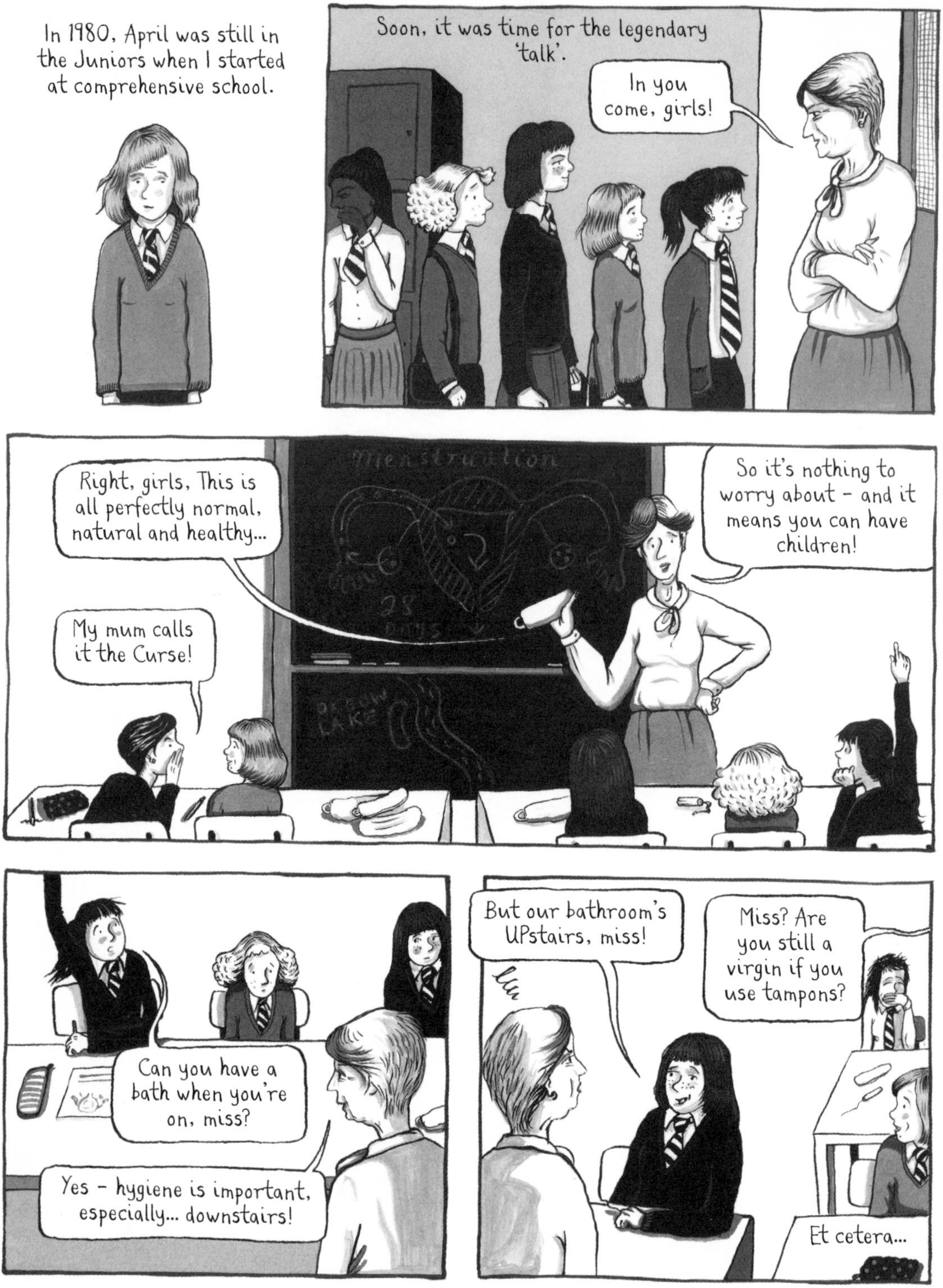

In 1980, April was still in the Juniors when I started at comprehensive school.
Soon, it was time for the legendary 'talk'.
In you come, girls!
Right, girls, This is all perfectly normal, natural and healthy...
So it's nothing to worry about - and it means you can have children!
My mum calls it the Curse!
Can you have a bath when you're on, miss?
Yes - hygiene is important, especially... downstairs!
But our bathroom's UPstairs, miss!
Miss? Are you still a virgin if you use tampons?
Et cetera...

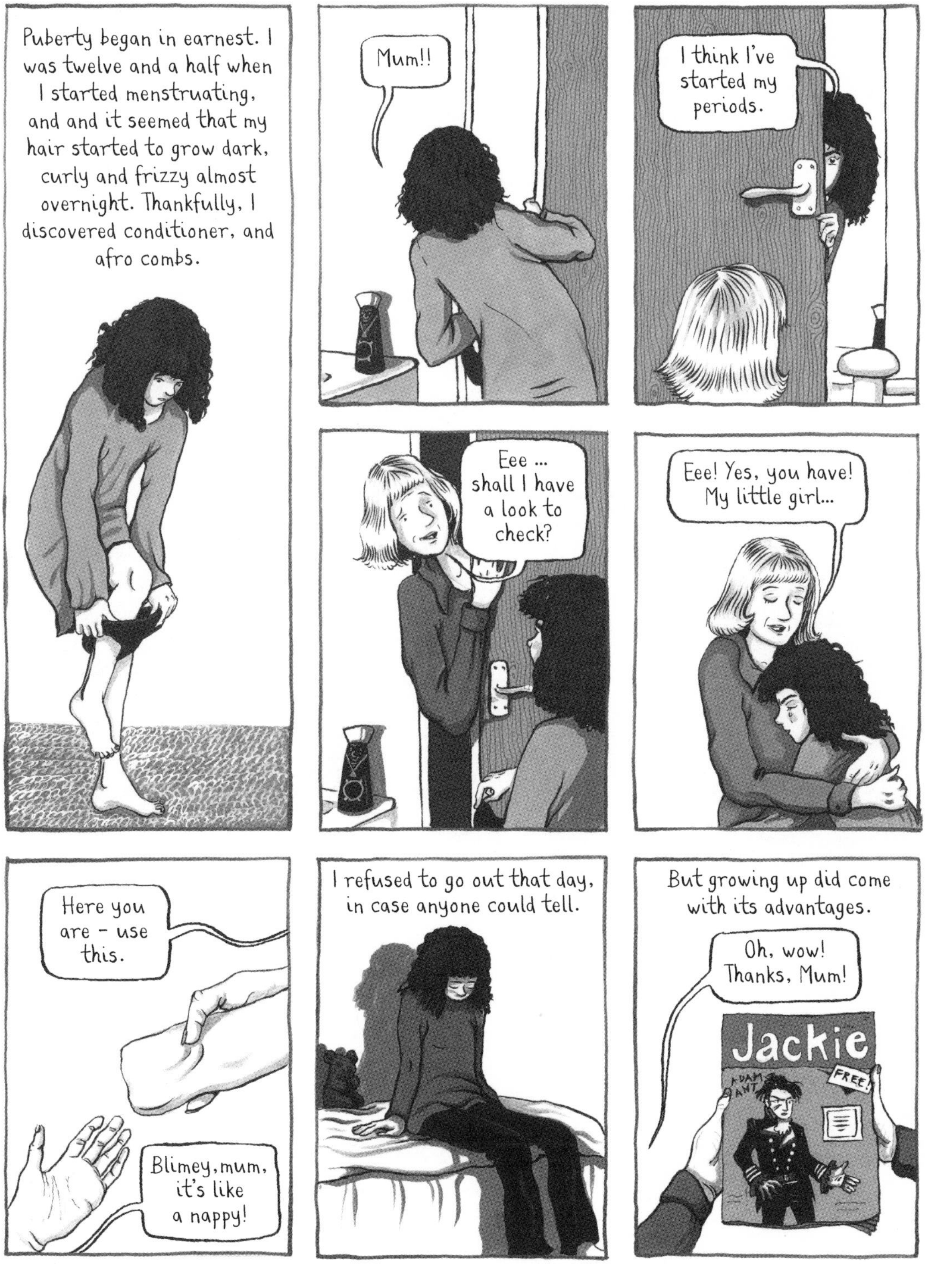

Puberty began in earnest. I was twelve and a half when I started menstruating, and and it seemed that my hair started to grow dark, curly and frizzy almost overnight. Thankfully, I discovered conditioner, and afro combs.
Mum!!
I think I've started my periods.
Eee ... shall I have a look to check?
Eee! Yes, you have! My little girl...
Here you are - use this.
Blimey, mum, it's like a nappy!
I refused to go out that day, in case anyone could tell.
But growing up did come with its advantages.
Oh, wow! Thanks, Mum!
Jackie
FREE!
ADAM ANT

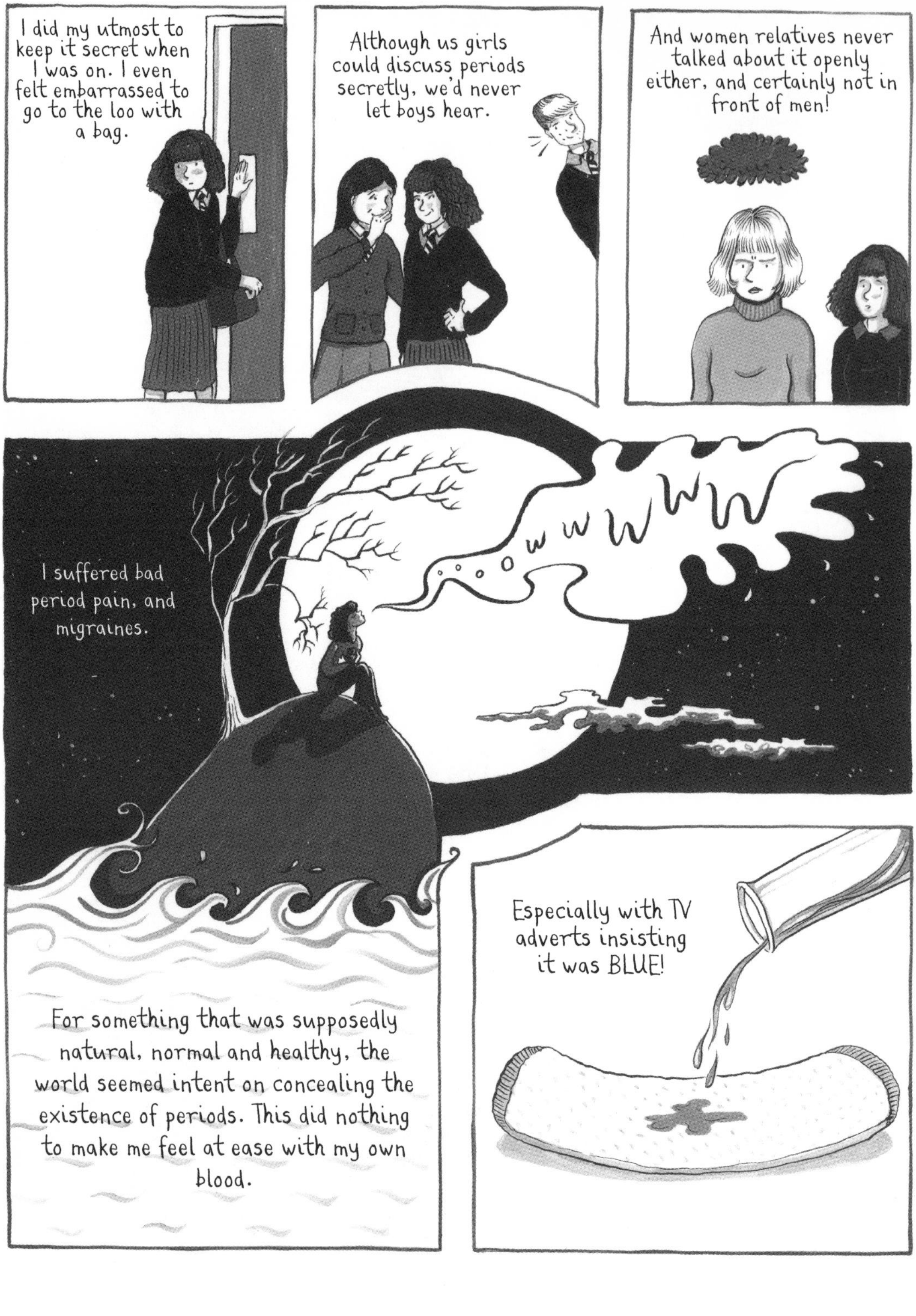
I did my utmost to keep it secret when I was on. I even felt embarrassed to go to the loo with a bag.
Although us girls could discuss periods secretly, we'd never let boys hear.
And women relatives never talked about it openly either, and certainly not in front of men!
I suffered bad period pain, and migraines.
OOwwwWWWW
For something that was supposedly natural, normal and healthy, the world seemed intent on concealing the existence of periods. This did nothing to make me feel at ease with my own blood.
Especially with TV adverts insisting it was BLUE!

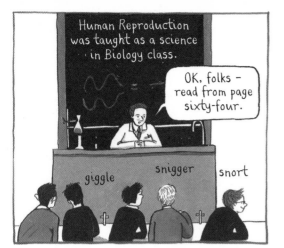

Human Reproduction was taught as a science in Biology class.

OK, folks – read from page sixty-four.

giggle   snigger   snort

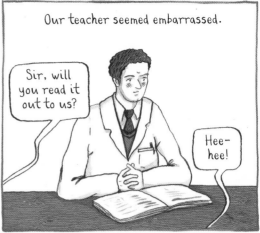

Our teacher seemed embarrassed.

Sir, will you read it out to us?

Hee-hee!

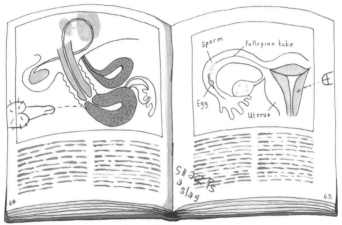

sperm   Fallopian tube

Egg   Uterus

slags slag

64   65

The male genitals were on top, impregnating the female genitals...

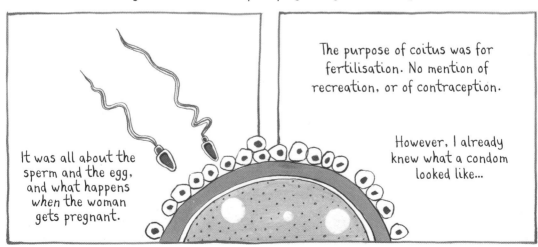

It was all about the sperm and the egg, and what happens when the woman gets pregnant.

The purpose of coitus was for fertilisation. No mention of recreation, or of contraception.

However, I already knew what a condom looked like...

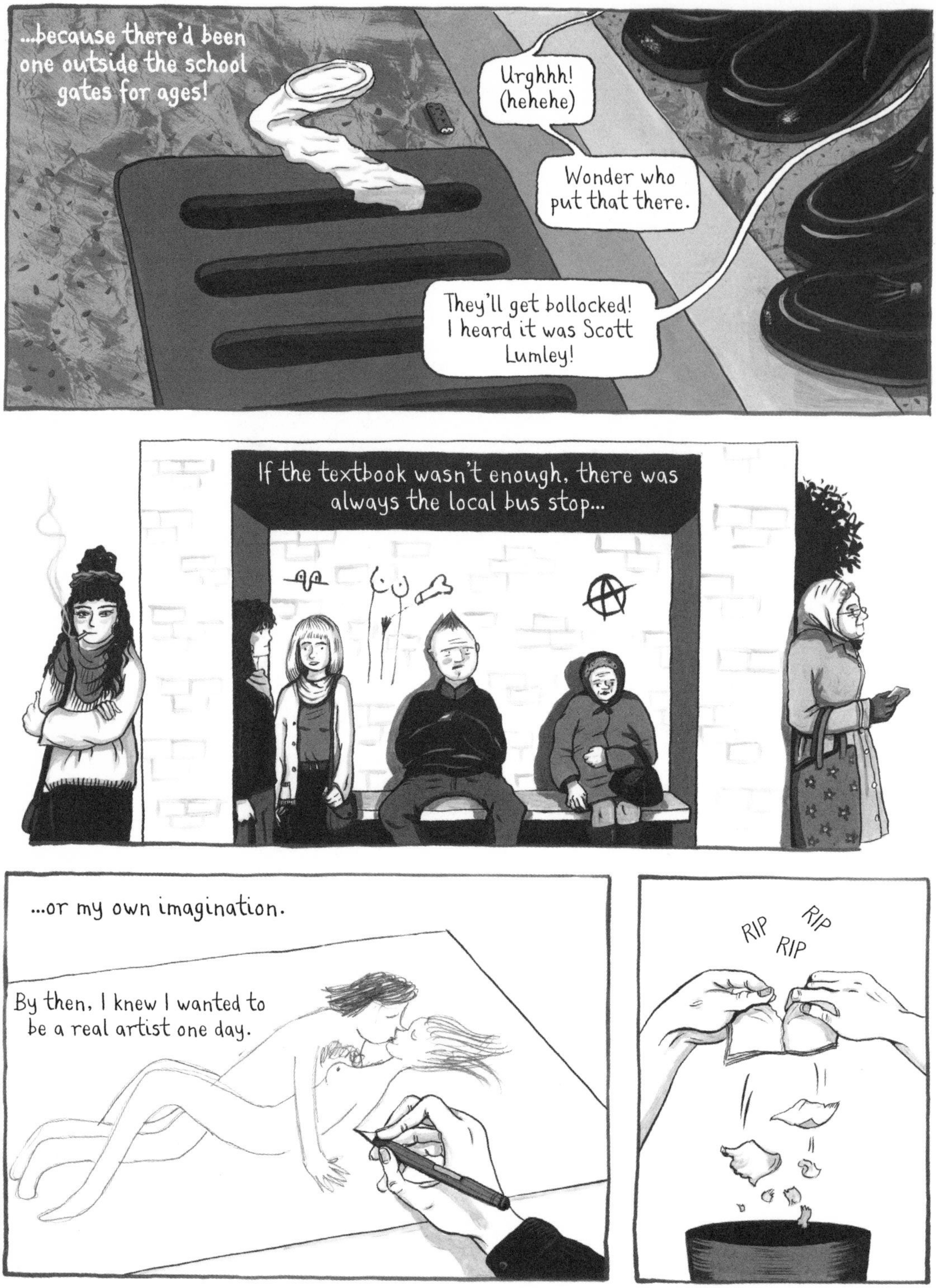
...because there'd been one outside the school gates for ages!
Urghhh! (hehehe)
Wonder who put that there.
They'll get bollocked! I heard it was Scott Lumley!
If the textbook wasn't enough, there was always the local bus stop...
...or my own imagination.
By then, I knew I wanted to be a real artist one day.
RIP
RIP
RIP

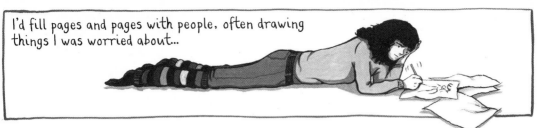
I'd fill pages and pages with people, often drawing things I was worried about...

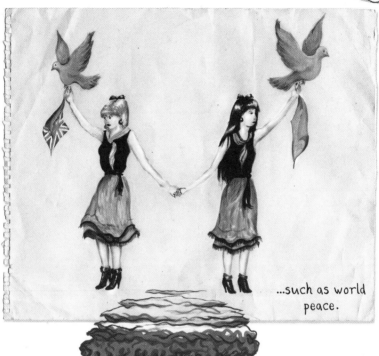
...such as world peace.

Would Ronald Reagan and Yuri Andropov...

...drop off anything nasty over our town?

There was the Falklands Crisis...

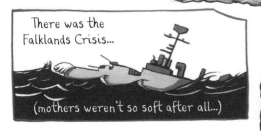
(mothers weren't so soft after all...)

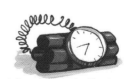
...and bombs exploding everywhere.

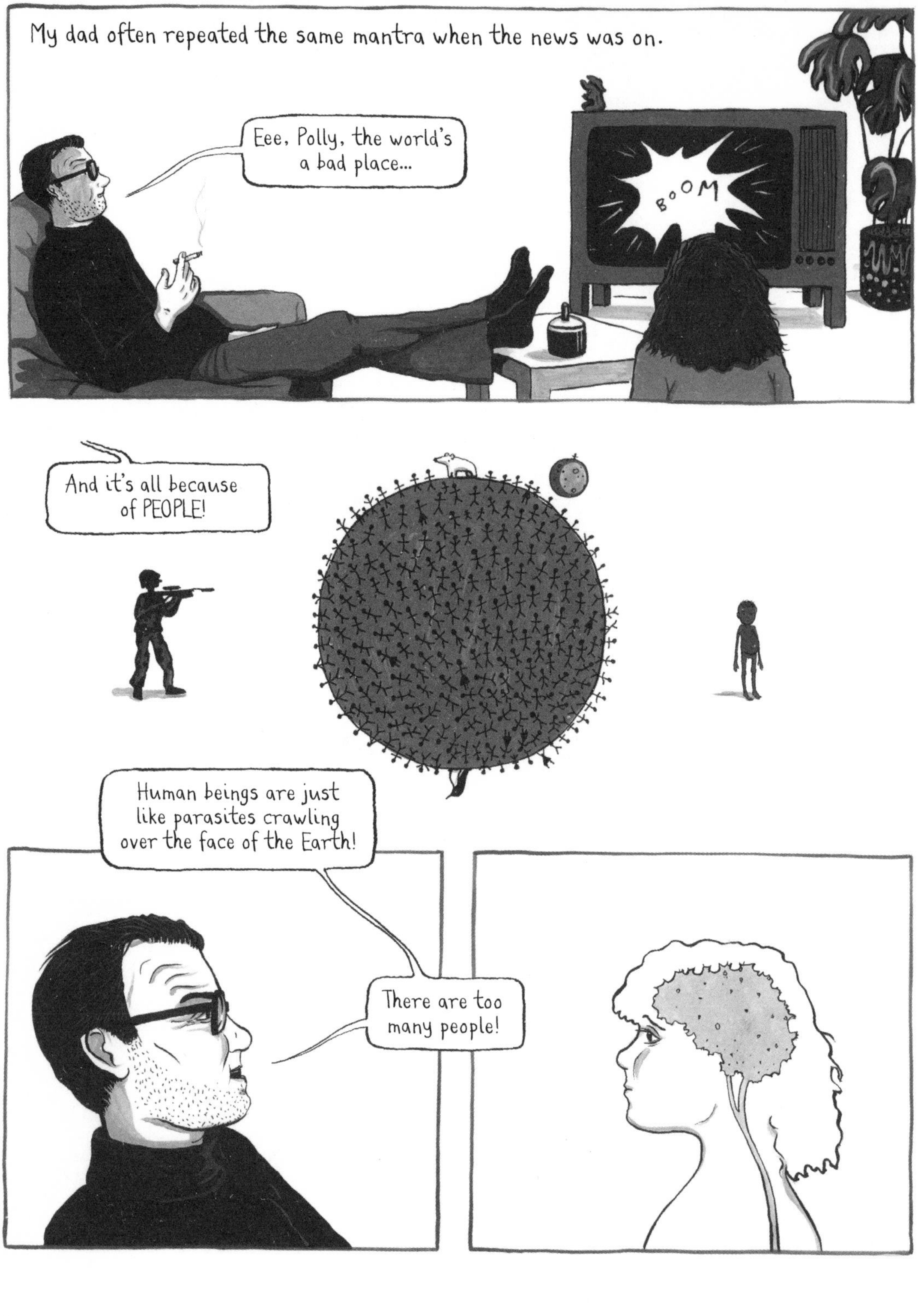
My dad often repeated the same mantra when the news was on.
Eee, Polly, the world's a bad place...
BOOM
And it's all because of PEOPLE!
Human beings are just like parasites crawling over the face of the Earth!
There are too many people!

It was a good job some people didn't have children, then!

In 1982, there was a very uncool song in the charts – but I secretly liked it.

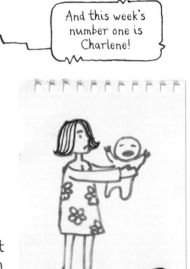

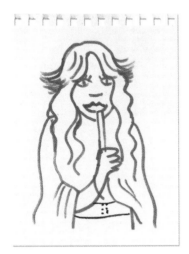

It was a lament by a lonely woman who had regrets about not having had kids.

And this week's number one is Charlene!

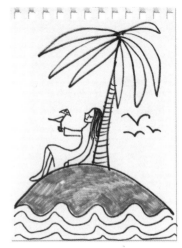

She was singing it to an unhappy housewife who felt like she was missing out on an exciting life, because she was a mother.

The lady in the song had travelled the world, 'had' lots of men and been to lots of parties.

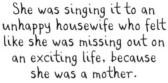

I couldn't work out if it meant she was a prostitute or not.

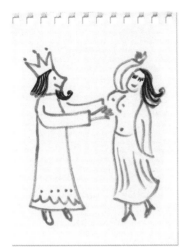

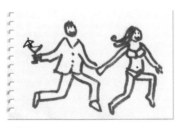

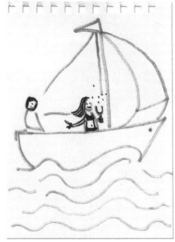

It sounded as if she'd had a great time – but now she was older she was lonely, because she hadn't settled down with a nice husband and had a baby.

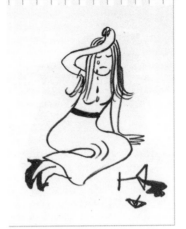

She thought that these were the most important things in life, but now it was too late for her to do that.

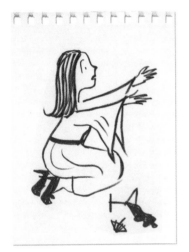

She wanted to tell the bored mother to be thankful that she had a baby and husband, because, if she didn't have them, then she'd only regret it and be lonely.

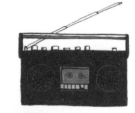

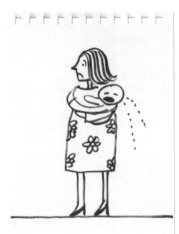

She was crying about children that she hadn't had – children who would have made her feel whole. I didn't know if she meant she'd had abortions or just that she'd never got pregnant.

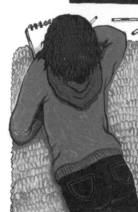

I thought it was all tragic and lovely, and even though she'd 'done it' with a vicar (and I fancied the local vicar's son), I felt I didn't want to end up like her, so maybe I should be careful of having too much fun, especially in California, or Nice.

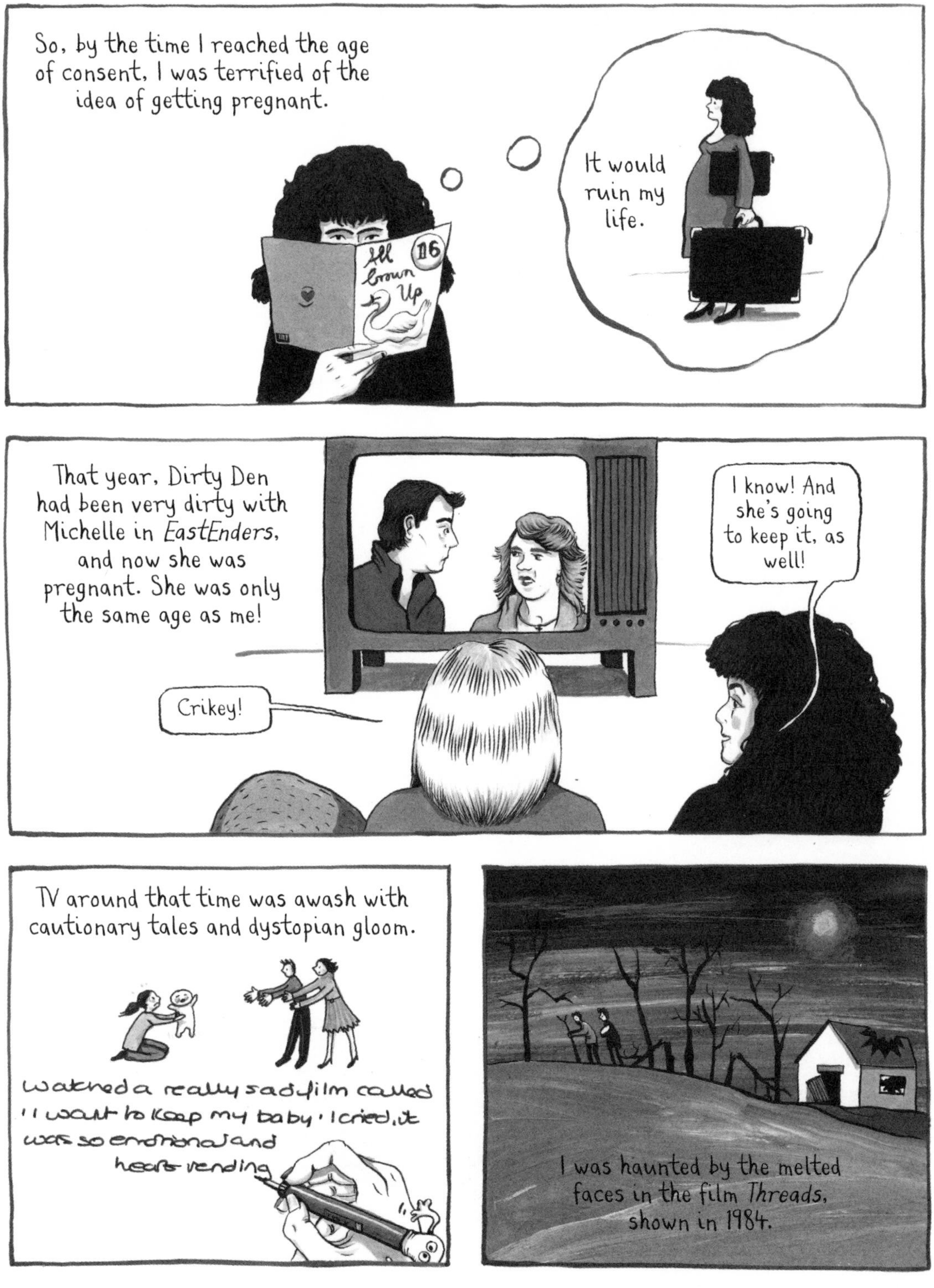
So, by the time I reached the age of consent, I was terrified of the idea of getting pregnant.
16
All Grown Up
It would ruin my life.
That year, Dirty Den had been very dirty with Michelle in *EastEnders*, and now she was pregnant. She was only the same age as me!
I know! And she's going to keep it, as well!
Crikey!
TV around that time was awash with cautionary tales and dystopian gloom.
watched a really sad film called 'I want to keep my baby' I cried, it was so emotional and heart rending
I was haunted by the melted faces in the film *Threads*, shown in 1984.

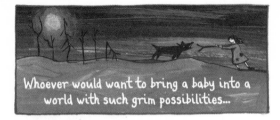

Whoever would want to bring a baby into a world with such grim possibilities...

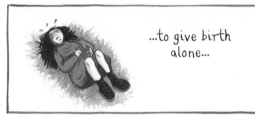

...to give birth alone...

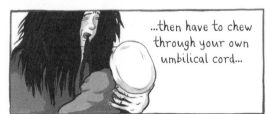

...then have to chew through your own umbilical cord...

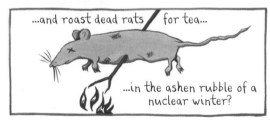

...and roast dead rats for tea...

...in the ashen rubble of a nuclear winter?

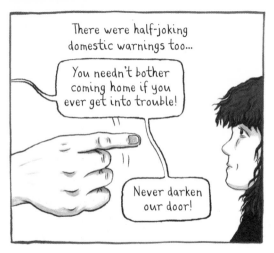

There were half-joking domestic warnings too...

You needn't bother coming home if you ever get into trouble!

Never darken our door!

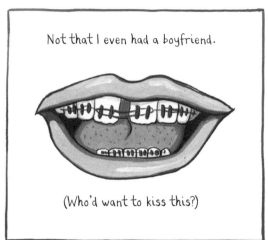

Not that I even had a boyfriend.

(Who'd want to kiss this?)

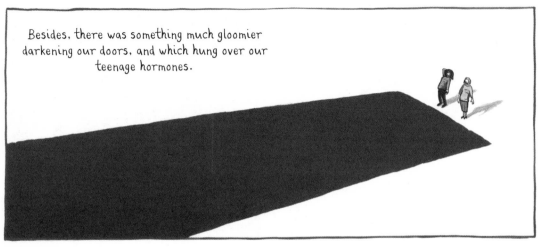

Besides, there was something much gloomier darkening our doors, and which hung over our teenage hormones.

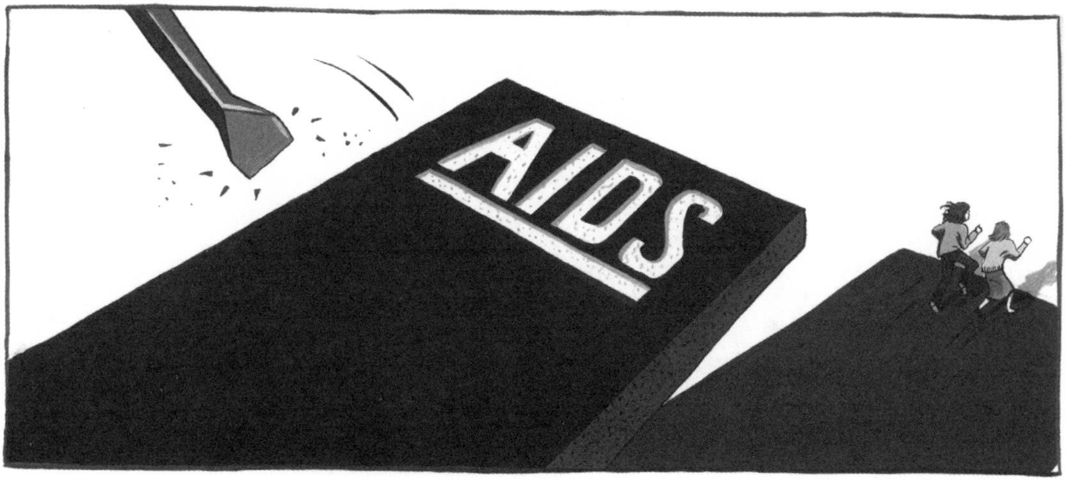
AIDS

My parents needn't have worried. Getting pregnant might have meant being a housewife!

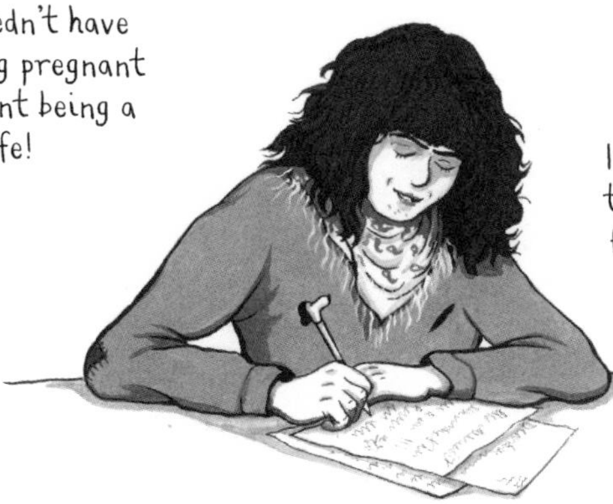

In one of my prolific letters to a pen friend, I vented my feelings on that particular matter...

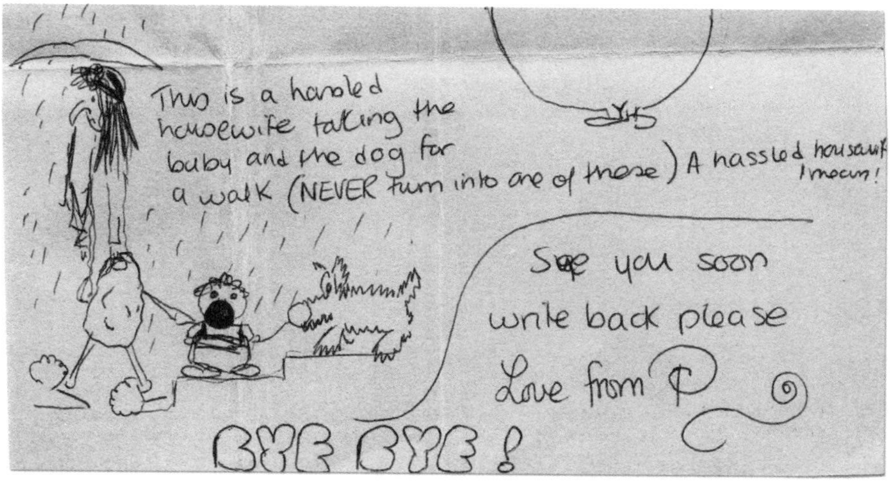
This is a hassled housewife taking the baby and the dog for a walk (NEVER turn into one of these) A hassled housewife I mean!
See you soon
write back please
Love from
BYE BYE!

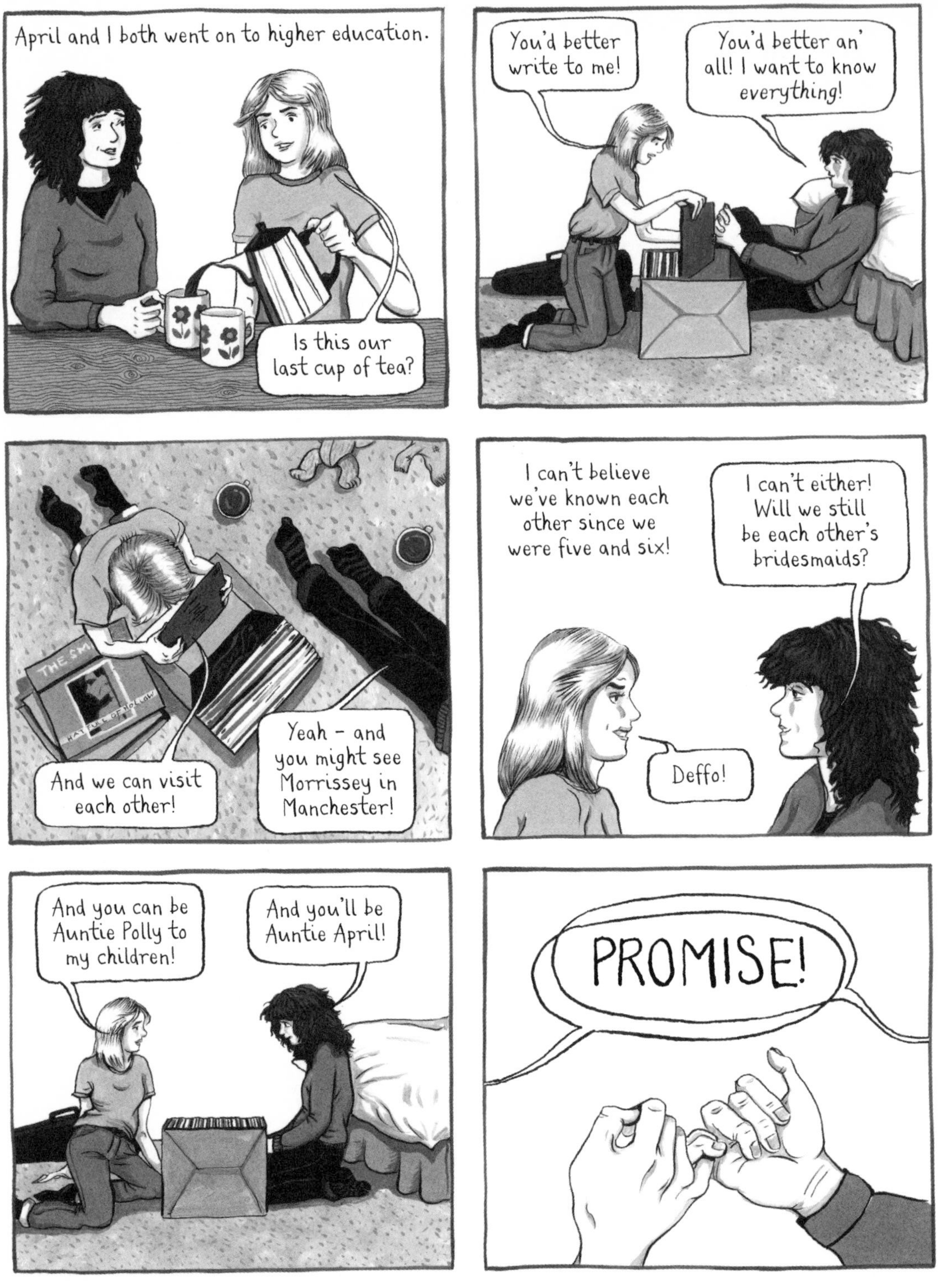
April and I both went on to higher education.
Is this our last cup of tea?
You'd better write to me!
You'd better an' all! I want to know everything!
And we can visit each other!
Yeah - and you might see Morrissey in Manchester!
I can't believe we've known each other since we were five and six!
I can't either! Will we still be each other's bridesmaids?
Deffo!
And you can be Auntie Polly to my children!
And you'll be Auntie April!
PROMISE!

April went the day before me.

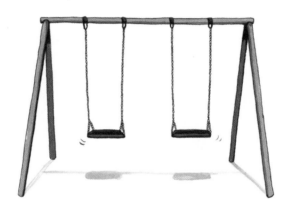

I hate being the last one left.

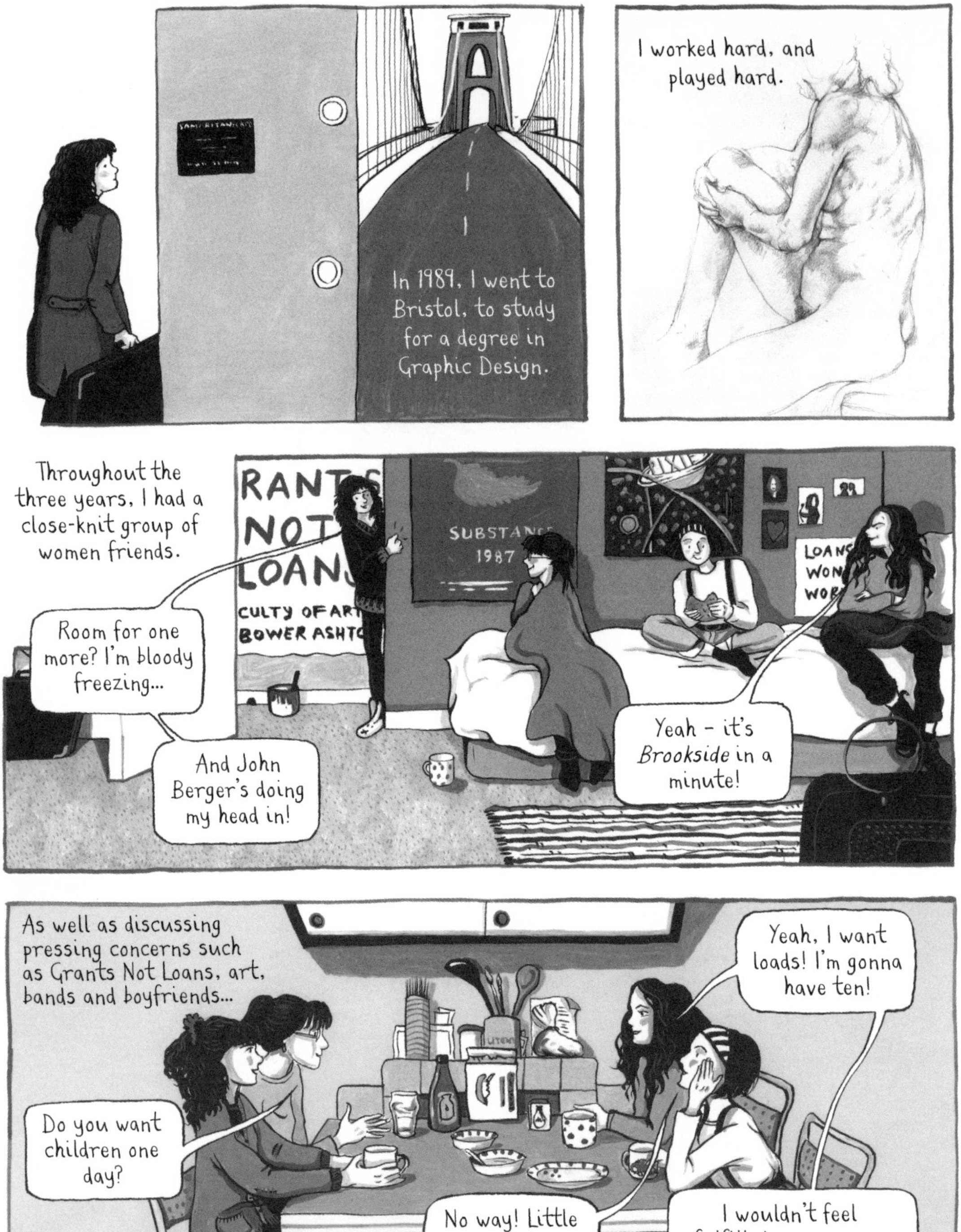
In 1989, I went to Bristol, to study for a degree in Graphic Design.
I worked hard, and played hard.
Throughout the three years, I had a close-knit group of women friends.
RANTS NOT LOANS
CULTY OF ART BOWER ASHTO
SUBSTANC 1987
Room for one more? I'm bloody freezing...
And John Berger's doing my head in!
Yeah – it's *Brookside* in a minute!
As well as discussing pressing concerns such as Grants Not Loans, art, bands and boyfriends...
Do you want children one day?
No way! Little ankle-biters!
Yeah, I want loads! I'm gonna have ten!
I wouldn't feel fulfilled as a woman if I didn't have any.

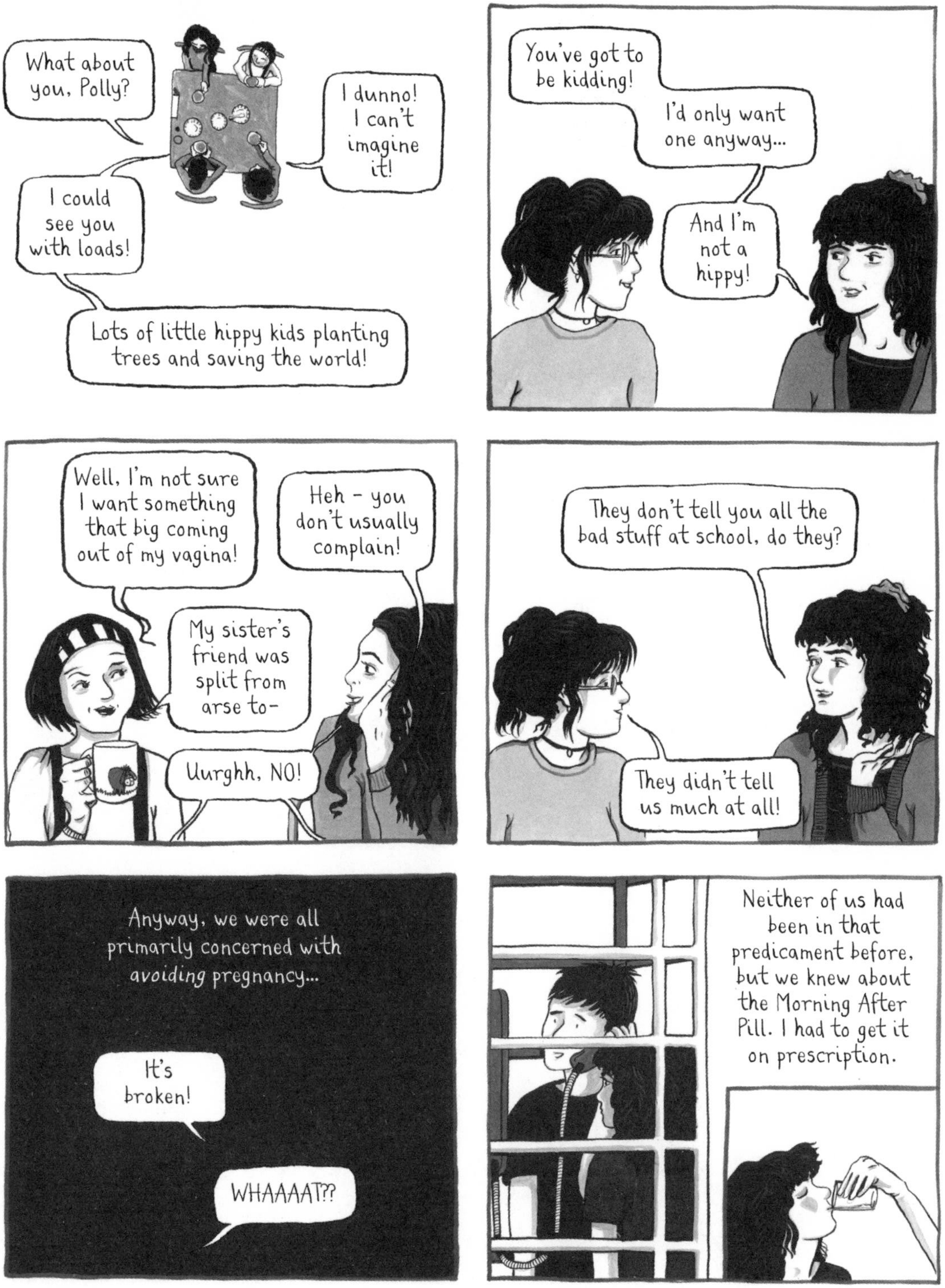
What about you, Polly?
I dunno! I can't imagine it!
I could see you with loads!
Lots of little hippy kids planting trees and saving the world!
You've got to be kidding!
I'd only want one anyway...
And I'm not a hippy!
Well, I'm not sure I want something that big coming out of my vagina!
Heh - you don't usually complain!
My sister's friend was split from arse to-
Uurghh, NO!
They don't tell you all the bad stuff at school, do they?
They didn't tell us much at all!
Anyway, we were all primarily concerned with avoiding pregnancy...
It's broken!
WHAAAAT??
Neither of us had been in that predicament before, but we knew about the Morning After Pill. I had to get it on prescription.

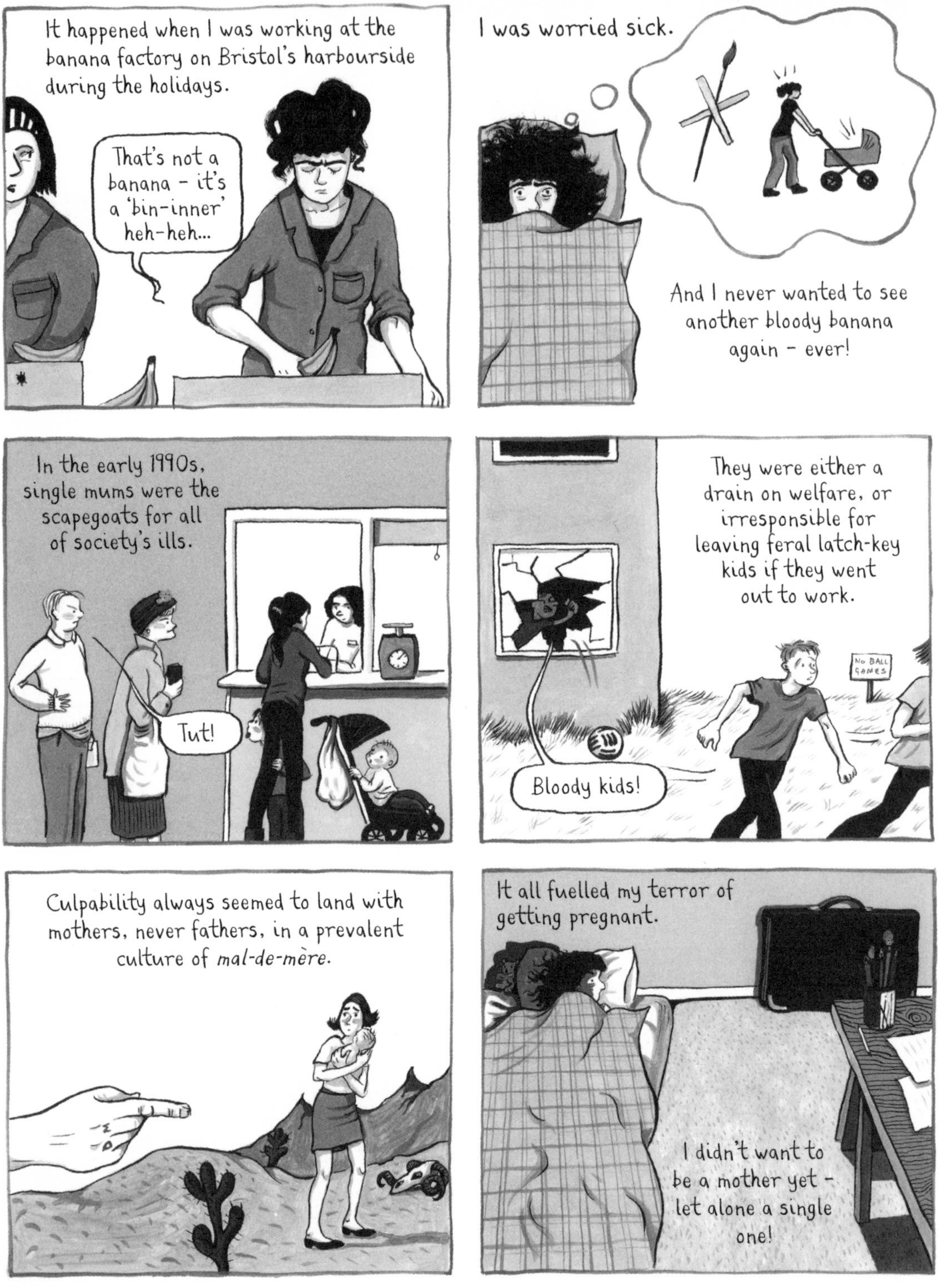
It happened when I was working at the banana factory on Bristol's harbourside during the holidays.
That's not a banana – it's a 'bin-inner' heh-heh...
I was worried sick.
And I never wanted to see another bloody banana again – ever!
In the early 1990s, single mums were the scapegoats for all of society's ills.
Tut!
They were either a drain on welfare, or irresponsible for leaving feral latch-key kids if they went out to work.
NO BALL GAMES
Bloody kids!
Culpability always seemed to land with mothers, never fathers, in a prevalent culture of *mal-de-mère*.
It all fuelled my terror of getting pregnant.
I didn't want to be a mother yet – let alone a single one!

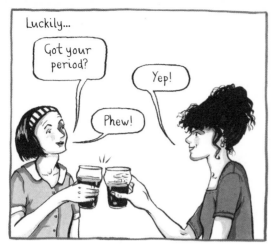

Luckily...

Got your period?

Yep!

Phew!

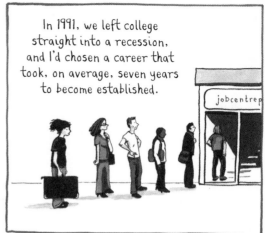

In 1991, we left college straight into a recession, and I'd chosen a career that took, on average, seven years to become established.

jobcentrep

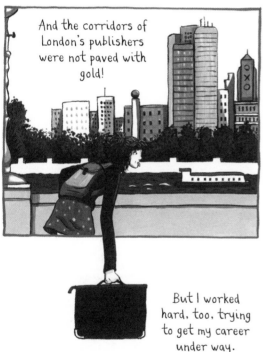

And the corridors of London's publishers were not paved with gold!

OXO

But I worked hard, too, trying to get my career under way.

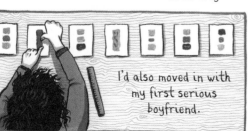

I'd also moved in with my first serious boyfriend.

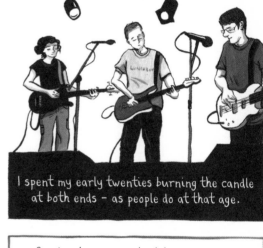

I spent my early twenties burning the candle at both ends – as people do at that age.

So, I put my persistent tiredness and stubborn sore throat down to a busy life and bad diet.

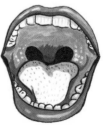

I resolved to eat more protein, and Vitamin C.

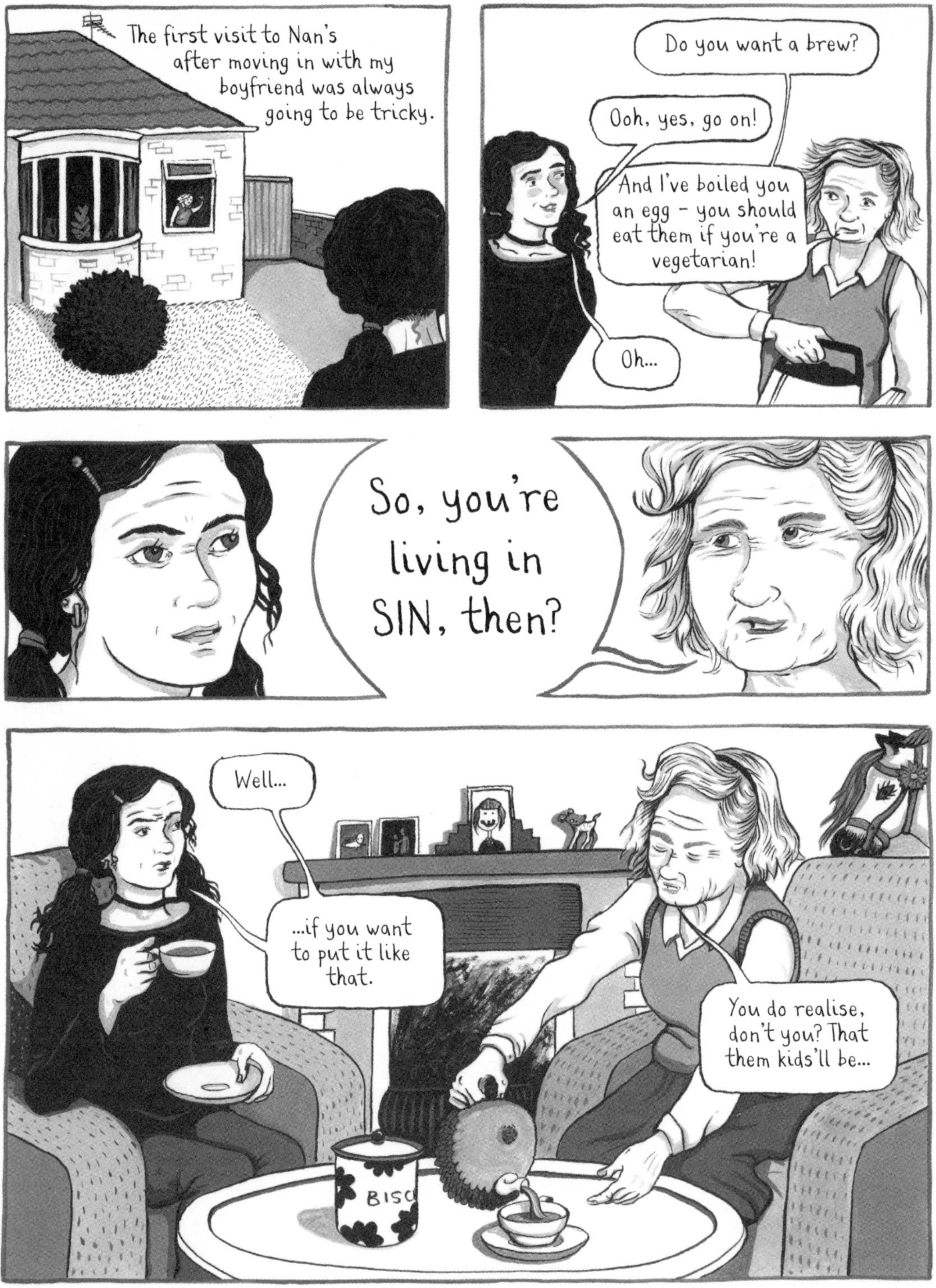
The first visit to Nan's after moving in with my boyfriend was always going to be tricky.
Do you want a brew?
Ooh, yes, go on!
And I've boiled you an egg – you should eat them if you're a vegetarian!
Oh...
So, you're living in SIN, then?
Well...
...if you want to put it like that.
You do realise, don't you? That them kids'll be...
BISC

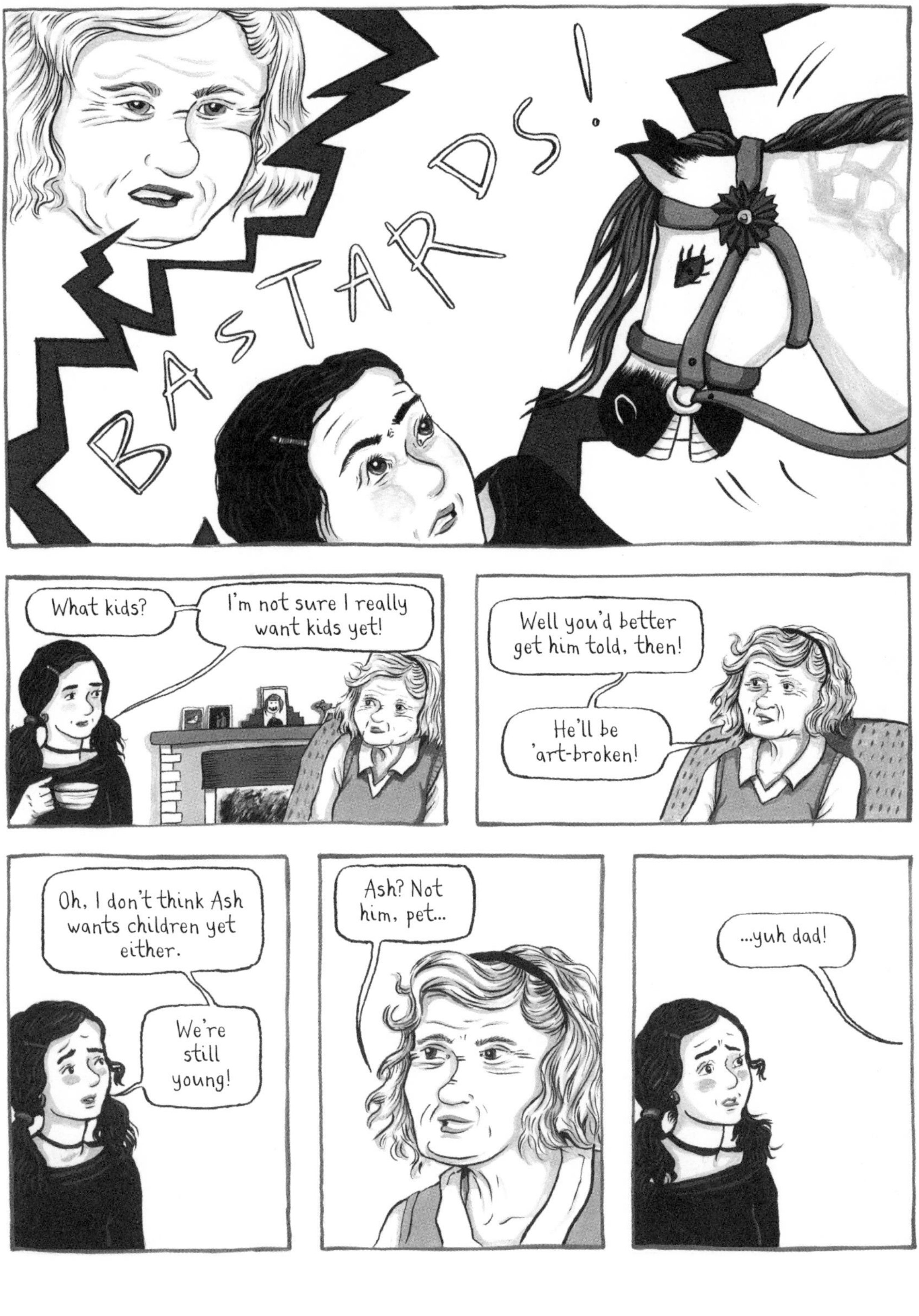
BASTARDS!
What kids?
I'm not sure I really want kids yet!
Well you'd better get him told, then!
He'll be 'art-broken!
Oh, I don't think Ash wants children yet either.
We're still young!
Ash? Not him, pet...
...yuh dad!

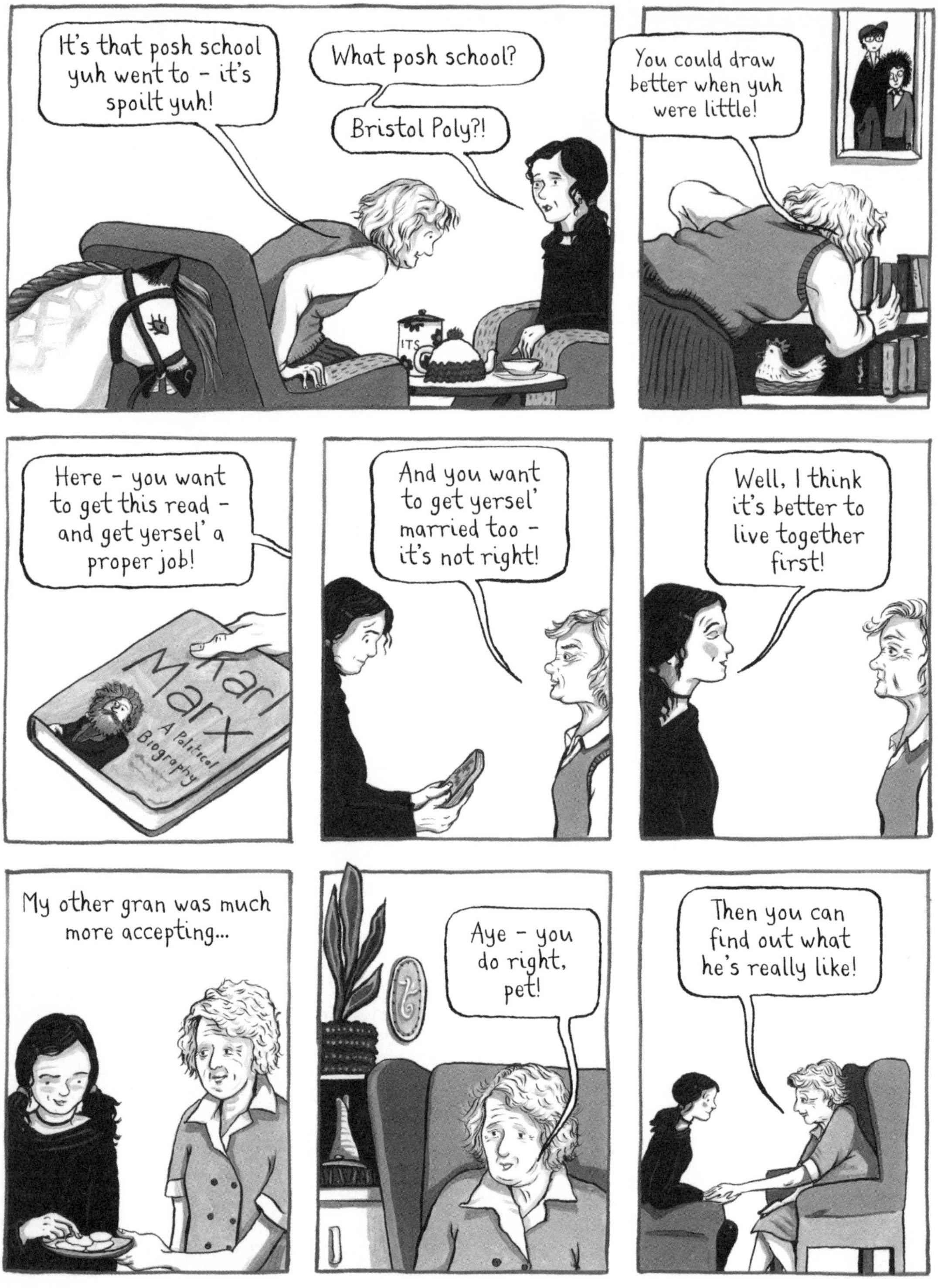
It's that posh school yuh went to - it's spoilt yuh!
What posh school?
Bristol Poly?!
ITS
You could draw better when yuh were little!
Here - you want to get this read - and get yersel' a proper job!
Karl Marx
A Political Biography
And you want to get yersel' married too - it's not right!
Well, I think it's better to live together first!
My other gran was much more accepting...
Aye - you do right, pet!
Then you can find out what he's really like!

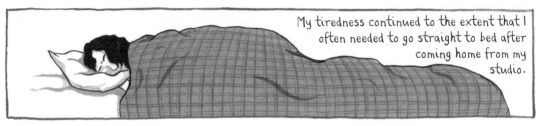

My tiredness continued to the extent that I often needed to go straight to bed after coming home from my studio.

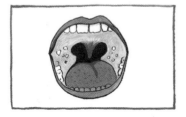

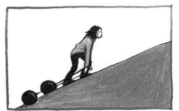

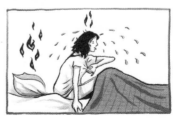

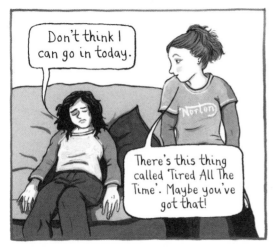

Don't think I can go in today.

There's this thing called 'Tired All The Time'. Maybe you've got that!

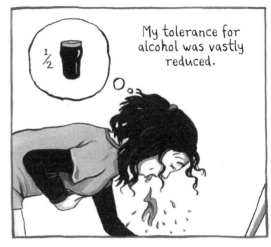

My tolerance for alcohol was vastly reduced.

½

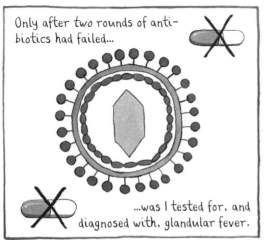

Only after two rounds of anti-biotics had failed...

...was I tested for, and diagnosed with, glandular fever.

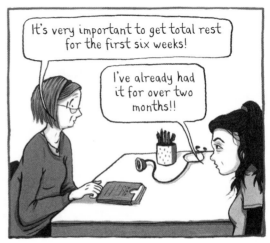

It's very important to get total rest for the first six weeks!

I've already had it for over two months!!

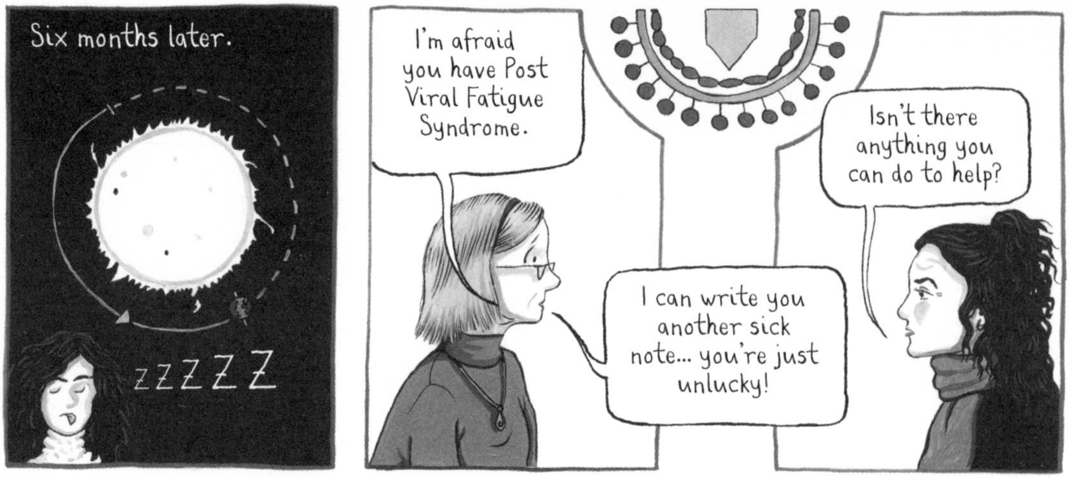
Six months later.
ZZZZZ
I'm afraid you have Post Viral Fatigue Syndrome.
Isn't there anything you can do to help?
I can write you another sick note... you're just unlucky!

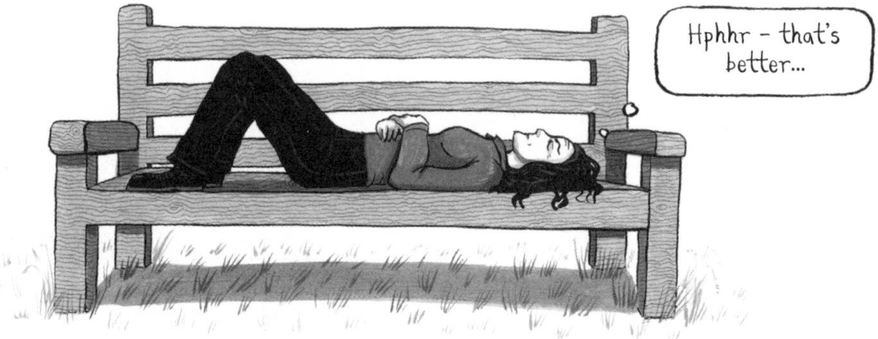
Hphhr - that's better...

I was 'unlucky' for the next few years. I became vertically challenged – the 'really boring' one who didn't drink or go out much – the 'hypochondriac'...

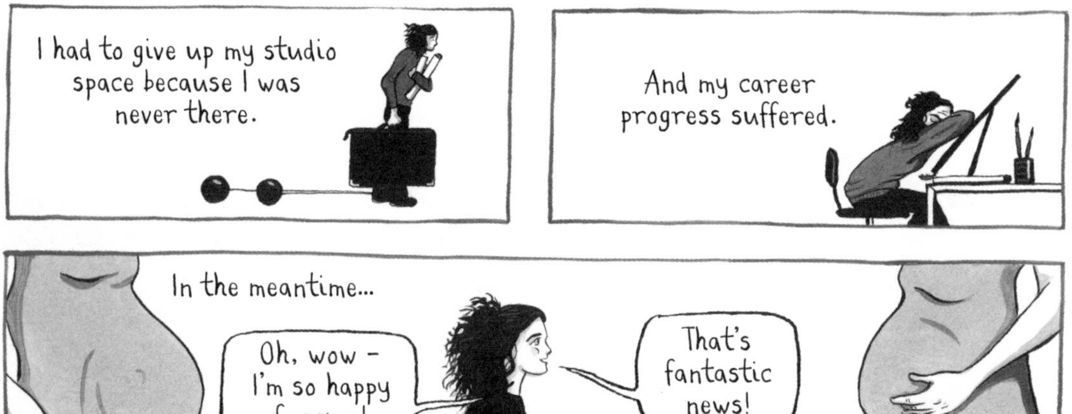
I had to give up my studio space because I was never there.
And my career progress suffered.
In the meantime...
Oh, wow - I'm so happy for you!
That's fantastic news!

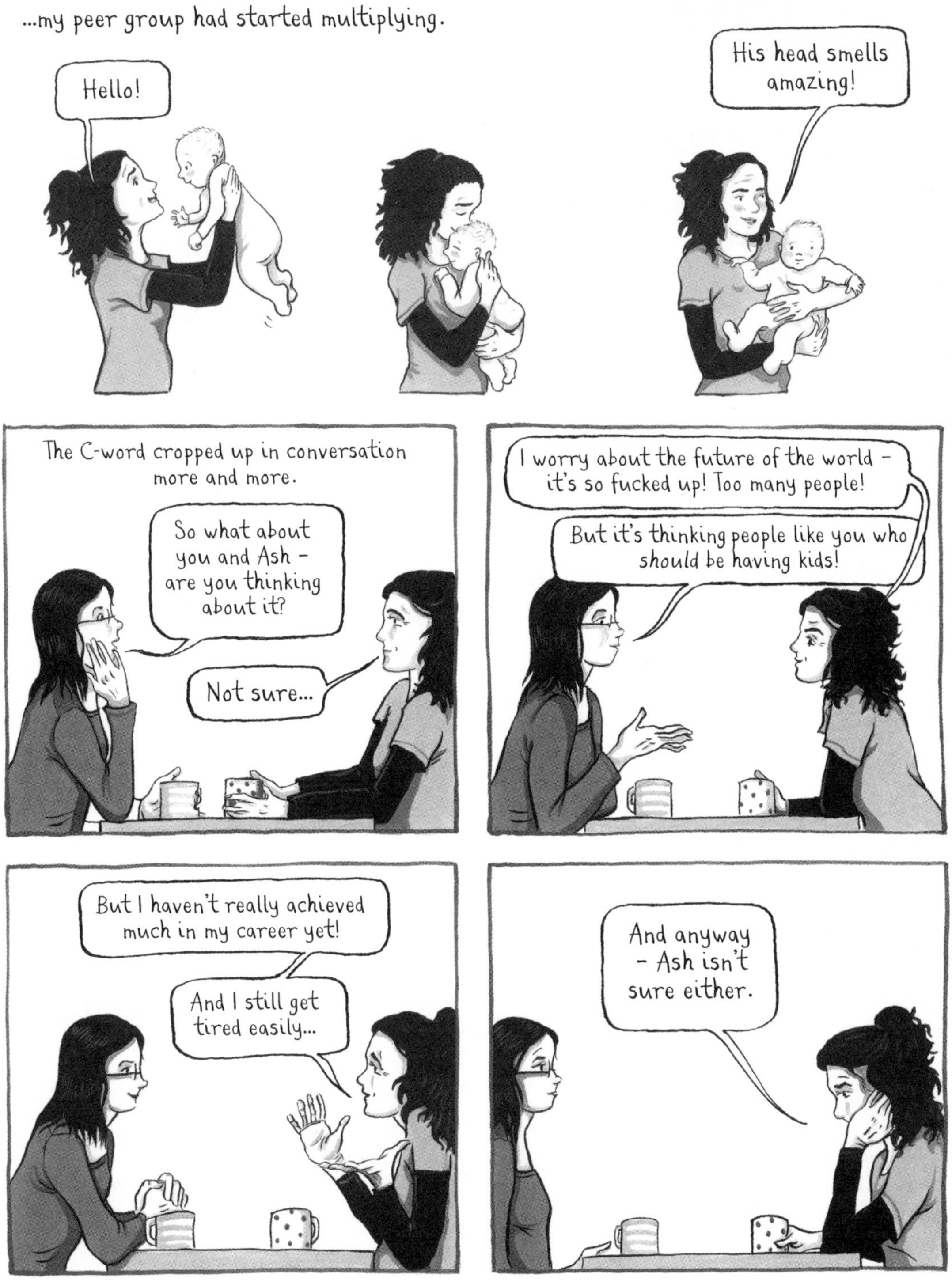
...my peer group had started multiplying.
Hello!
His head smells amazing!
The C-word cropped up in conversation more and more.
So what about you and Ash - are you thinking about it?
Not sure...
I worry about the future of the world - it's so fucked up! Too many people!
But it's thinking people like you who *should* be having kids!
But I haven't really achieved much in my career yet!
And I still get tired easily...
And anyway - Ash isn't sure either.

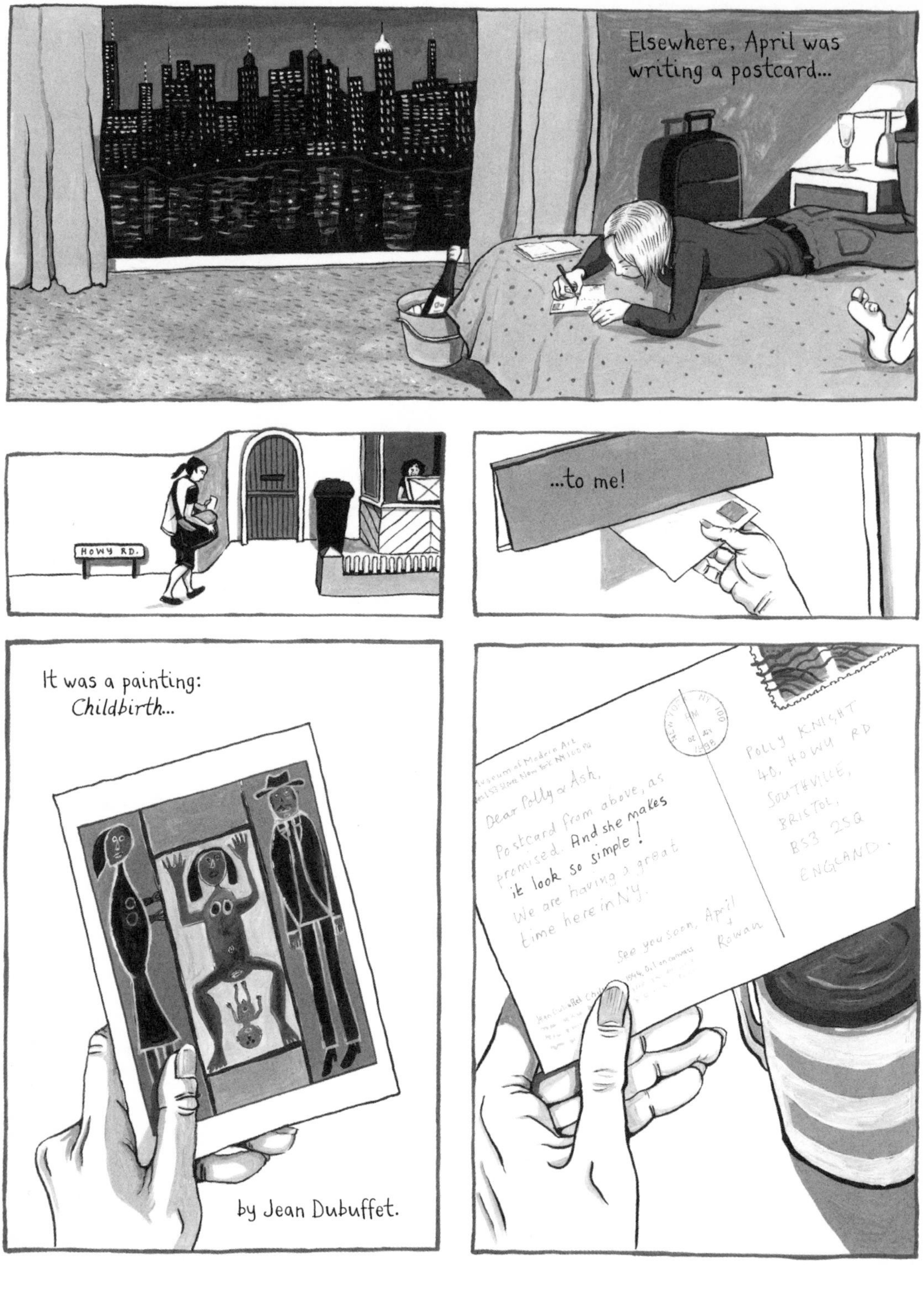
Elsewhere, April was writing a postcard...
HOWY RD.
...to me!
It was a painting: *Childbirth*...
by Jean Dubuffet.
Museum of Modern Art
Dear Polly & Ash,
Postcard from above, as promised. And she makes it look so simple!
We are having a great time here in NY.
See you soon, April + Rowan
POLLY KNIGHT
40, HOWY RD
SOUTHVILLE,
BRISTOL,
BS3 2SQ
ENGLAND.

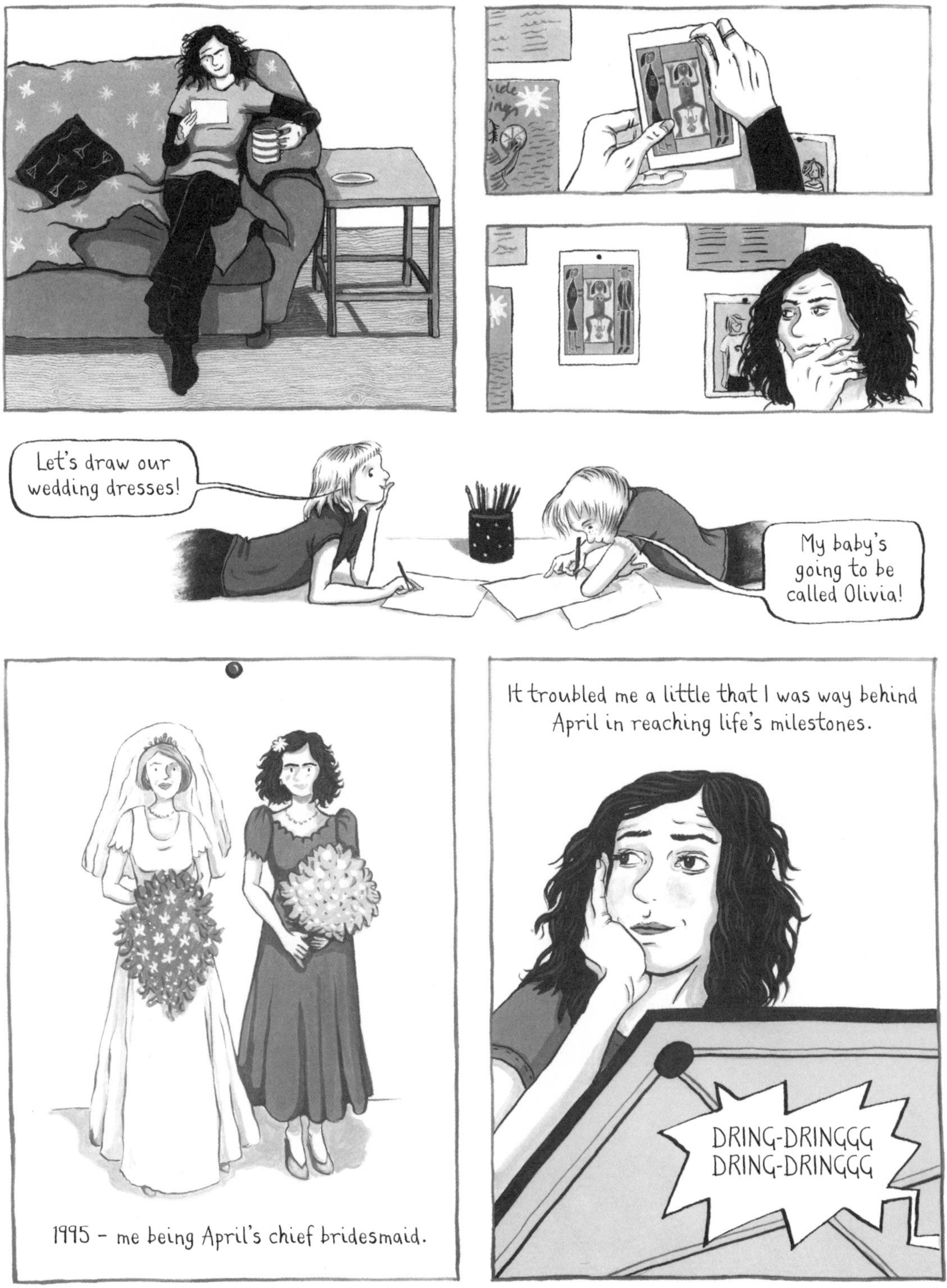
Let's draw our wedding dresses!
My baby's going to be called Olivia!
1995 – me being April's chief bridesmaid.
It troubled me a little that I was way behind April in reaching life's milestones.
DRING-DRINGGG DRING-DRINGGG

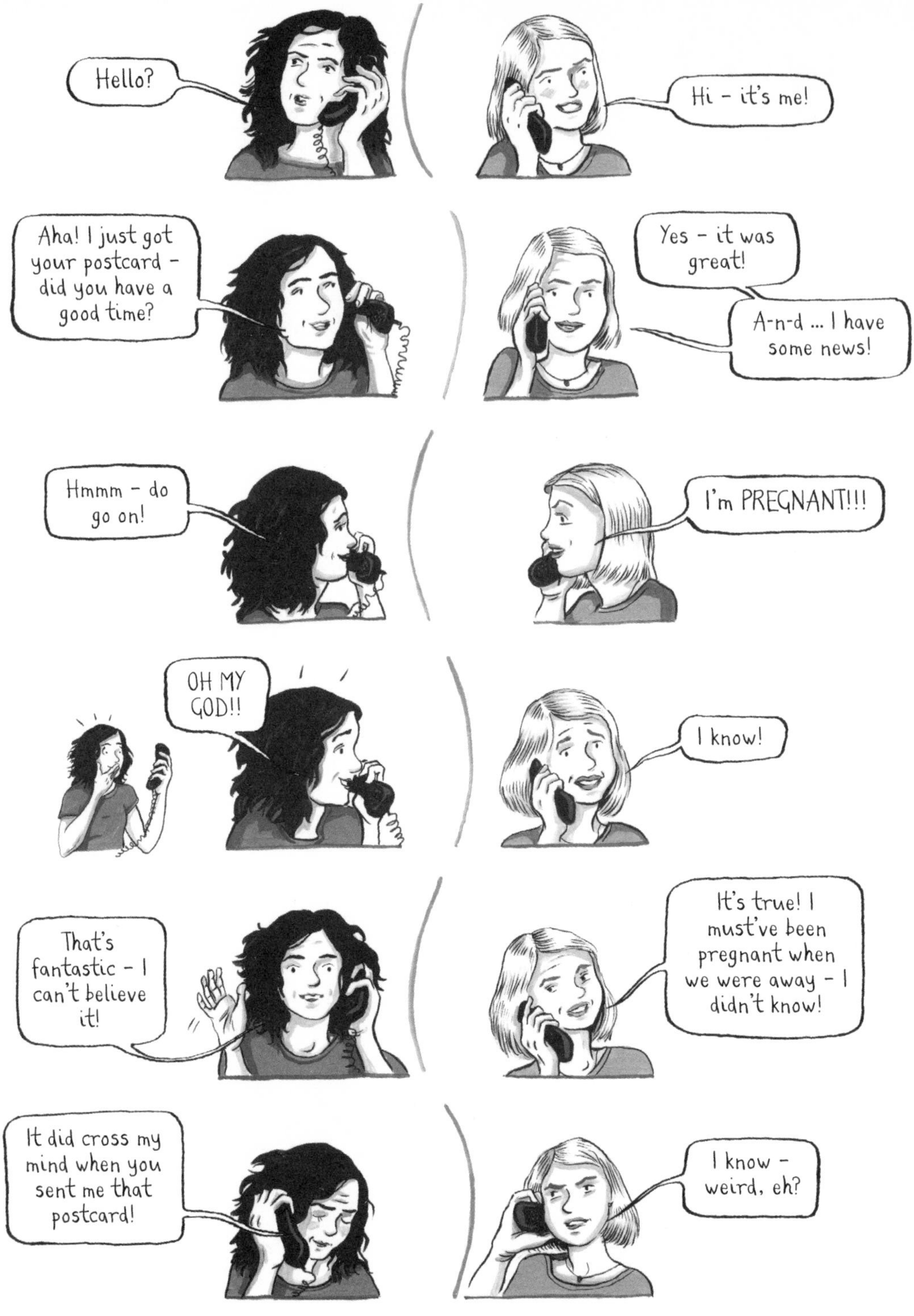
Hello?
Hi - it's me!
Aha! I just got your postcard - did you have a good time?
Yes - it was great!
A-n-d ... I have some news!
Hmmm - do go on!
I'm PREGNANT!!!
OH MY GOD!!
I know!
That's fantastic - I can't believe it!
It's true! I must've been pregnant when we were away - I didn't know!
It did cross my mind when you sent me that postcard!
I know - weird, eh?

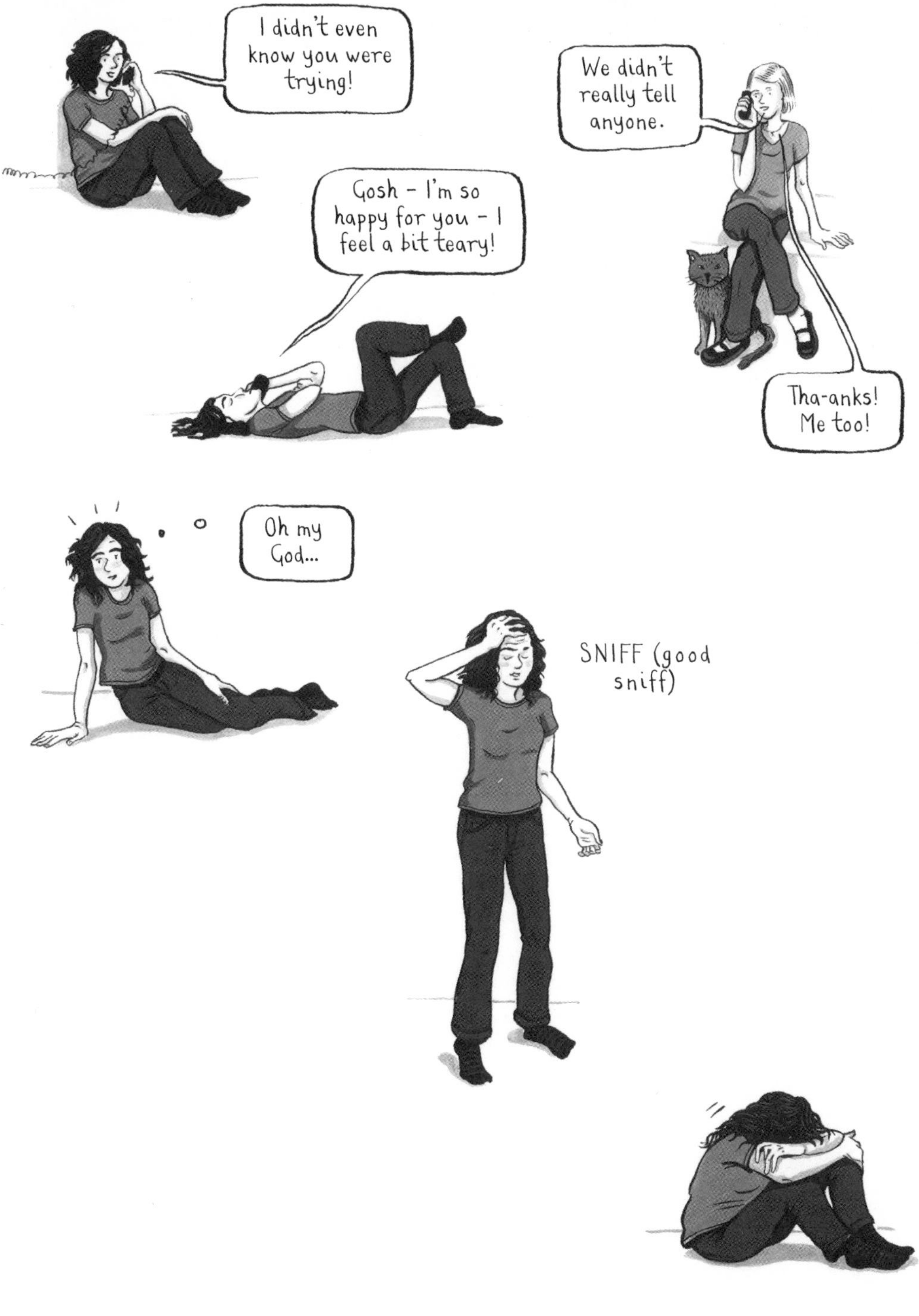
I didn't even know you were trying!
We didn't really tell anyone.
Gosh - I'm so happy for you - I feel a bit teary!
Tha-anks! Me too!
Oh my God...
SNIFF (good sniff)

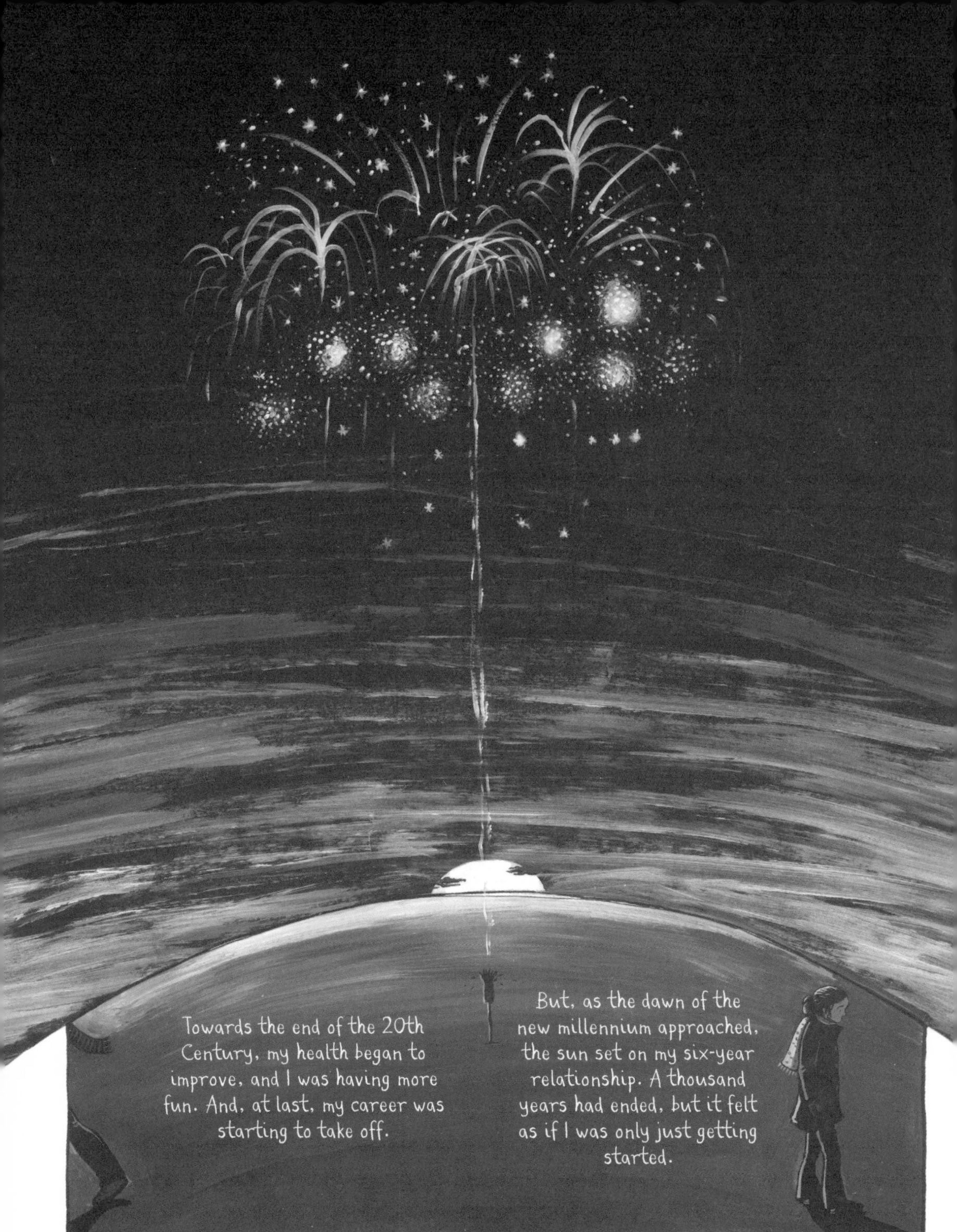
Towards the end of the 20th Century, my health began to improve, and I was having more fun. And, at last, my career was starting to take off.
But, as the dawn of the new millennium approached, the sun set on my six-year relationship. A thousand years had ended, but it felt as if I was only just getting started.

TWO

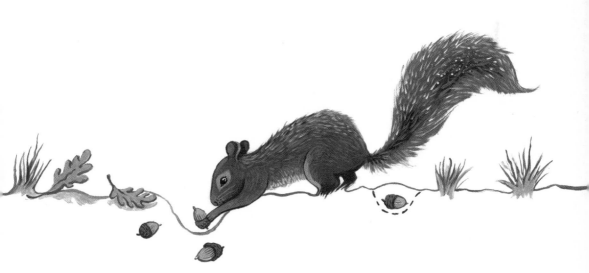

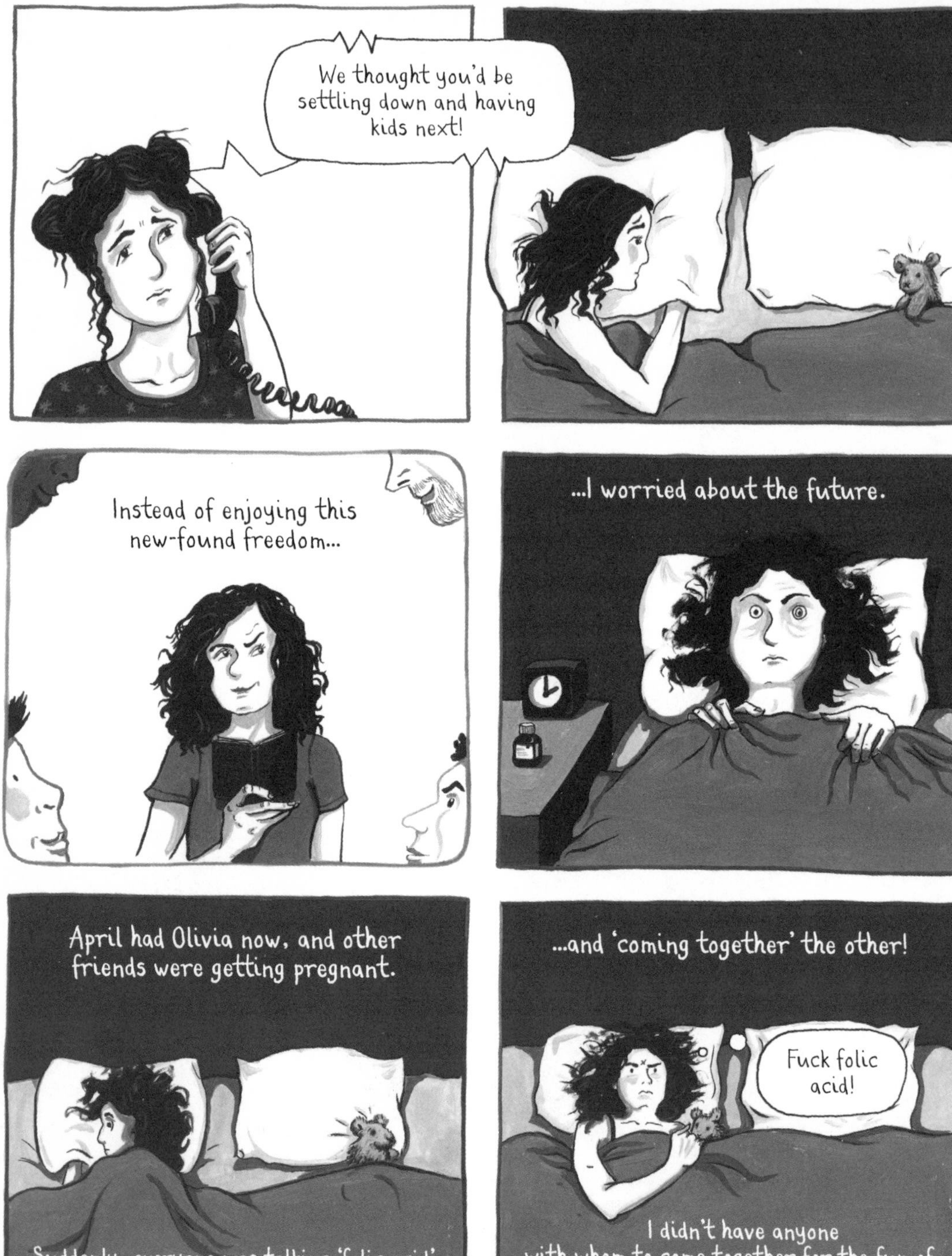

We thought you'd be settling down and having kids next!
Instead of enjoying this new-found freedom...
...I worried about the future.
April had Olivia now, and other friends were getting pregnant.
Suddenly, everyone was talking 'folic acid' this, 'ovulation' that...
...and 'coming together' the other!
Fuck folic acid!
I didn't have anyone with whom to come together for the fun of it, let alone to expedite sperm to egg!

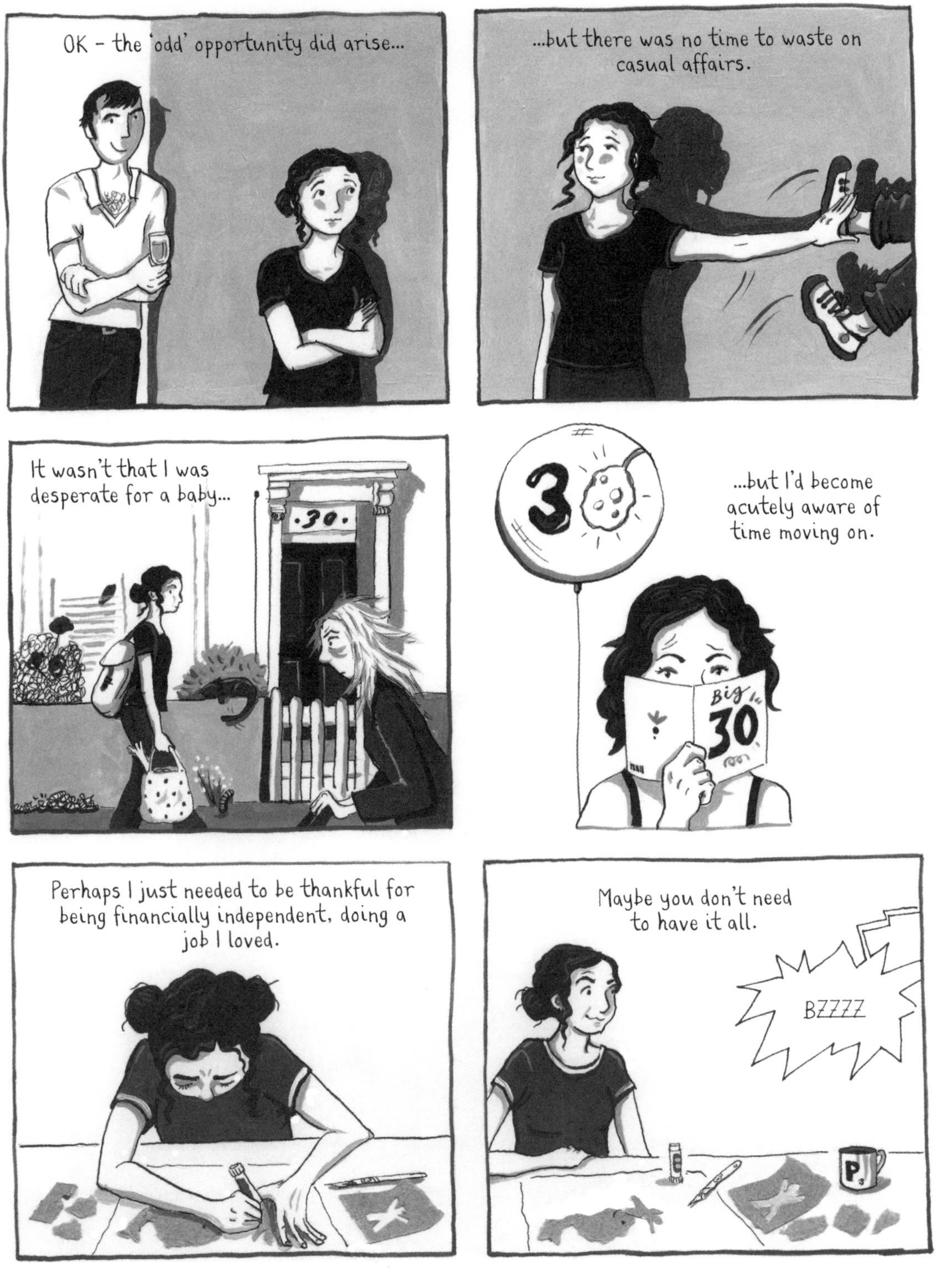
OK – the 'odd' opportunity did arise...
...but there was no time to waste on casual affairs.
It wasn't that I was desperate for a baby...
·30·
30
...but I'd become acutely aware of time moving on.
Big 30
Perhaps I just needed to be thankful for being financially independent, doing a job I loved.
Maybe you don't need to have it all.
BZZZZ
P

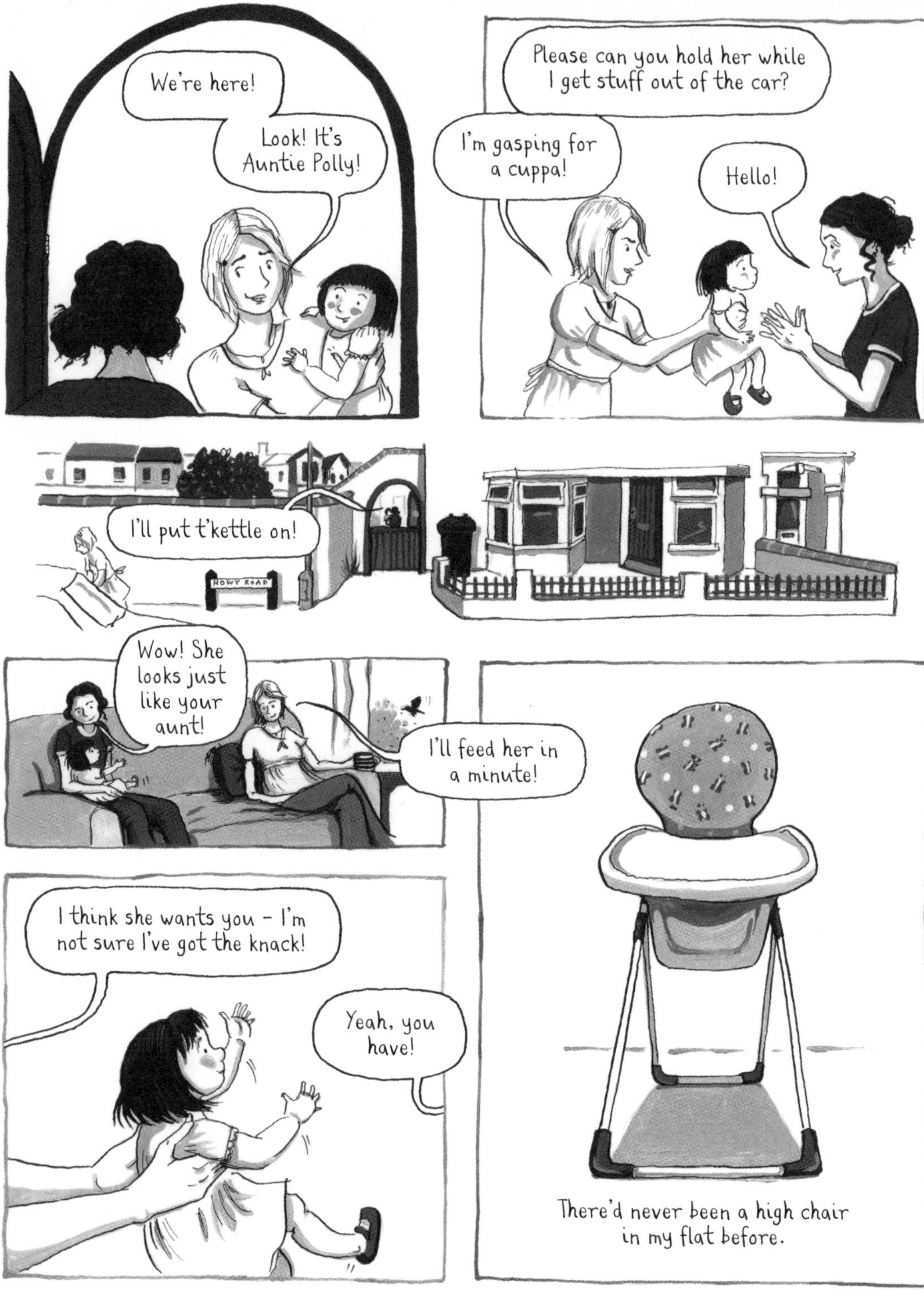
We're here!
Look! It's Auntie Polly!
Please can you hold her while I get stuff out of the car?
I'm gasping for a cuppa!
Hello!
I'll put t'kettle on!
Wow! She looks just like your aunt!
I'll feed her in a minute!
I think she wants you – I'm not sure I've got the knack!
Yeah, you have!
There'd never been a high chair in my flat before.

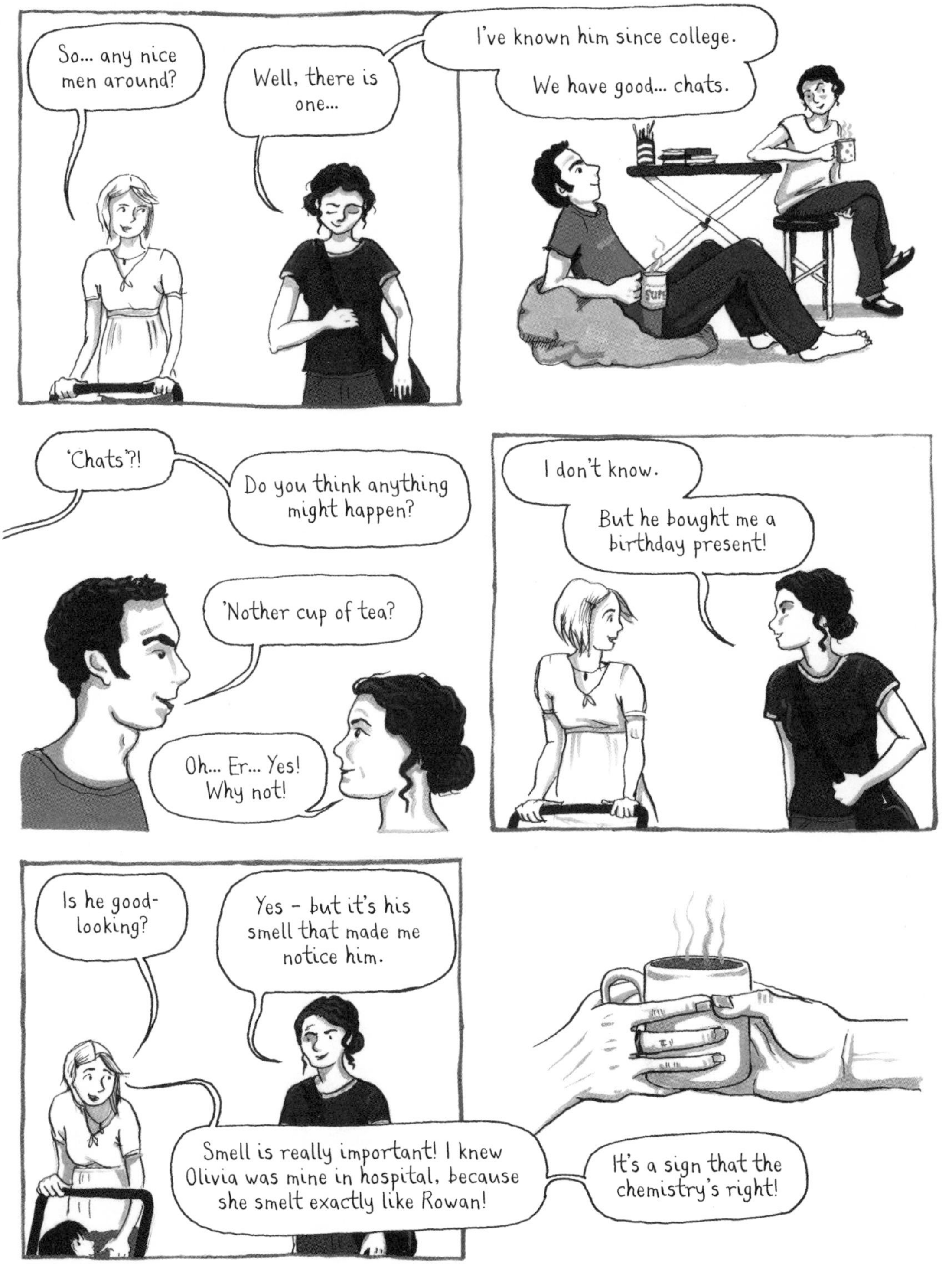
So... any nice men around?
Well, there is one...
I've known him since college.
We have good... chats.
'Chats'?!
Do you think anything might happen?
'Nother cup of tea?
Oh... Er... Yes! Why not!
I don't know.
But he bought me a birthday present!
Is he good-looking?
Yes - but it's his smell that made me notice him.
Smell is really important! I knew Olivia was mine in hospital, because she smelt exactly like Rowan!
It's a sign that the chemistry's right!

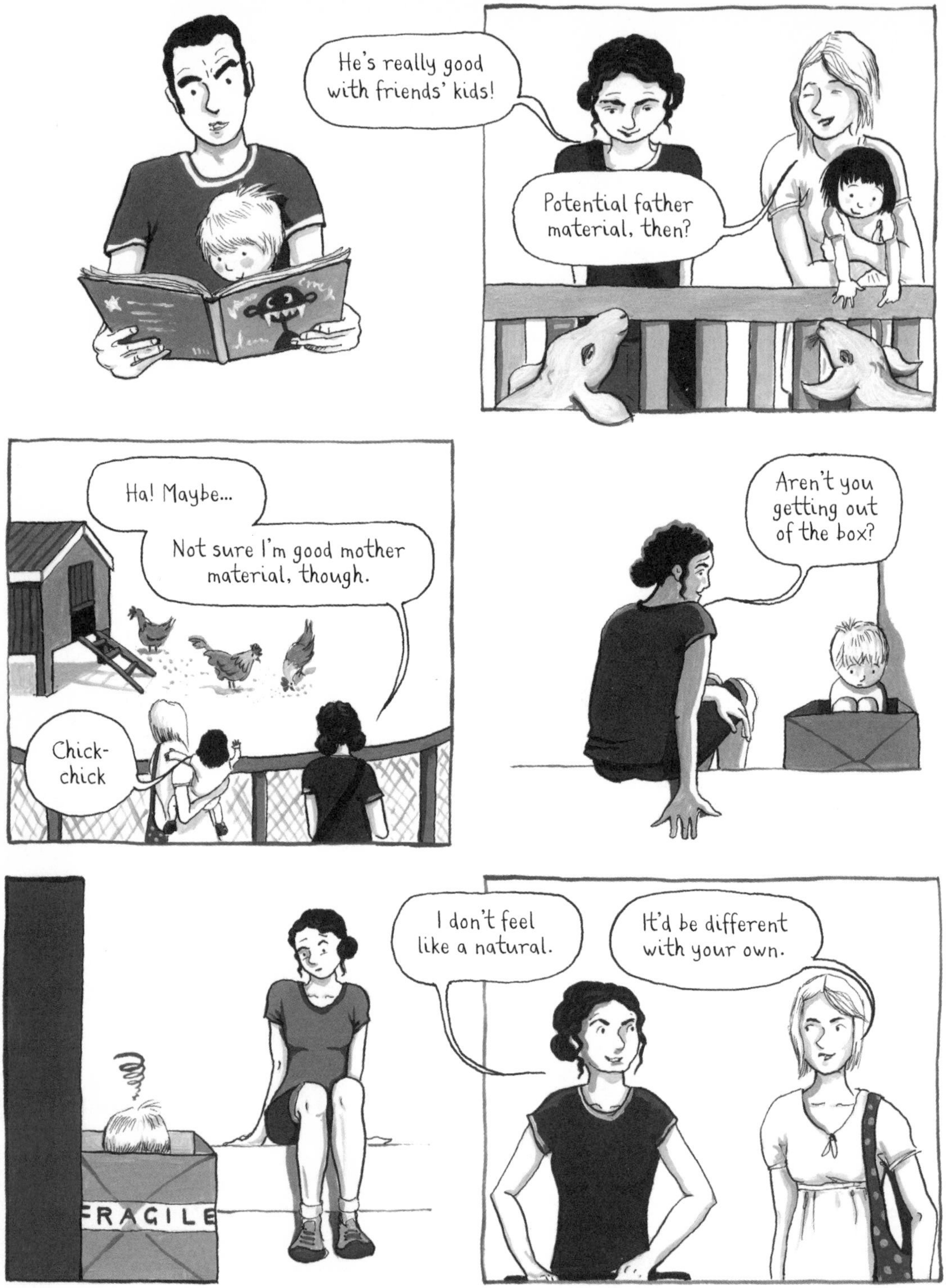
He's really good with friends' kids!
Potential father material, then?
Ha! Maybe...
Not sure I'm good mother material, though.
Chick-chick
Aren't you getting out of the box?
FRAGILE
I don't feel like a natural.
It'd be different with your own.

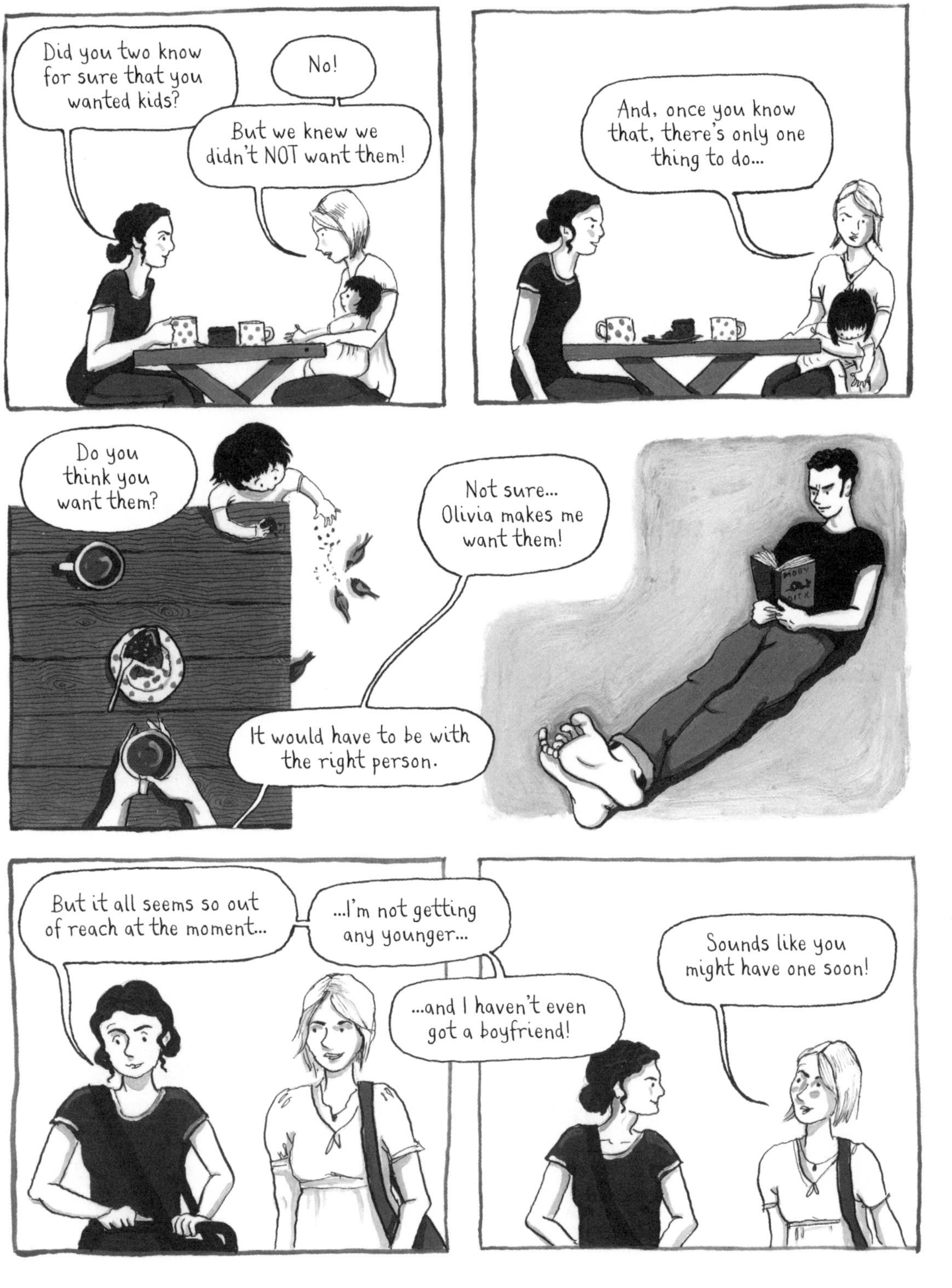

Did you two know for sure that you wanted kids?
No!
But we knew we didn't NOT want them!
And, once you know that, there's only one thing to do...
Do you think you want them?
Not sure... Olivia makes me want them!
It would have to be with the right person.
MOBY DICK
But it all seems so out of reach at the moment...
...I'm not getting any younger...
...and I haven't even got a boyfriend!
Sounds like you might have one soon!

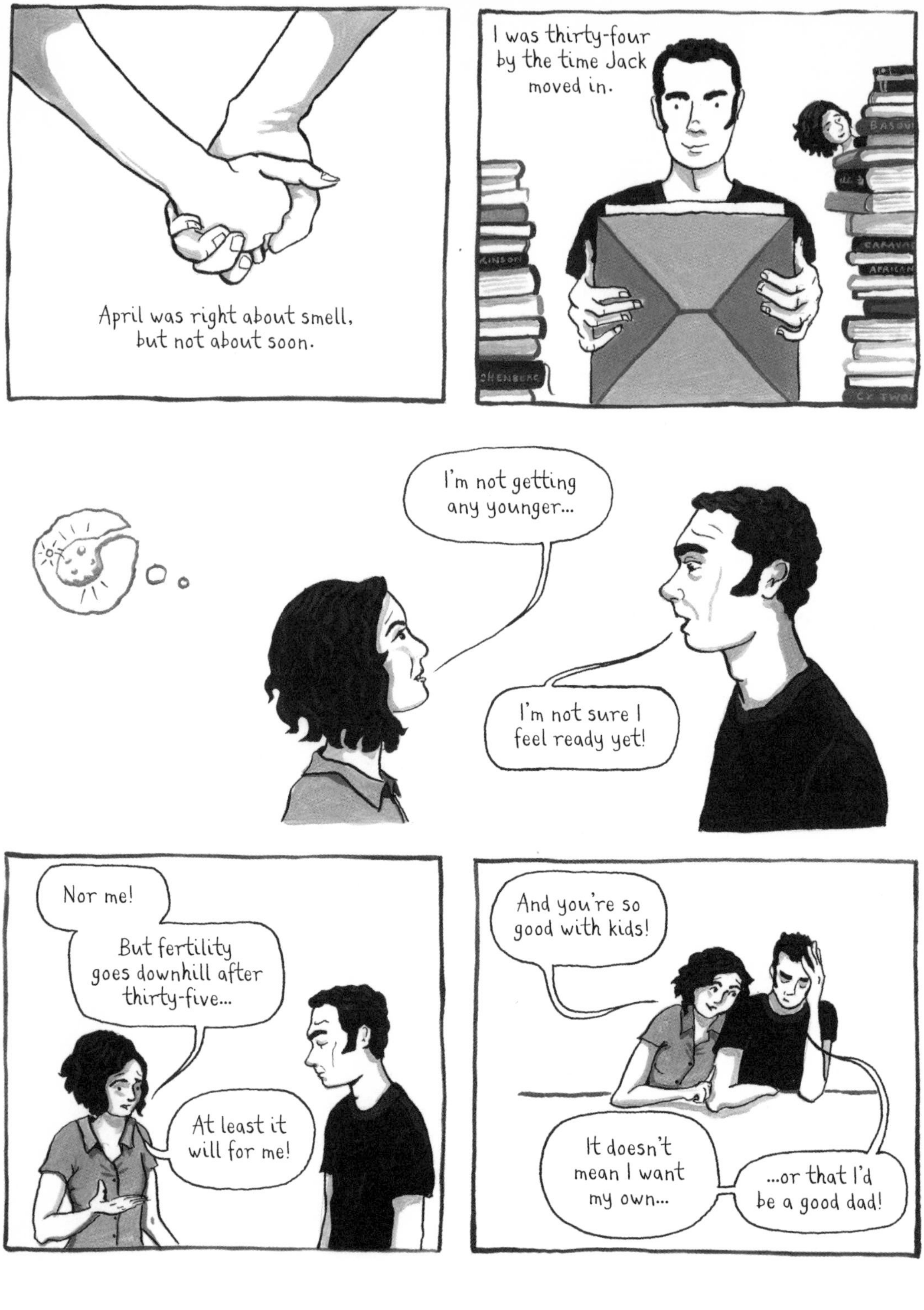
April was right about smell, but not about soon.
I was thirty-four by the time Jack moved in.
I'm not getting any younger...
I'm not sure I feel ready yet!
Nor me!
But fertility goes downhill after thirty-five...
At least it will for me!
And you're so good with kids!
It doesn't mean I want my own...
...or that I'd be a good dad!

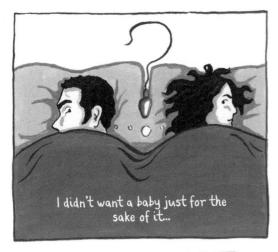

I didn't want a baby just for the sake of it...

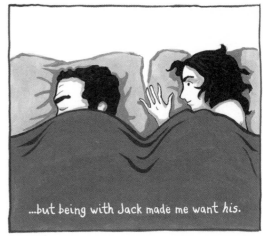

...but being with Jack made me want *his*.

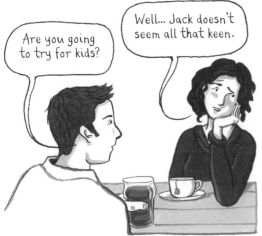

Are you going to try for kids?

Well... Jack doesn't seem all that keen.

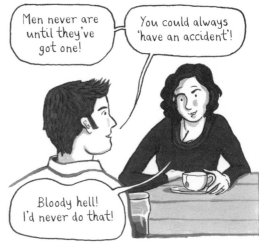

Men never are until they've got one!

You could always 'have an accident'!

Bloody hell! I'd never do that!

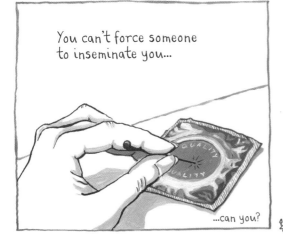

You can't force someone to inseminate you...

...can you?

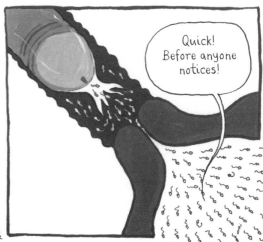

Quick! Before anyone notices!

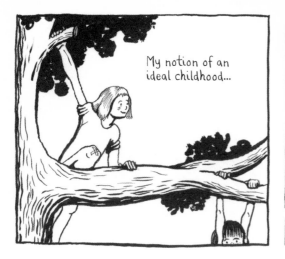

My notion of an ideal childhood...

...was opposed to what modern...

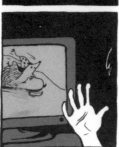

...childhood seemed to resemble.

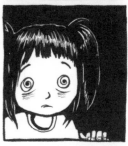

And besides, the illness I'd had made me feel less confident - what if it were to return?

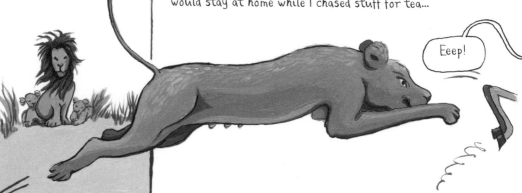

If only I were a lioness! I'd be strong - and the lion would stay at home while I chased stuff for tea...

Eeep!

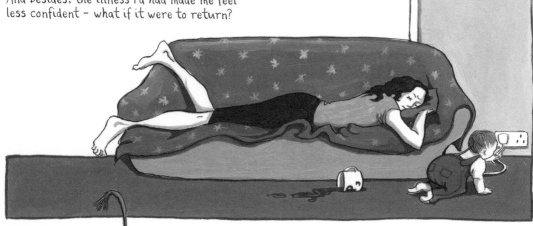

78

Whatever happened to the mantra from my formative years: having it all?

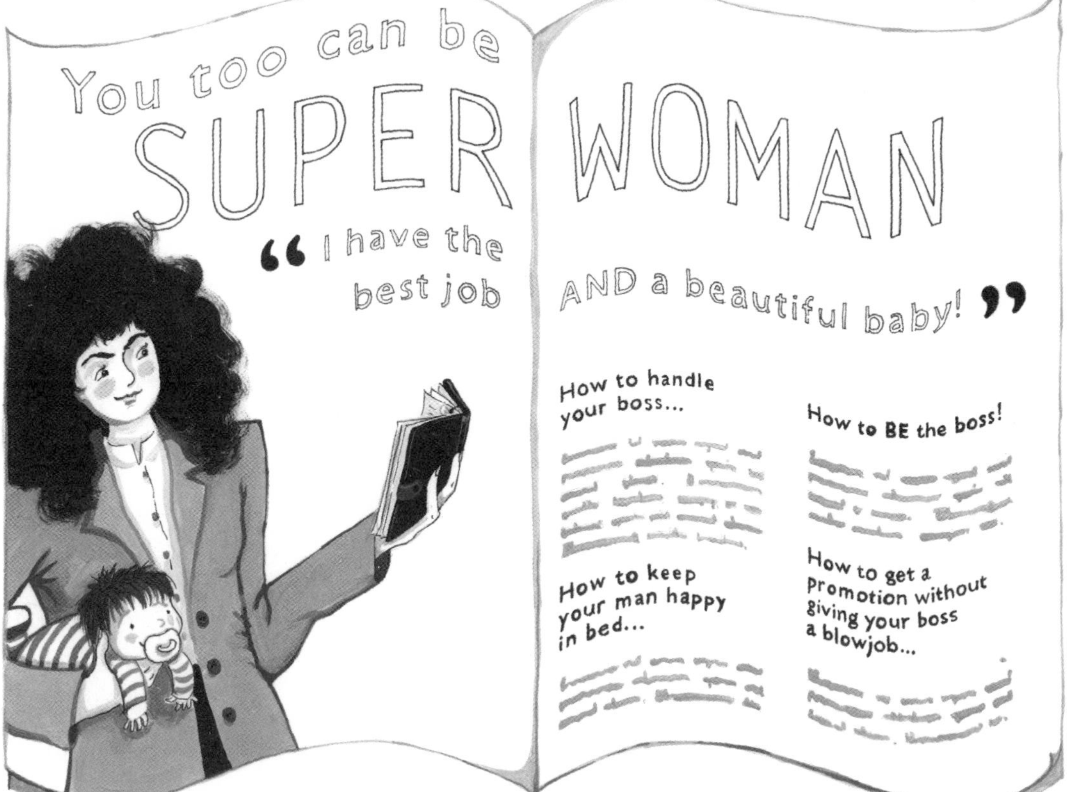
You too can be
SUPER WOMAN
"I have the best job AND a beautiful baby!"
How to handle your boss...
How to BE the boss!
How to keep your man happy in bed...
How to get a promotion without giving your boss a blowjob...

As an 80s teenager plotting my future, the world was telling me it was ALL possible.

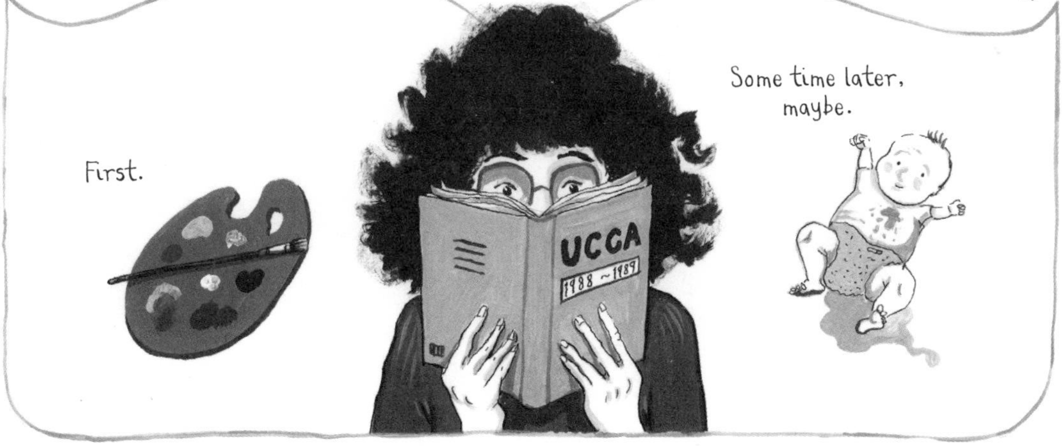
First.
UCCA
1988 ~ 1989
Some time later, maybe.

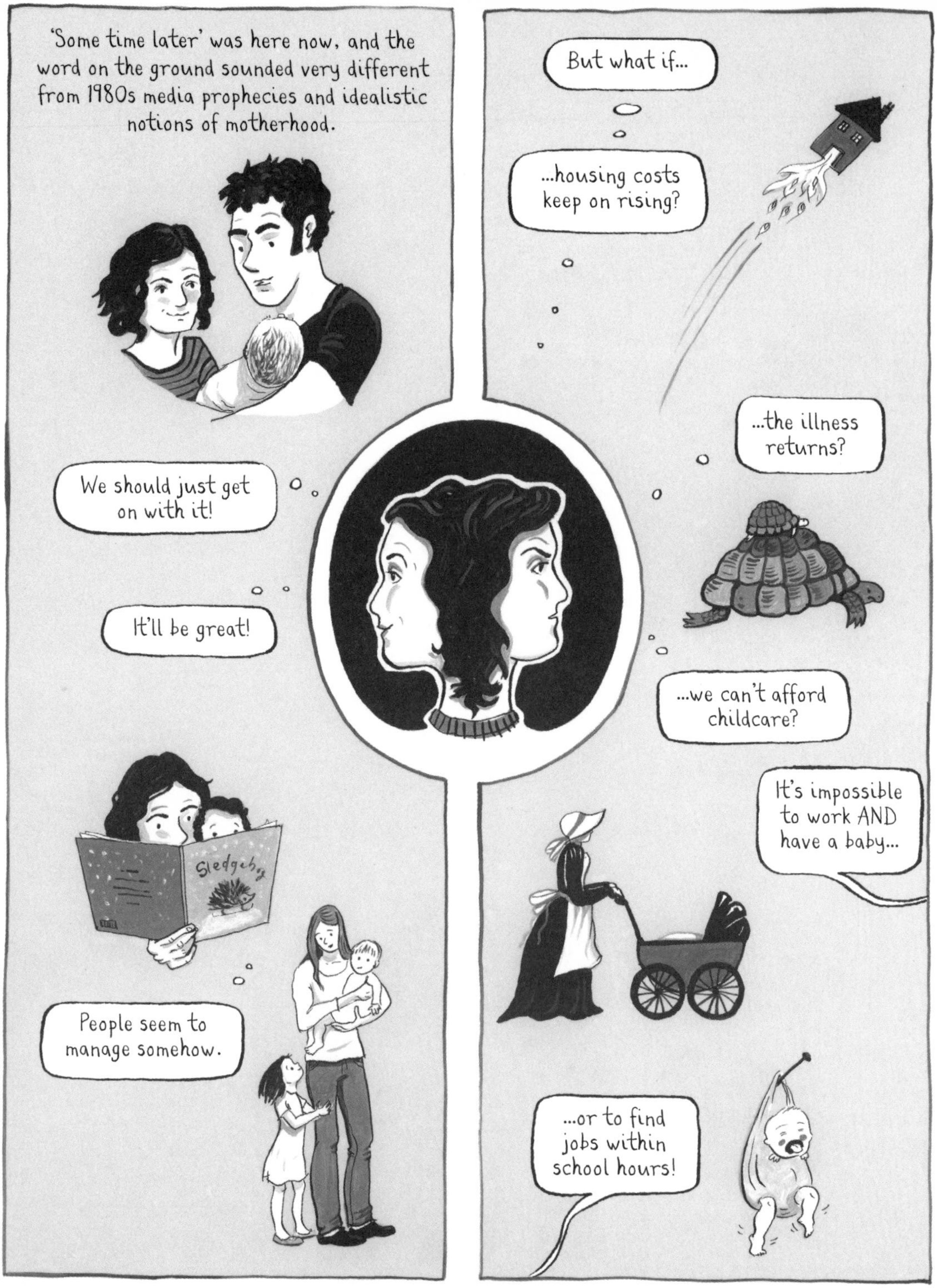
'Some time later' was here now, and the word on the ground sounded very different from 1980s media prophecies and idealistic notions of motherhood.
We should just get on with it!
It'll be great!
Sledgehog
People seem to manage somehow.
But what if...
...housing costs keep on rising?
...the illness returns?
...we can't afford childcare?
It's impossible to work AND have a baby...
...or to find jobs within school hours!

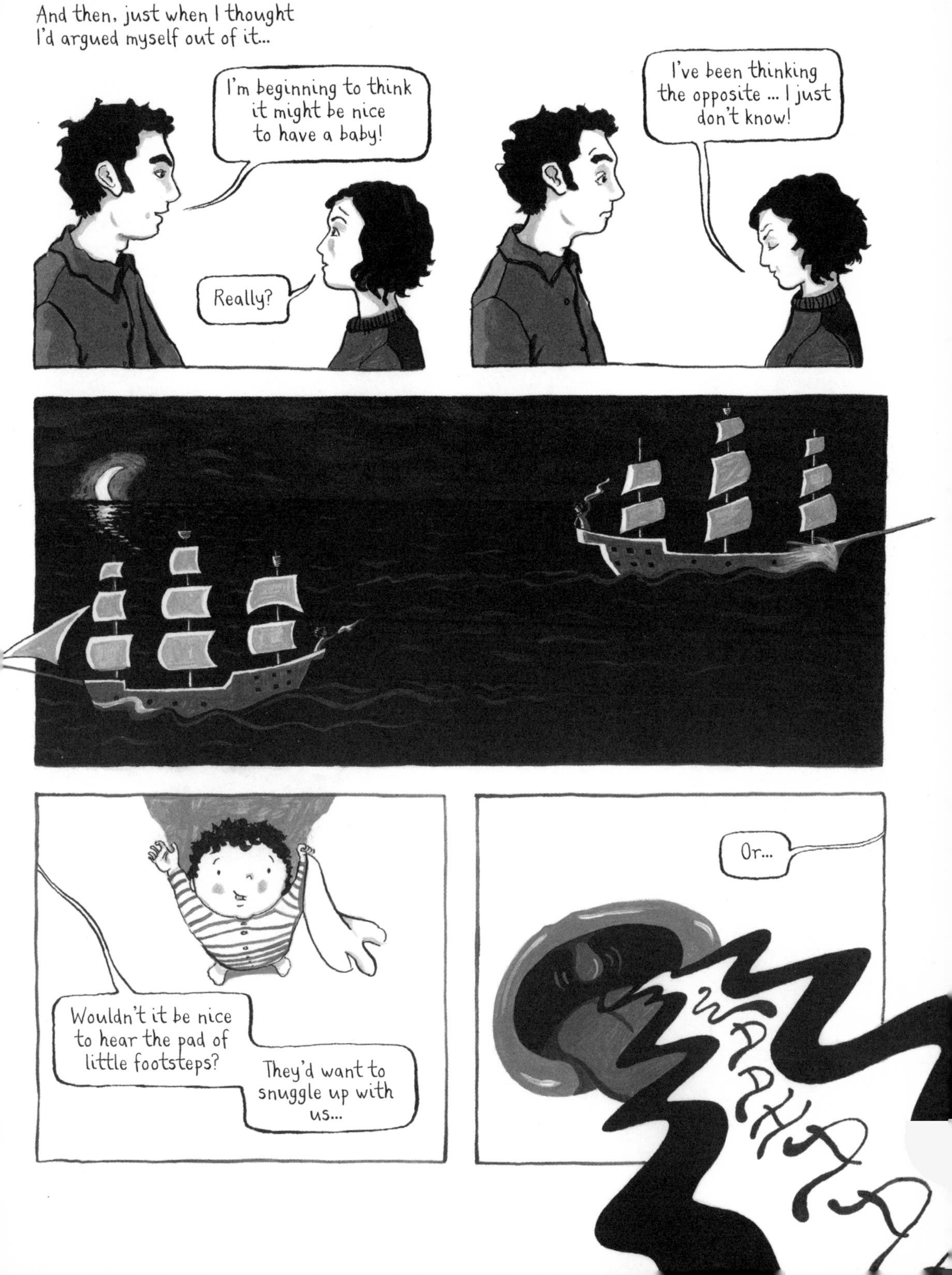
And then, just when I thought I'd argued myself out of it...
I'm beginning to think it might be nice to have a baby!
Really?
I've been thinking the opposite ... I just don't know!
Wouldn't it be nice to hear the pad of little footsteps?
They'd want to snuggle up with us...
Or...
WAAHH

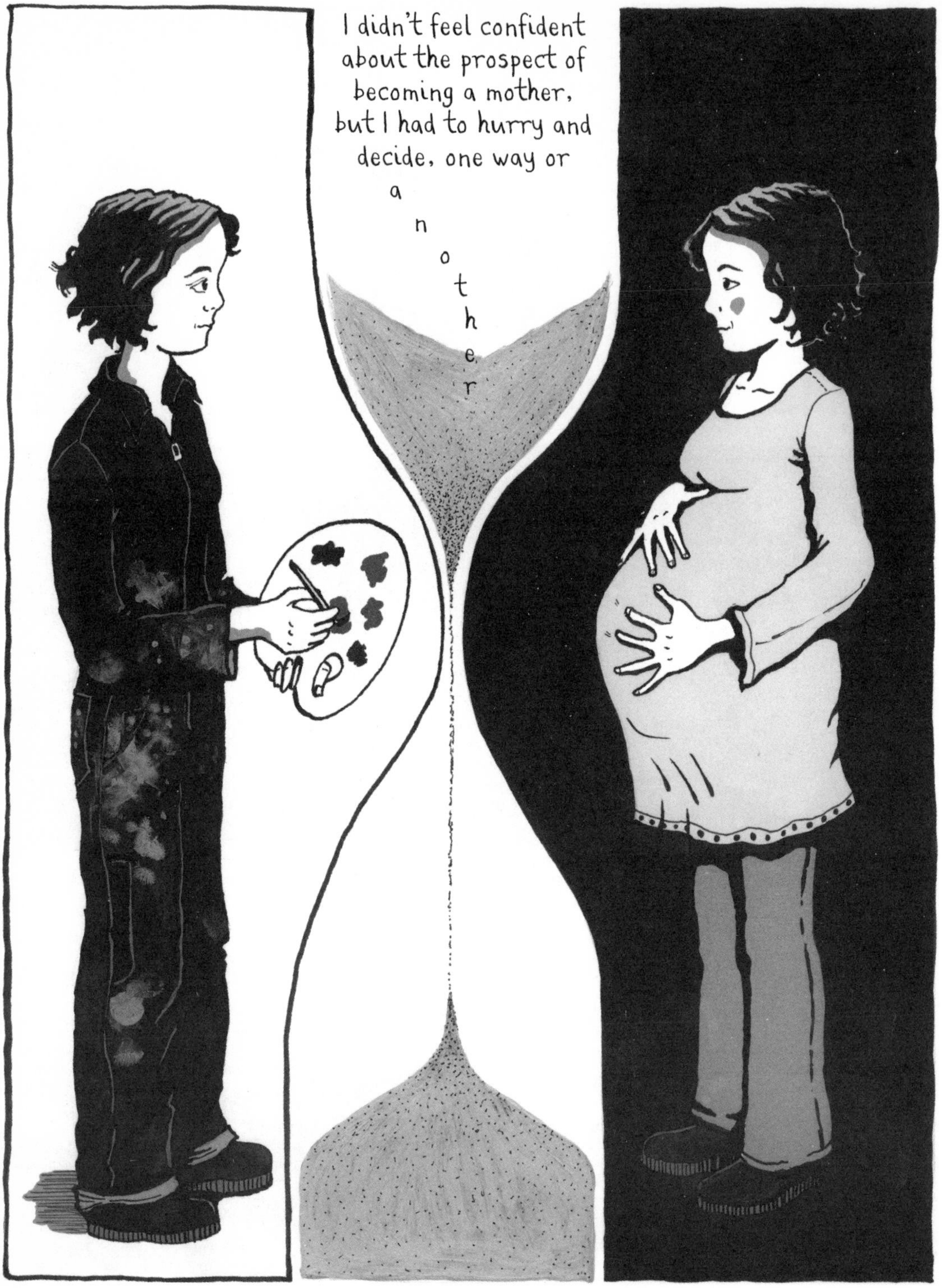
I didn't feel confident about the prospect of becoming a mother, but I had to hurry and decide, one way or a n o t h e r

Cervical screening:

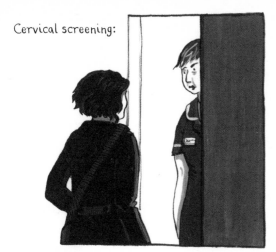

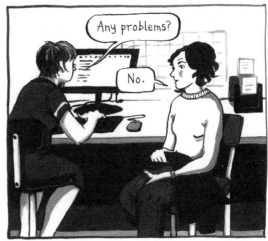

Any problems?

No.

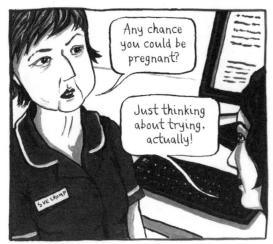

Any chance you could be pregnant?

Just thinking about trying, actually!

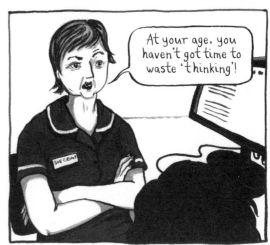

At your age, you haven't got time to waste 'thinking'!

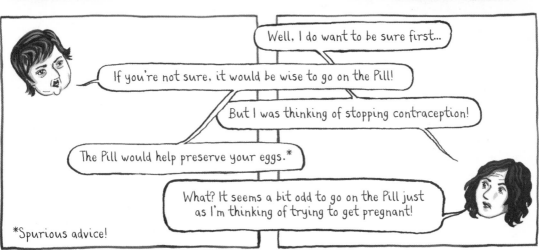

Well, I do want to be sure first...

If you're not sure, it would be wise to go on the Pill!

But I was thinking of stopping contraception!

The Pill would help preserve your eggs.*

What? It seems a bit odd to go on the Pill just as I'm thinking of trying to get pregnant!

*Spurious advice!

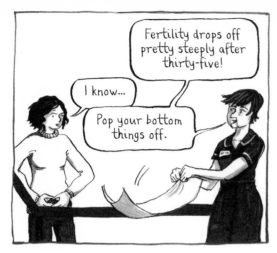

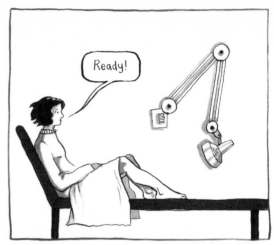

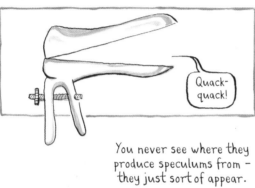

Fertility drops off pretty steeply after thirty-five!
I know...
Pop your bottom things off.
Ready!
Quack-quack!
You never see where they produce speculums from – they just sort of appear.
BRRNNNG BRN
BRRNNNGBRNG
fumble twist
SIGH Just got to get that!

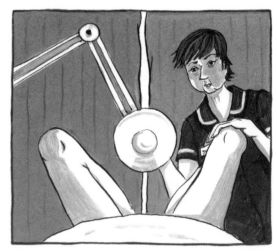

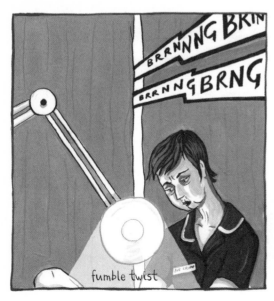

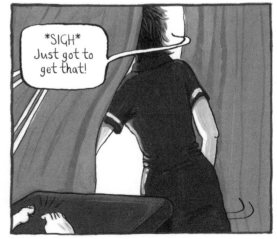

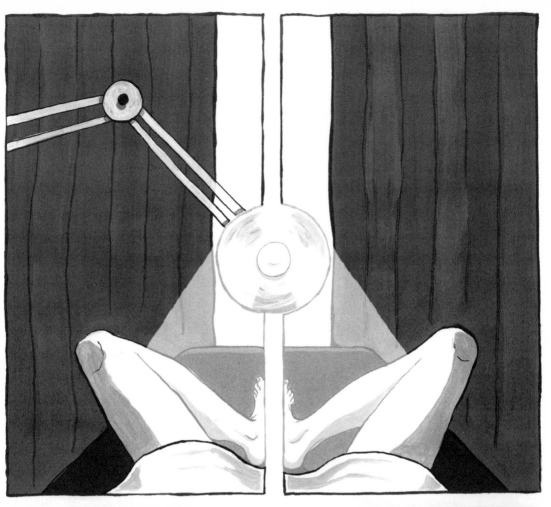

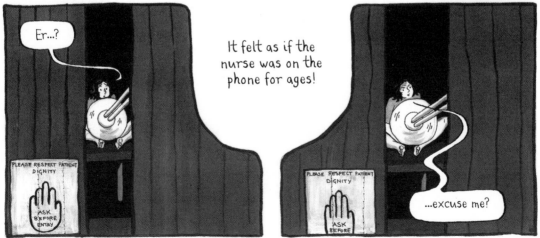

Er...?

It felt as if the nurse was on the phone for ages!

PLEASE RESPECT PATIENT DIGNITY

ASK BEFORE ENTRY

PLEASE RESPECT PATIENT DIGNITY

ASK BEFORE

...excuse me?

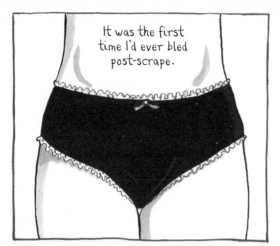

It was the first time I'd ever bled post-scrape.

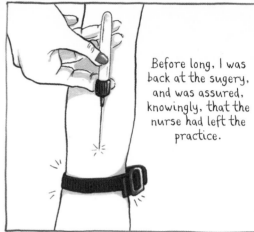

Before long, I was back at the sugery, and was assured, knowingly, that the nurse had left the practice.

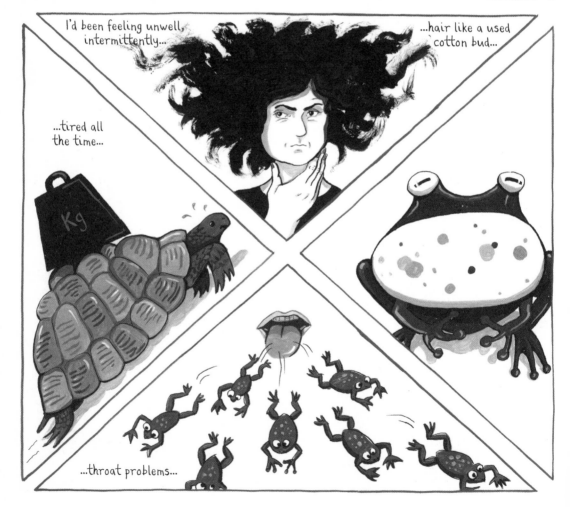

I'd been feeling unwell, intermittently...

...hair like a used cotton bud...

...tired all the time...

...throat problems...

They kept testing my thyroid function, but the result was always 'no further action'.

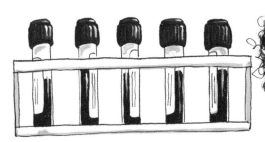

Please can you tell me the numbers?

They're within range – but I could send you to an endocrinologist, given your symptoms.

It might be worth trying you on a small dose of thyroxine.

I discovered that if I was in the USA, with my test results, I'd be treated for hypothyroidism – and that the UK lab ranges were wider.

Endocrinology appointment:

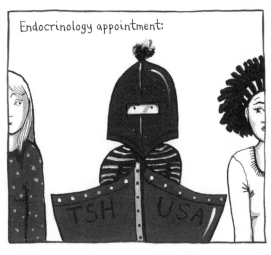

The consultant treated me like a time-waster.

I don't really know why you're here!

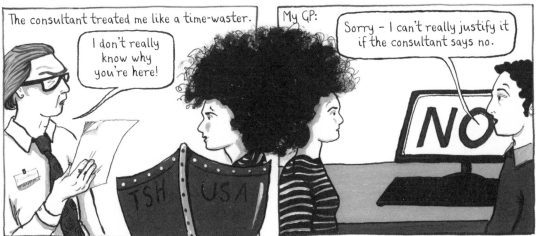

My GP:

Sorry – I can't really justify it if the consultant says no.

NO

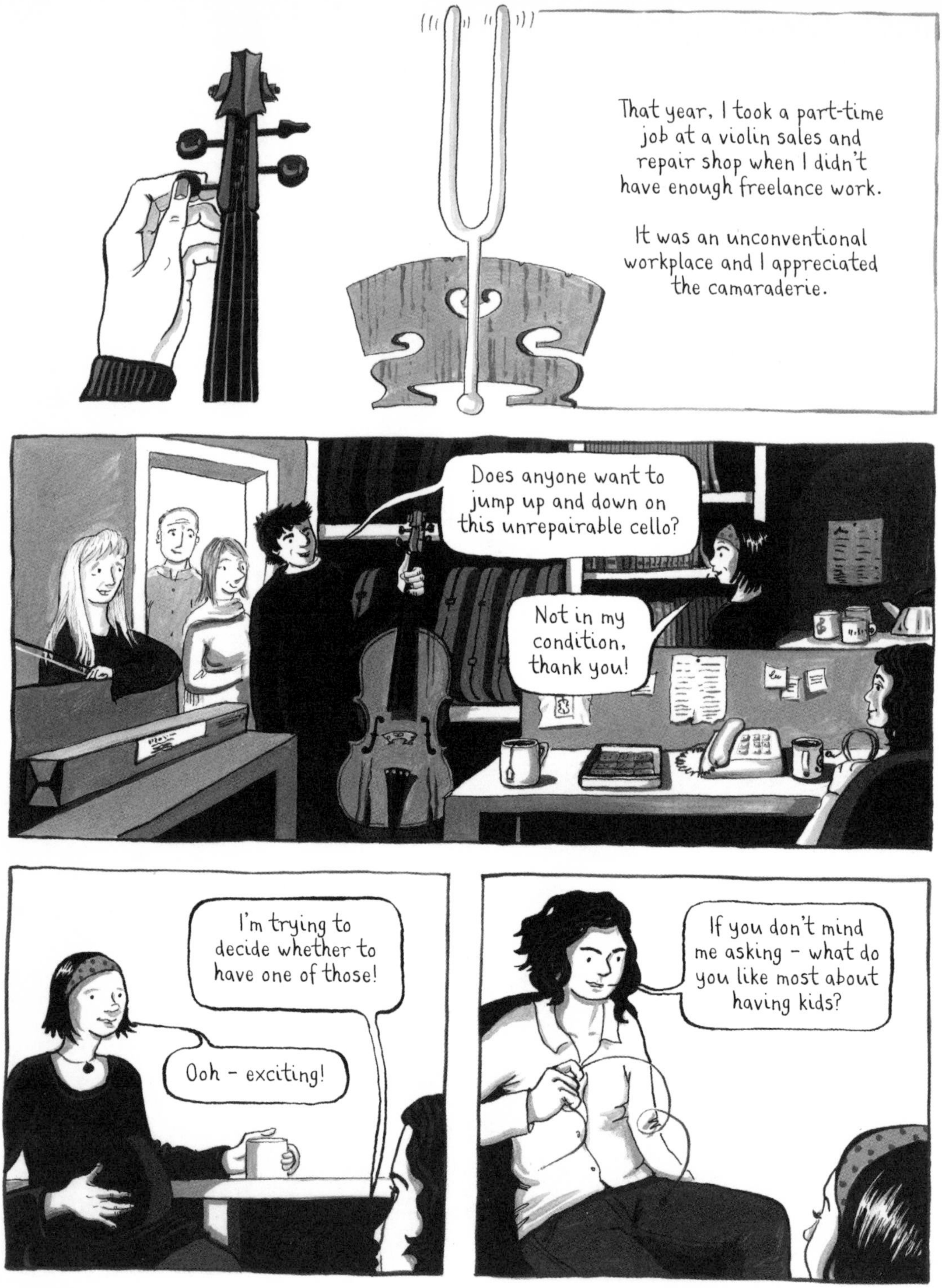
That year, I took a part-time job at a violin sales and repair shop when I didn't have enough freelance work.
It was an unconventional workplace and I appreciated the camaraderie.
Does anyone want to jump up and down on this unrepairable cello?
Not in my condition, thank you!
I'm trying to decide whether to have one of those!
Ooh - exciting!
If you don't mind me asking - what do you like most about having kids?

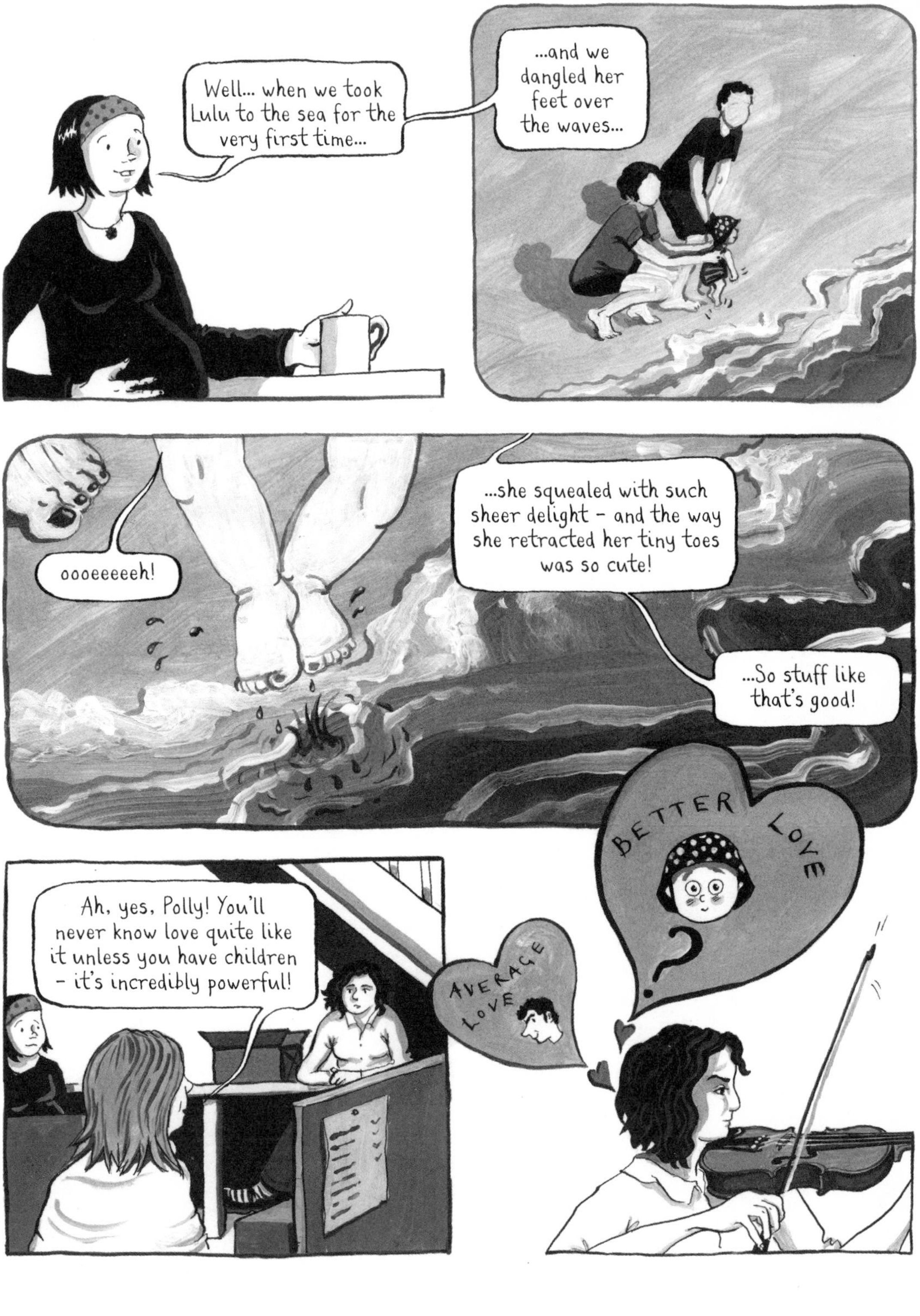

Well... when we took Lulu to the sea for the very first time...
...and we dangled her feet over the waves...
oooeeeeeh!
...she squealed with such sheer delight – and the way she retracted her tiny toes was so cute!
...So stuff like that's good!
Ah, yes, Polly! You'll never know love quite like it unless you have children – it's incredibly powerful!
AVERAGE LOVE
BETTER LOVE
?

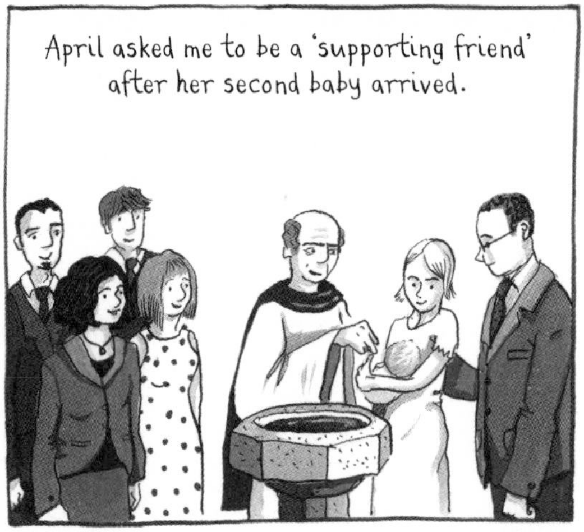
April asked me to be a 'supporting friend' after her second baby arrived.

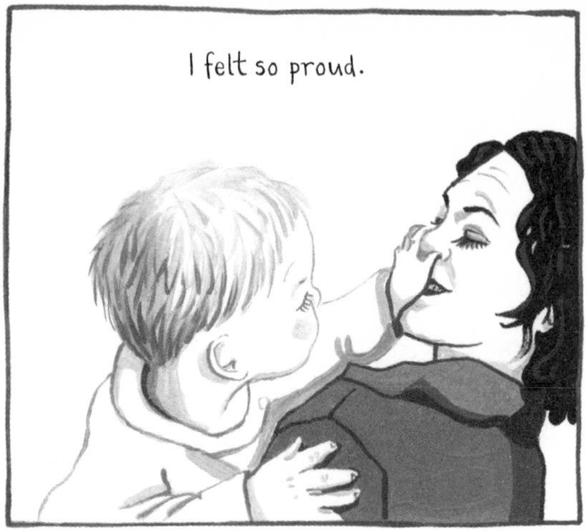
I felt so proud.

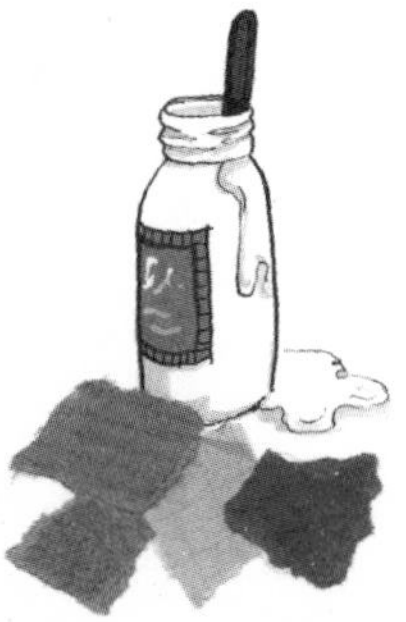

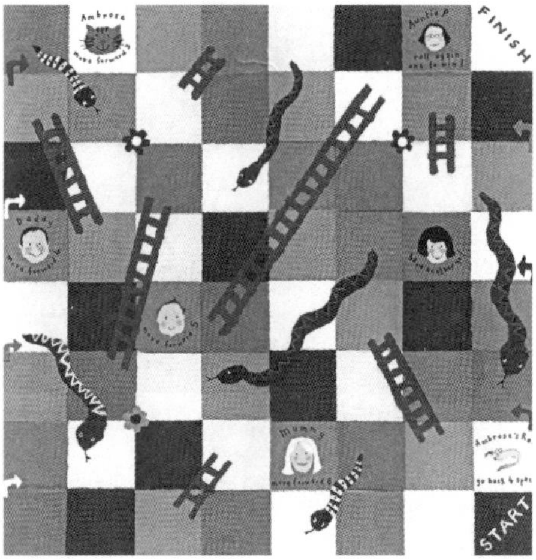
FINISH
START

I made Amber a game, with drawings of her family.

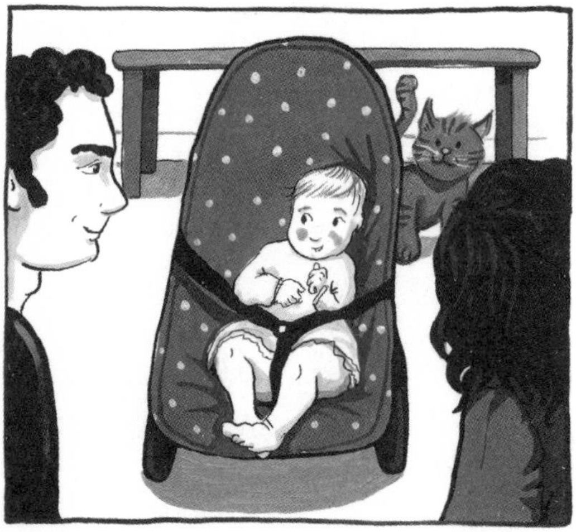

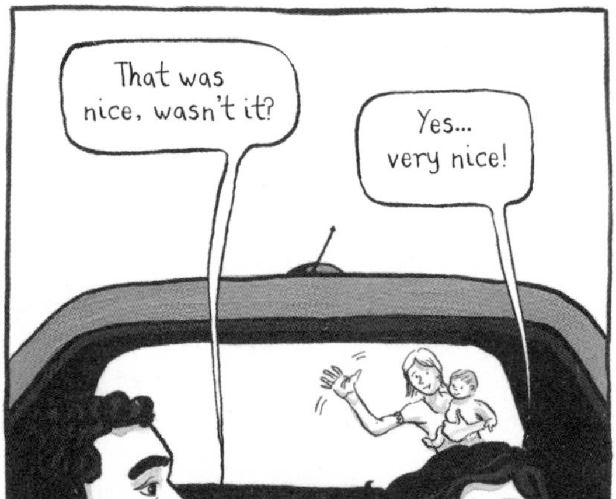
That was nice, wasn't it?
Yes... very nice!

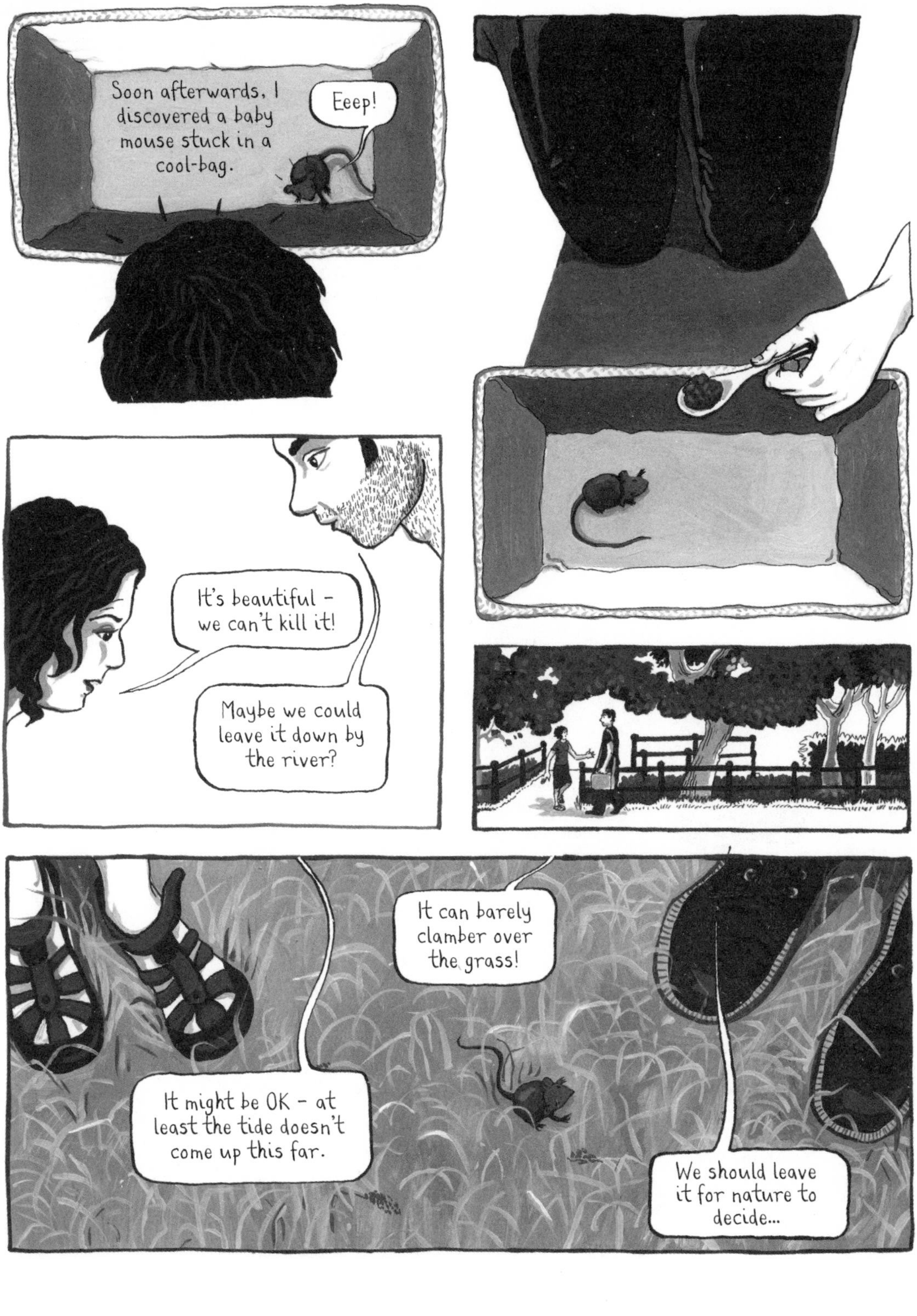

Soon afterwards, I discovered a baby mouse stuck in a cool-bag.
Eeep!
It's beautiful - we can't kill it!
Maybe we could leave it down by the river?
It might be OK - at least the tide doesn't come up this far.
It can barely clamber over the grass!
We should leave it for nature to decide...

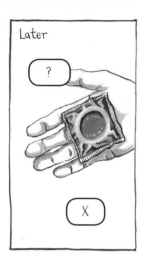

Later
?
X
I was thirty-five when we decided to 'leave it for nature to decide'. Not everyone has the chance to try for a baby within the ideal fertility window.
Eventually, when nothing happened, we were referred to the Reproductive Medicine Clinic.
In the meantime, I referred us to a naturopath.
MONTH
DATE
DAY OF CYCLE
TEMPERATURE
CELSIUS
38.0
37.0
36.0
BLEEDING
INTERCOURSE
We both quit alcohol.
We necked an array of sperm- and egg-loving supplements.
I recorded my basal body temperature, to help pinpoint ovulation.
Salmon for dinner again!
We tried to avoid stress, but, while on holiday, we found out that my mum had breast cancer.

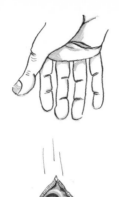

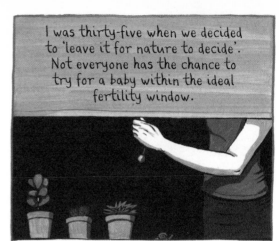

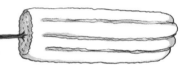

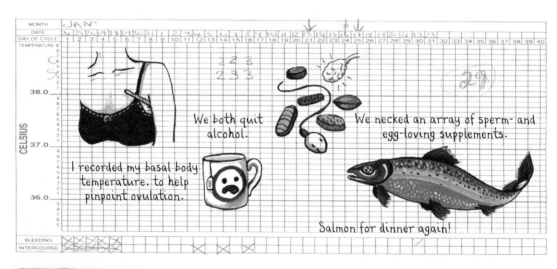

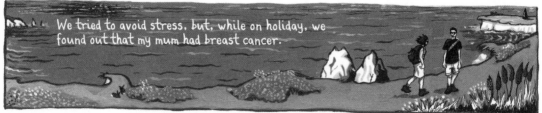

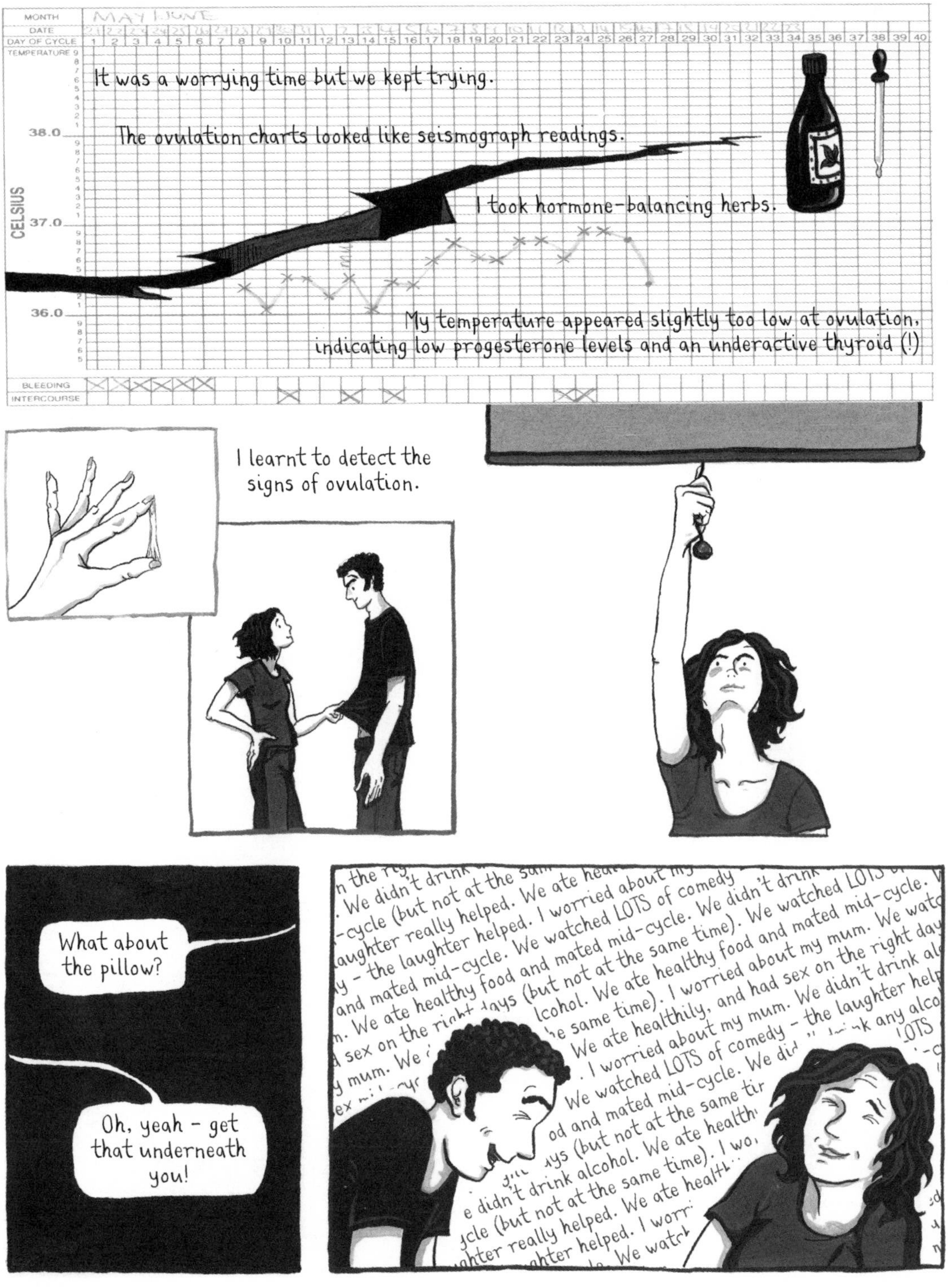
MONTH
MAY / JUNE
DATE
DAY OF CYCLE
TEMPERATURE
CELSIUS
BLEEDING
INTERCOURSE
It was a worrying time but we kept trying.
The ovulation charts looked like seismograph readings.
I took hormone-balancing herbs.
My temperature appeared slightly too low at ovulation, indicating low progesterone levels and an underactive thyroid (!)
I learnt to detect the signs of ovulation.
What about the pillow?
Oh, yeah - get that underneath you!
We watched LOTS of comedy - the laughter really helped.
We ate healthy food and mated mid-cycle.
We didn't drink alcohol.
I worried about my mum.

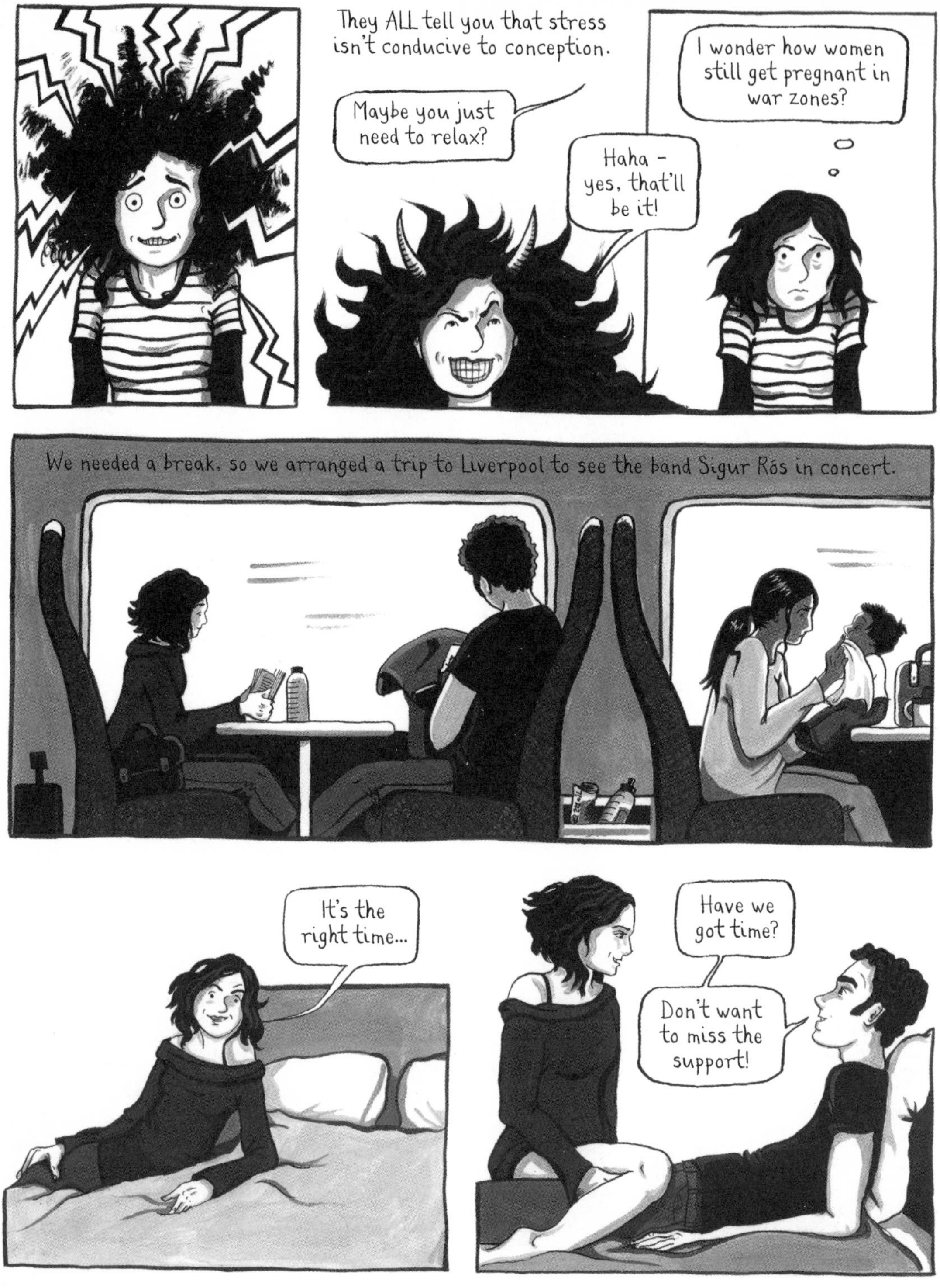
They ALL tell you that stress isn't conducive to conception.
Maybe you just need to relax?
Haha - yes, that'll be it!
I wonder how women still get pregnant in war zones?
We needed a break, so we arranged a trip to Liverpool to see the band Sigur Rós in concert.
It's the right time...
Have we got time?
Don't want to miss the support!

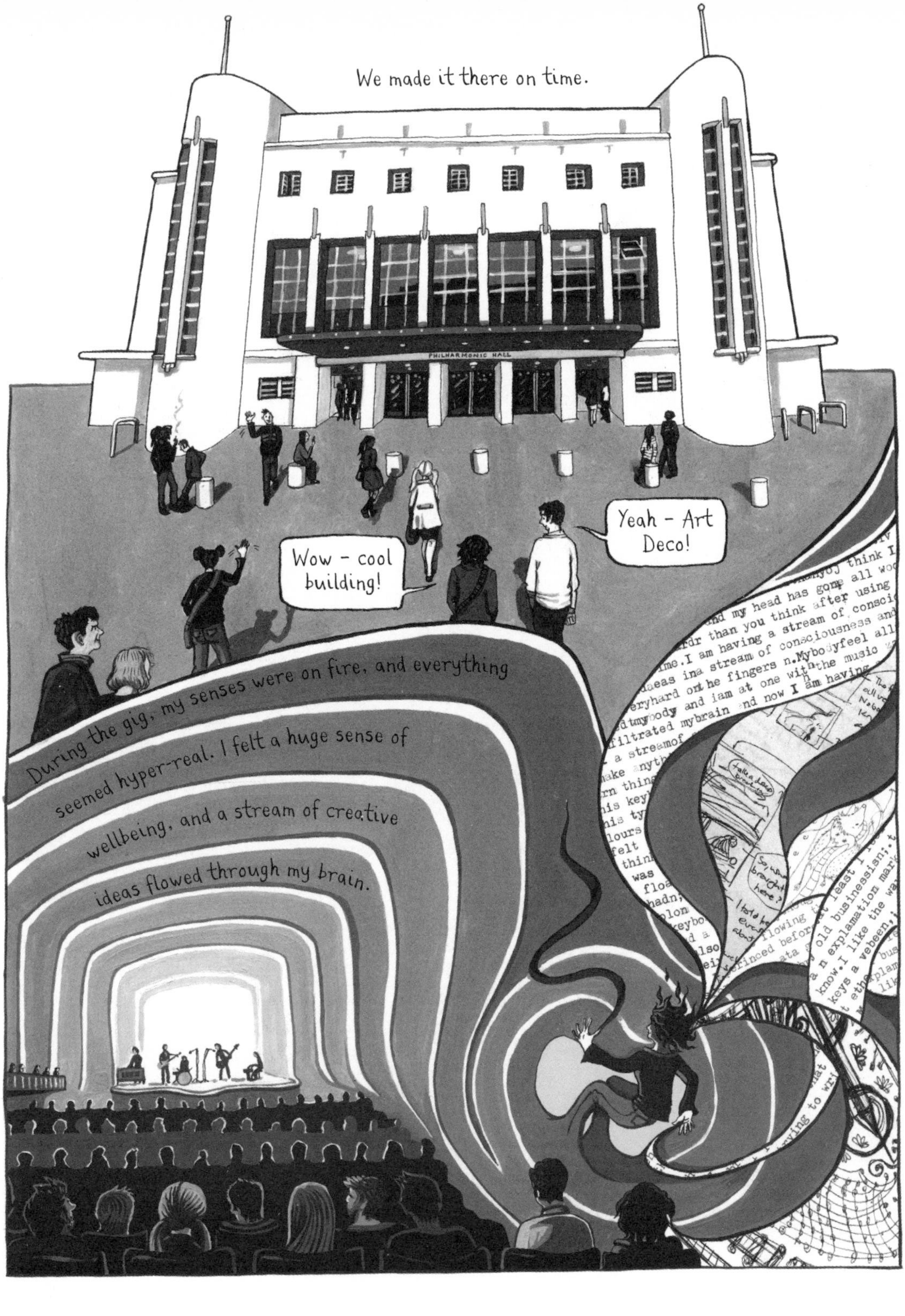
We made it there on time.
PHILHARMONIC HALL
Yeah - Art Deco!
Wow - cool building!
During the gig, my senses were on fire, and everything seemed hyper-real. I felt a huge sense of wellbeing, and a stream of creative ideas flowed through my brain.

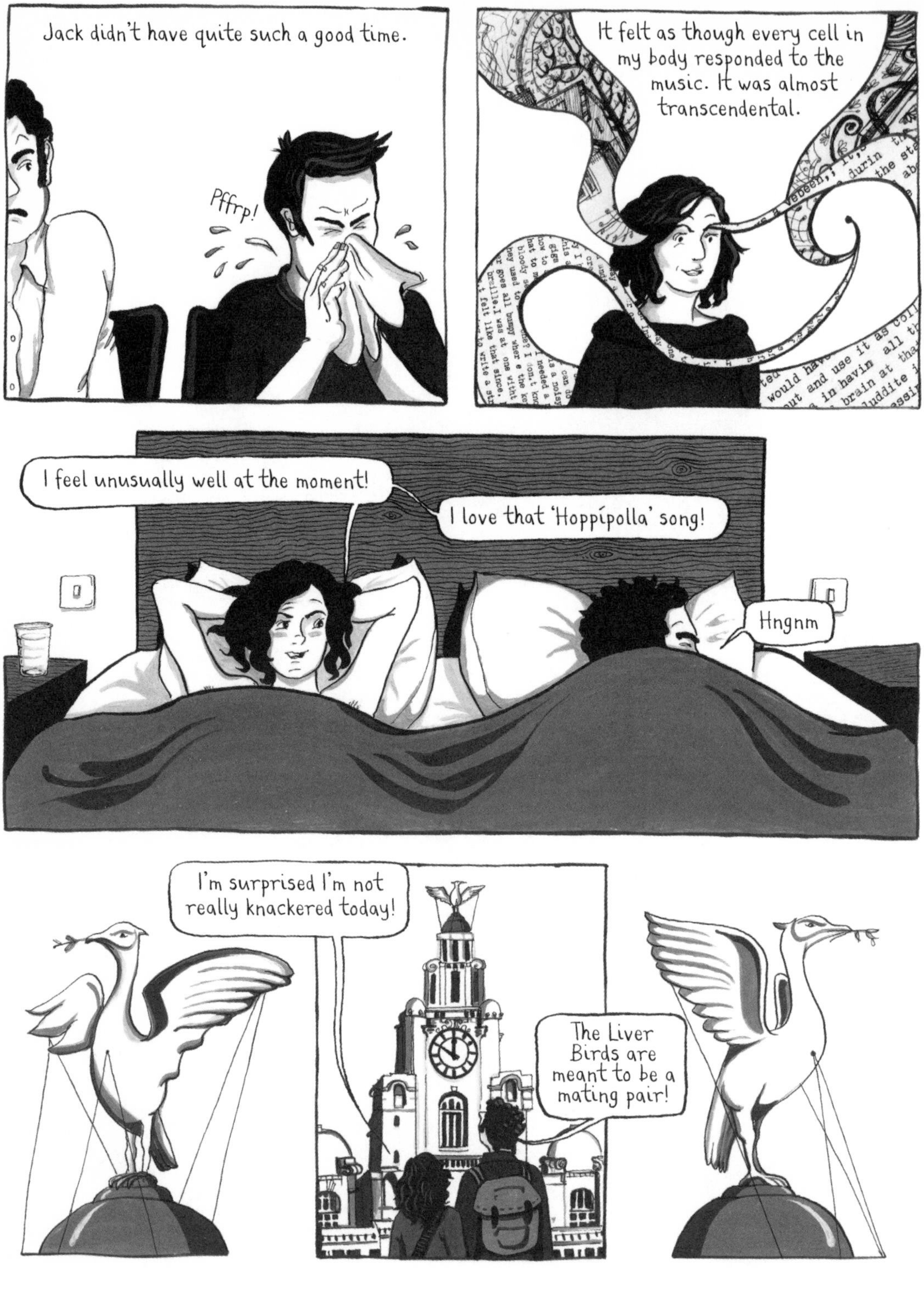
Jack didn't have quite such a good time.
Pffrp!
It felt as though every cell in my body responded to the music. It was almost transcendental.
I feel unusually well at the moment!
I love that 'Hoppípolla' song!
Hngnm
I'm surprised I'm not really knackered today!
The Liver Birds are meant to be a mating pair!

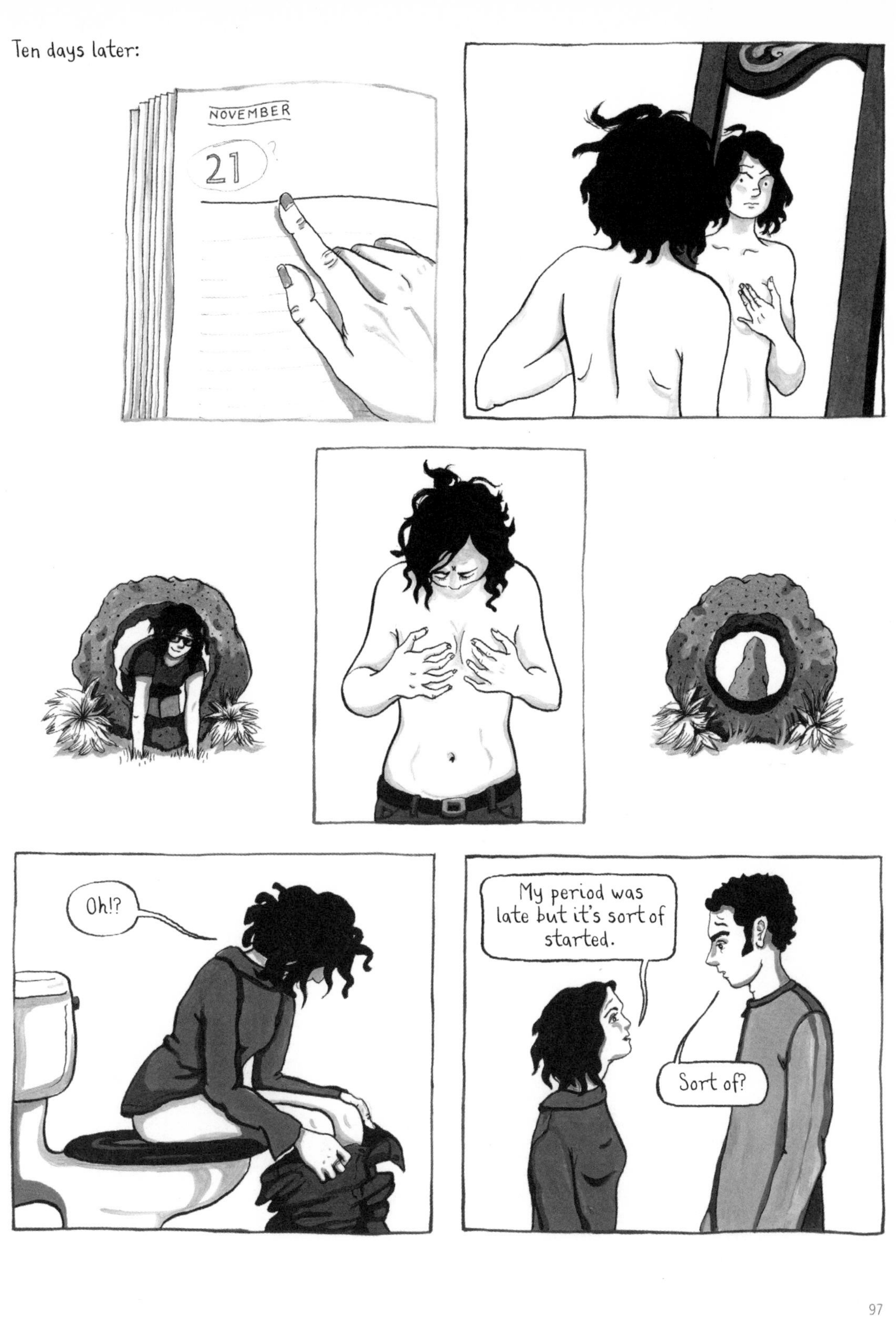
Ten days later:
NOVEMBER
21
?
Oh!?
My period was late but it's sort of started.
Sort of?

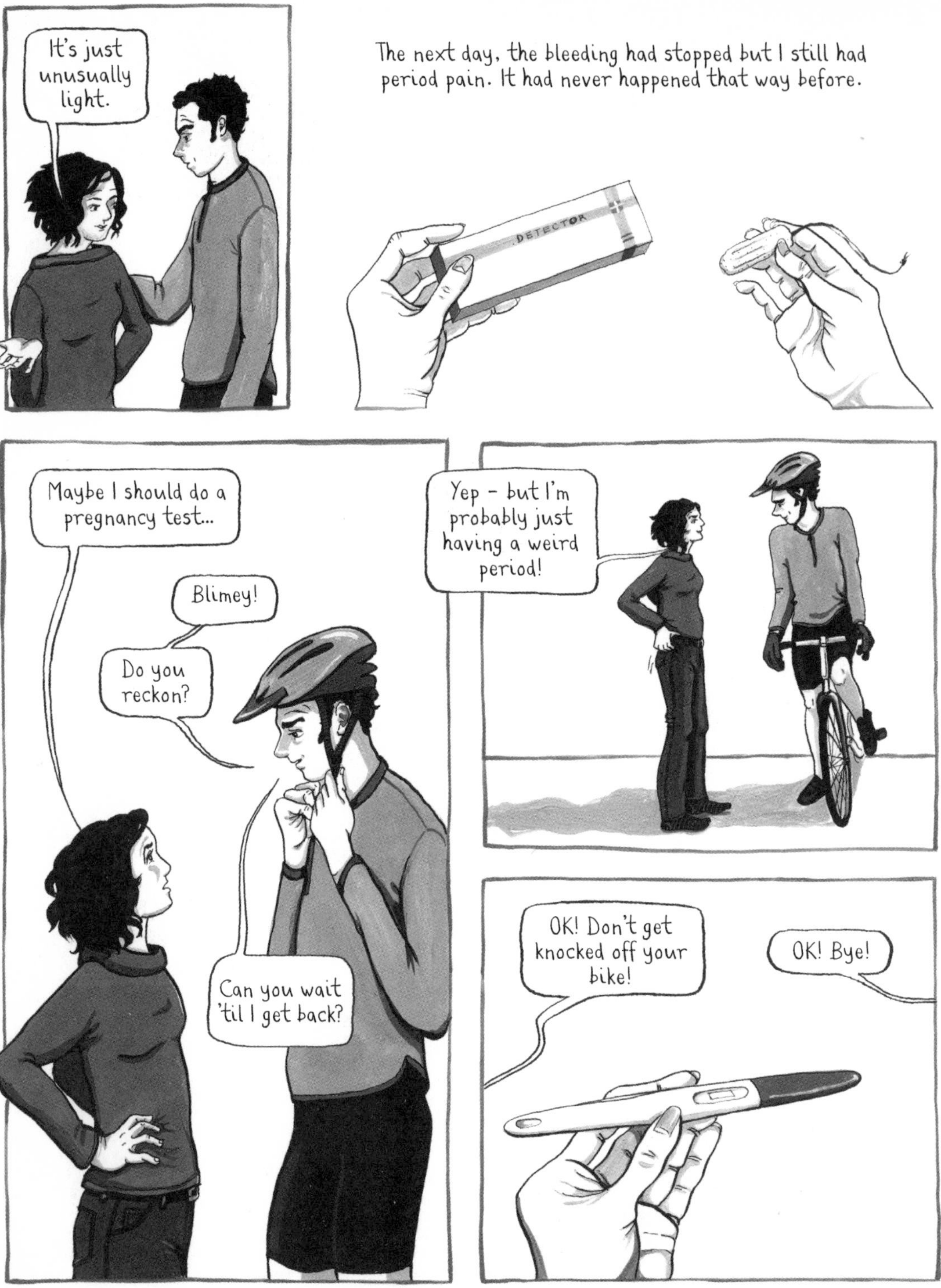
It's just unusually light.
The next day, the bleeding had stopped but I still had period pain. It had never happened that way before.
DETECTOR
Maybe I should do a pregnancy test...
Blimey!
Do you reckon?
Can you wait 'til I get back?
Yep - but I'm probably just having a weird period!
OK! Don't get knocked off your bike!
OK! Bye!

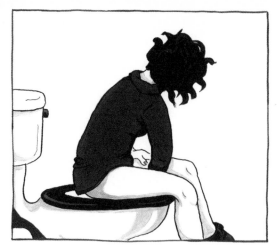

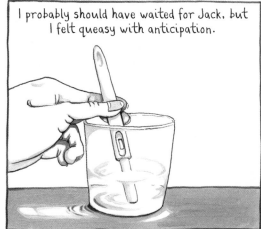
I probably should have waited for Jack, but I felt queasy with anticipation.

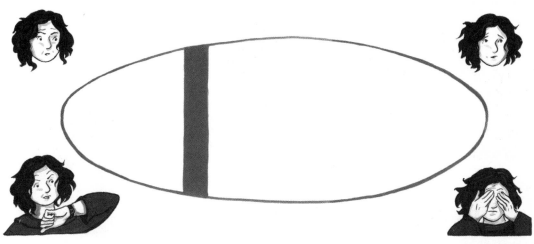

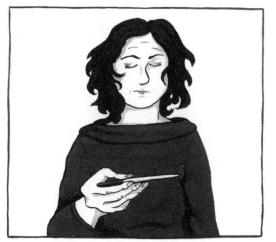

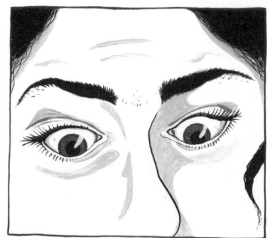

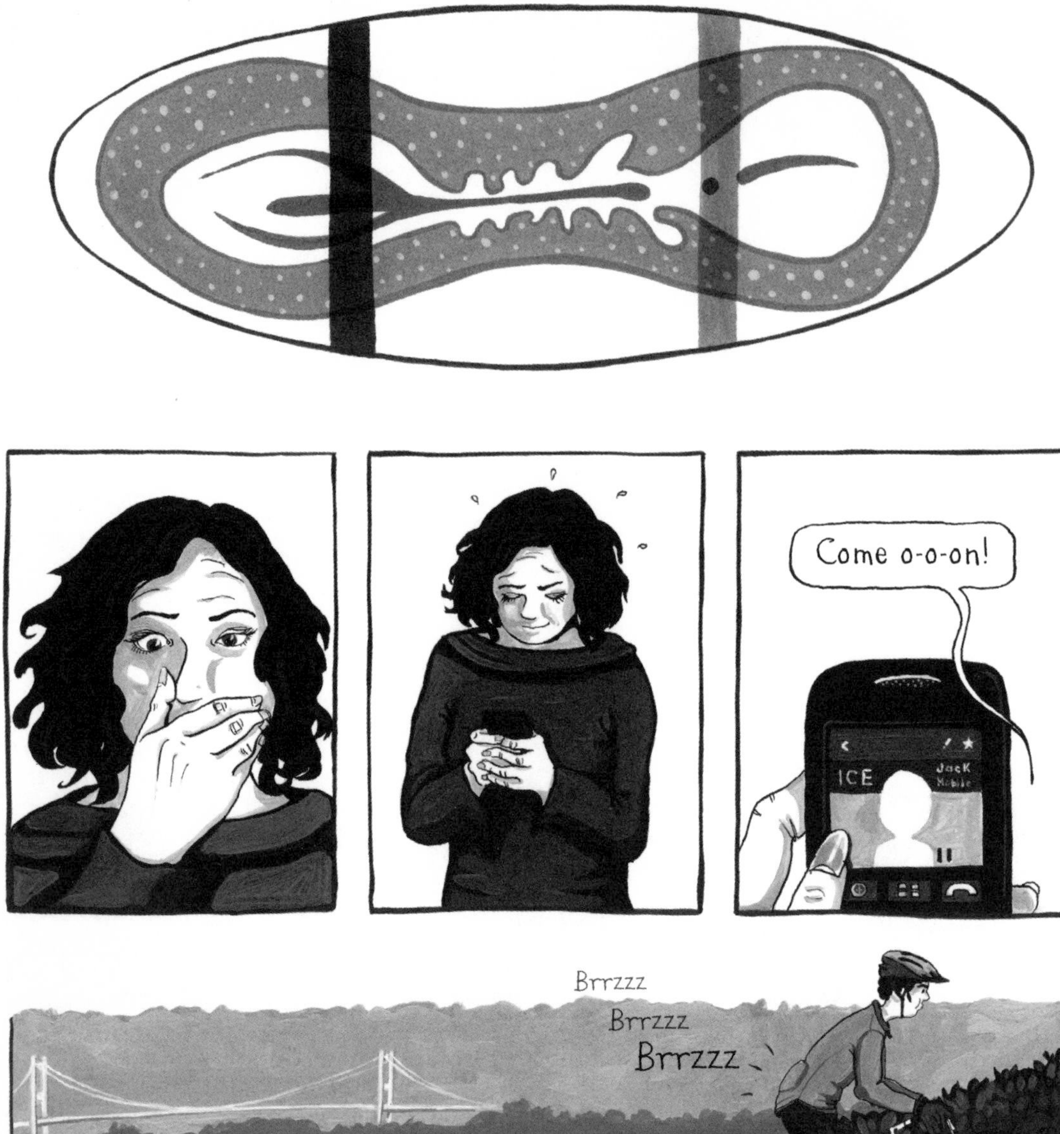
Come o-o-on!
ICE
Jack
Mobile
Brrzzz
Brrzzz
Brrzzz

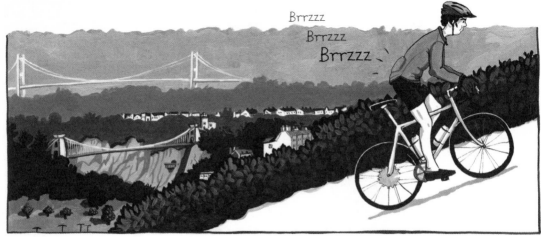

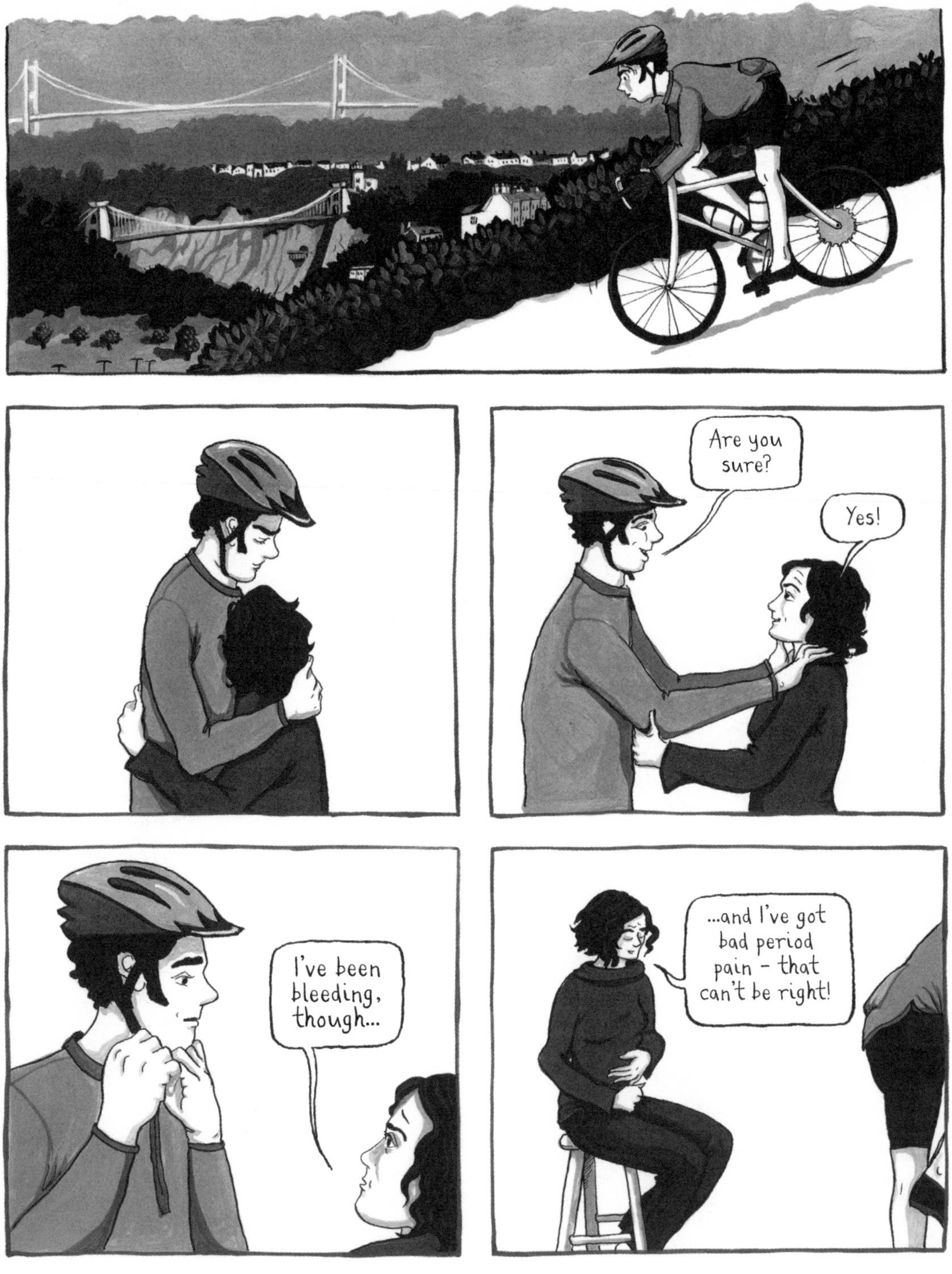
Are you sure?
Yes!
I've been bleeding, though...
...and I've got bad period pain – that can't be right!

Later:

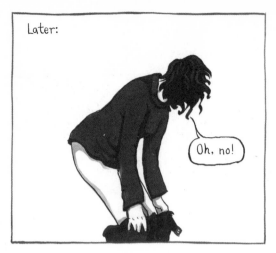

Oh, no!

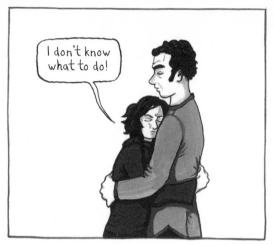

I don't know what to do!

We took a taxi to the NHS Walk-in Centre.

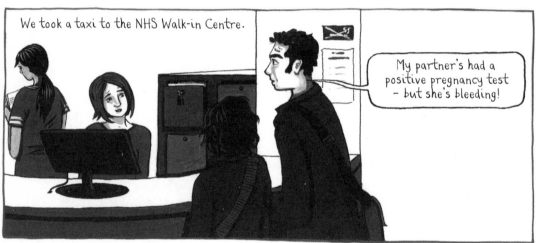

My partner's had a positive pregnancy test – but she's bleeding!

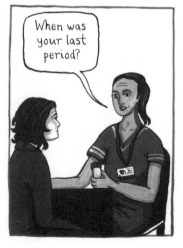

When was your last period?

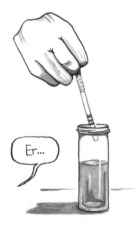

Er...

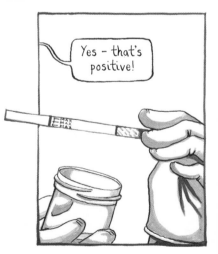

Yes – that's positive!

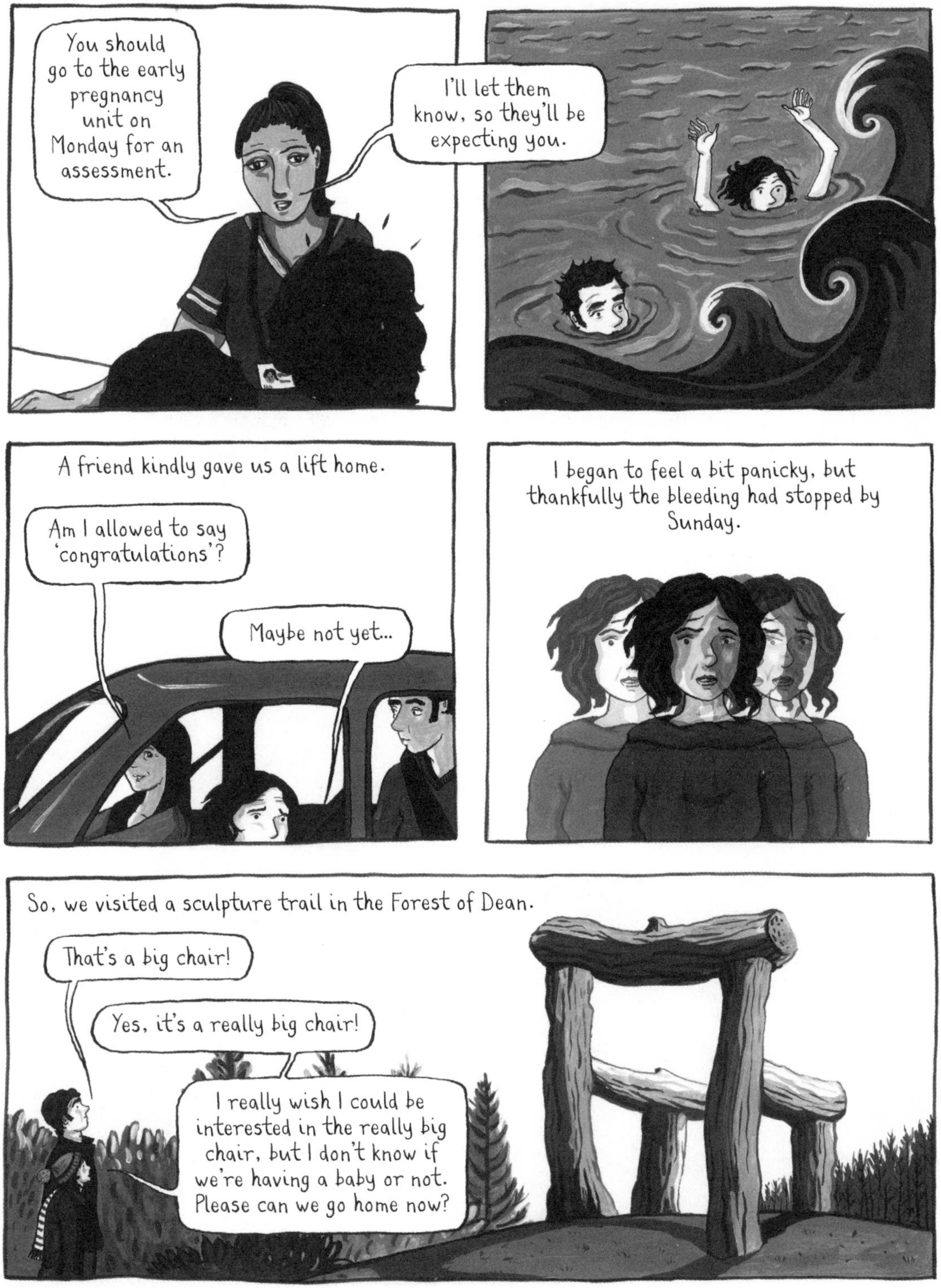
You should go to the early pregnancy unit on Monday for an assessment.
I'll let them know, so they'll be expecting you.
A friend kindly gave us a lift home.
Am I allowed to say 'congratulations'?
Maybe not yet...
I began to feel a bit panicky, but thankfully the bleeding had stopped by Sunday.
So, we visited a sculpture trail in the Forest of Dean.
That's a big chair!
Yes, it's a really big chair!
I really wish I could be interested in the really big chair, but I don't know if we're having a baby or not. Please can we go home now?

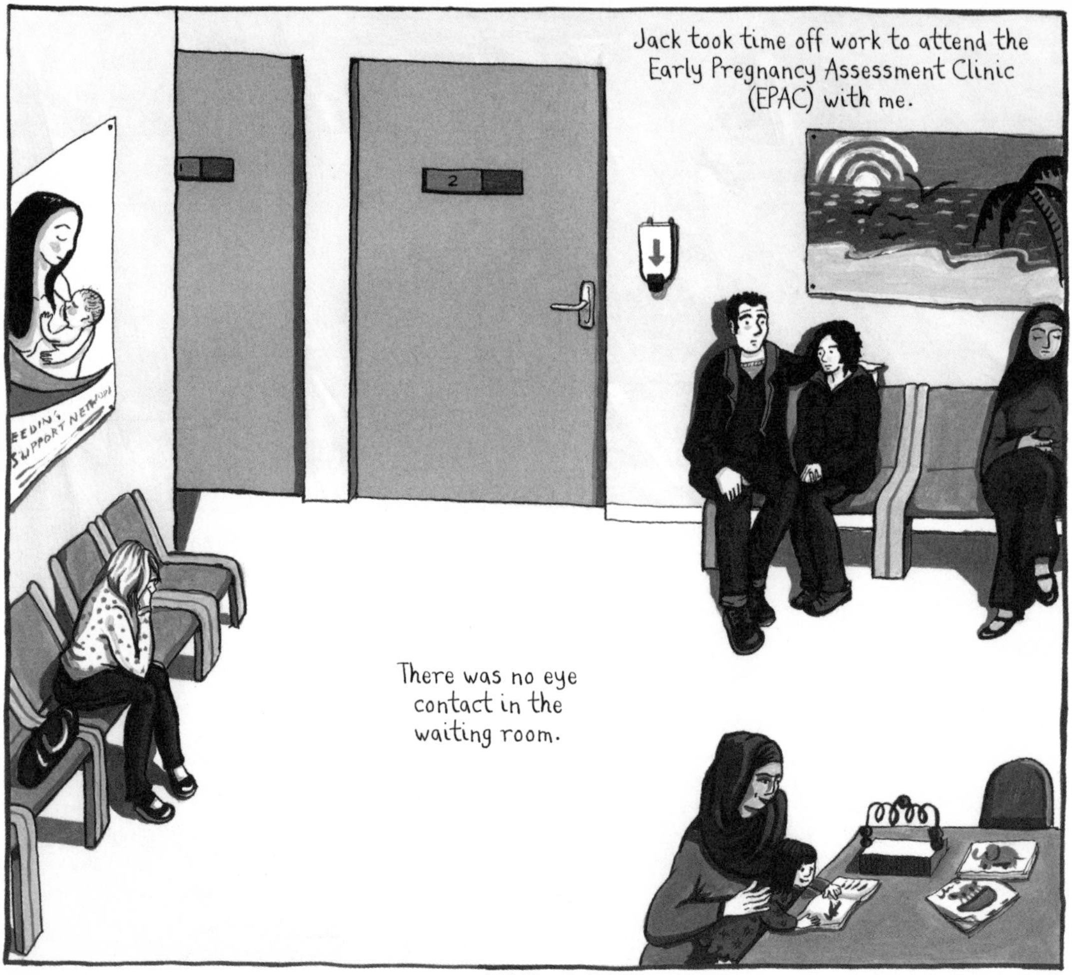
Jack took time off work to attend the Early Pregnancy Assessment Clinic (EPAC) with me.
There was no eye contact in the waiting room.

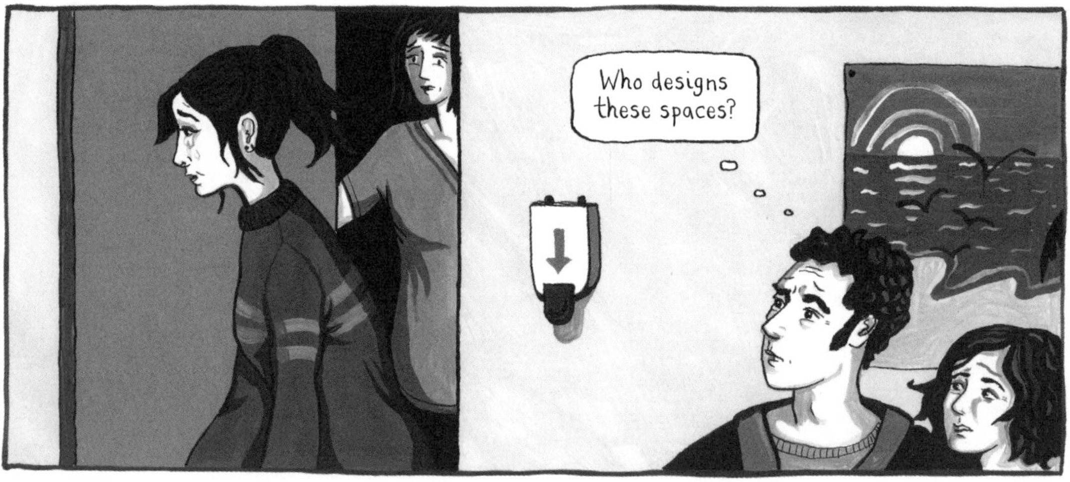
Who designs these spaces?

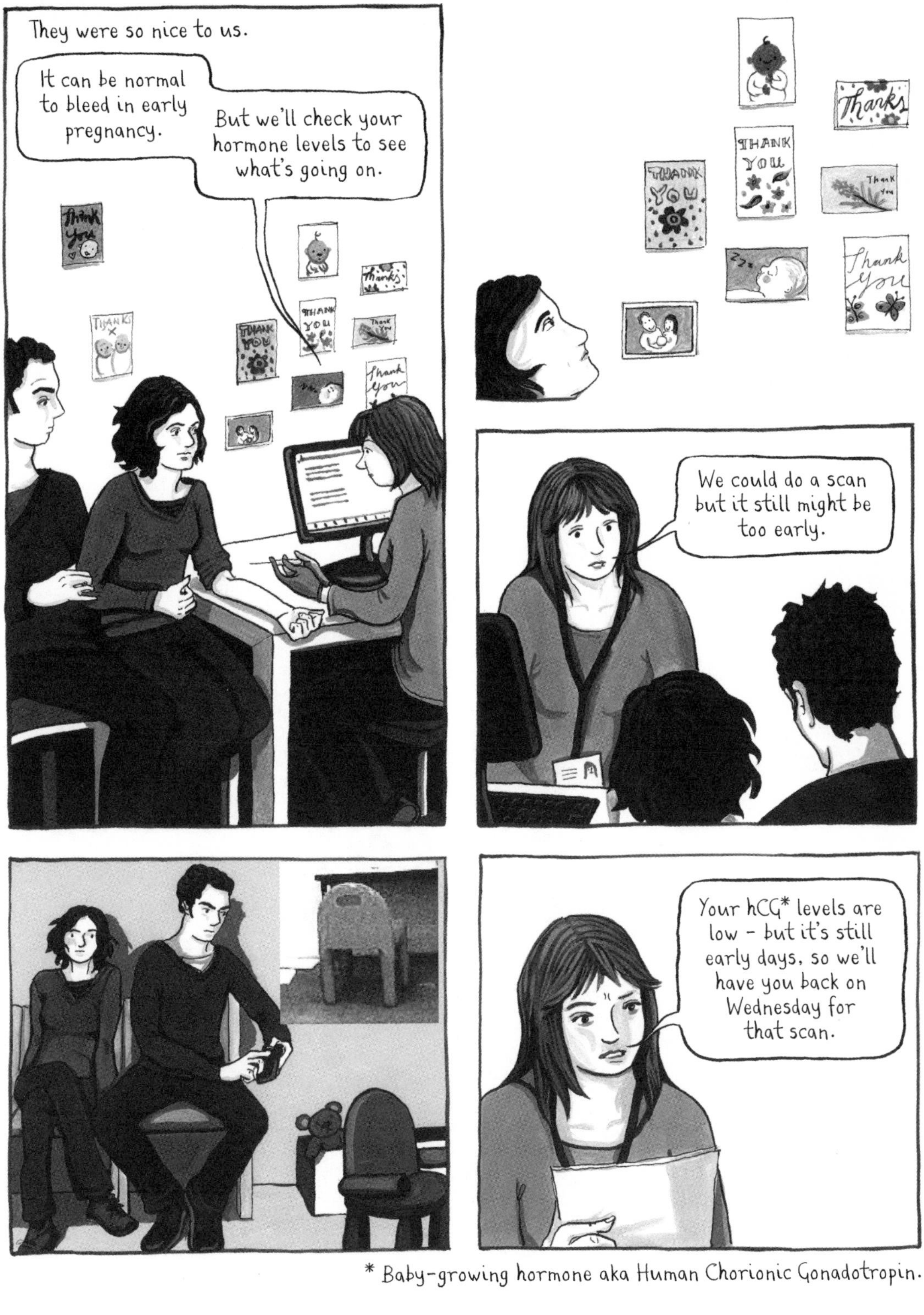
They were so nice to us.
It can be normal to bleed in early pregnancy.
But we'll check your hormone levels to see what's going on.
We could do a scan but it still might be too early.
Your hCG* levels are low - but it's still early days, so we'll have you back on Wednesday for that scan.

* Baby-growing hormone aka Human Chorionic Gonadotropin.

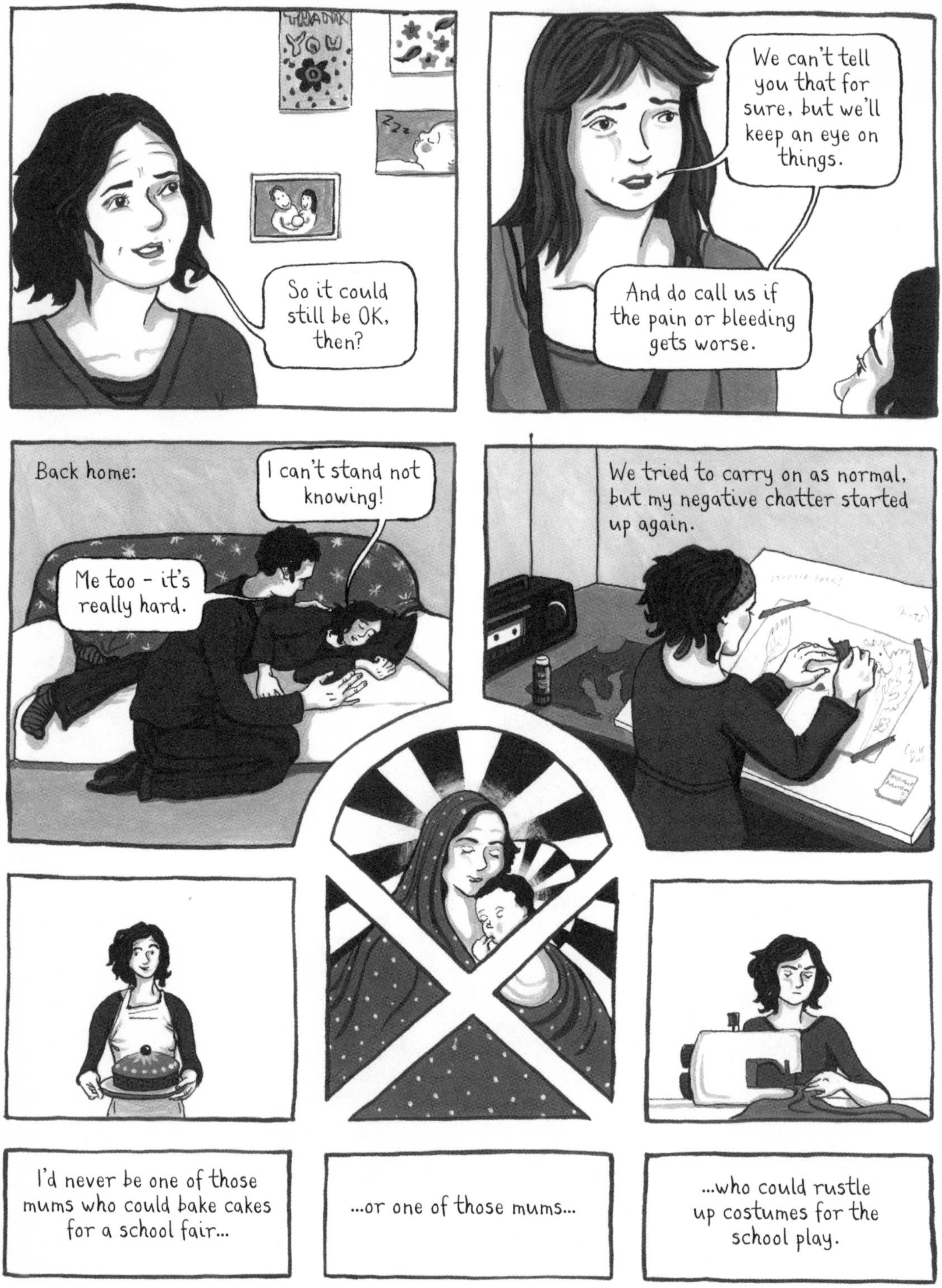
So it could still be OK, then?
We can't tell you that for sure, but we'll keep an eye on things.
And do call us if the pain or bleeding gets worse.
Back home:
I can't stand not knowing!
Me too – it's really hard.
We tried to carry on as normal, but my negative chatter started up again.
I'd never be one of those mums who could bake cakes for a school fair...
...or one of those mums...
...who could rustle up costumes for the school play.

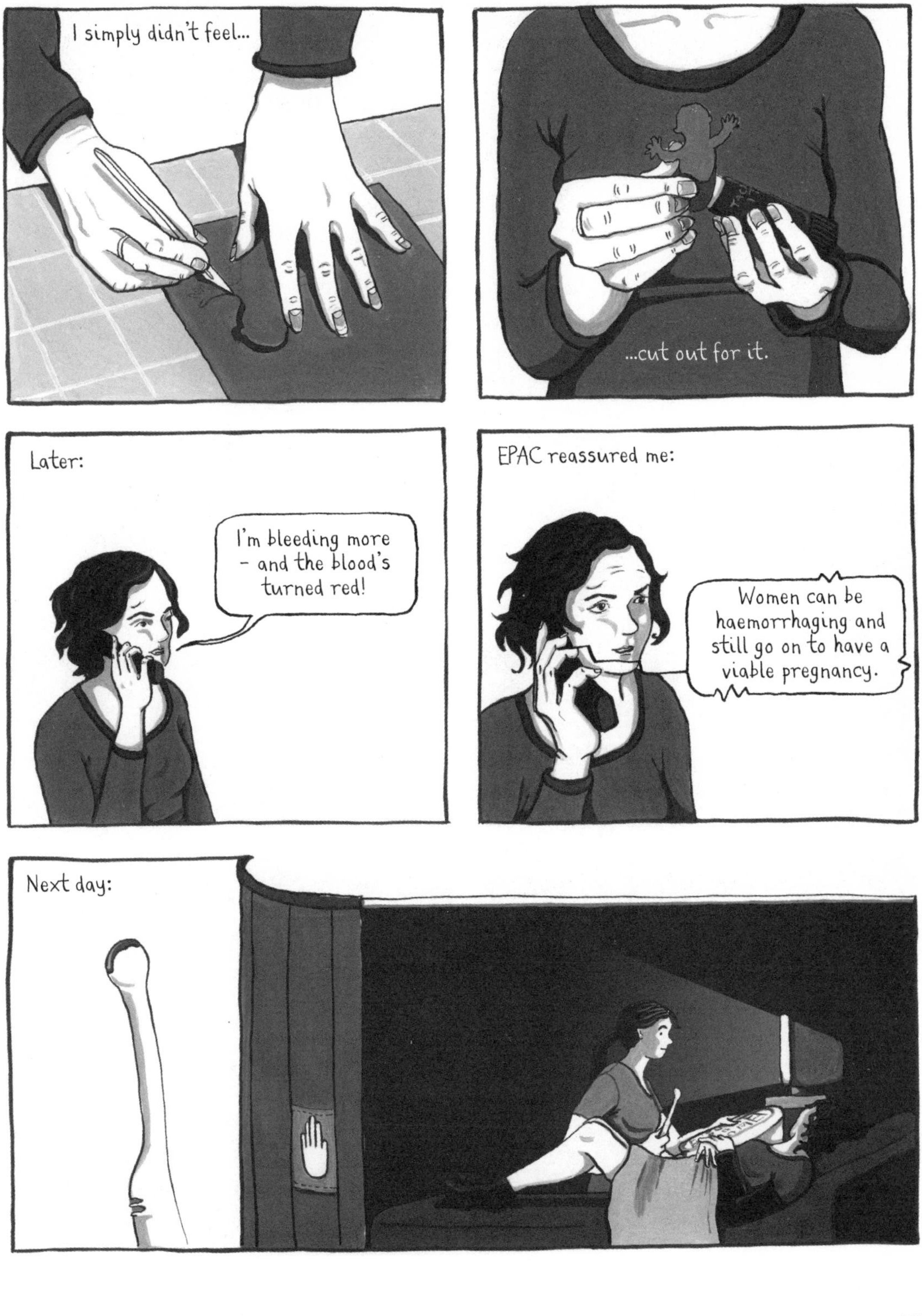

I simply didn't feel...
...cut out for it.
Later:
I'm bleeding more - and the blood's turned red!
EPAC reassured me:
Women can be haemorrhaging and still go on to have a viable pregnancy.
Next day:

ARE YOU OK
WITH LATEX?
Yes.
THIS'LL BE
A BIT COLD...
...
...?
I CAN'T... SEE ANYTHING.
IT COULD BE
TOO EARLY...
...OR IT'S ALREADY
PASSED...
...AND THERE'S SOME FREE FLUID IN
THE PELVIC CAVITY. THIS MIGHT
INDICATE A
LOSS.
Oh, right -
I see...

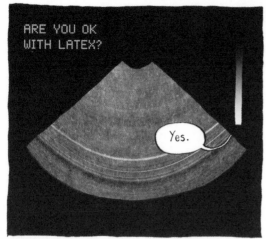

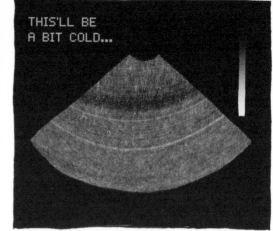

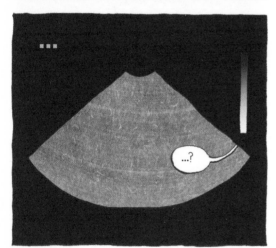

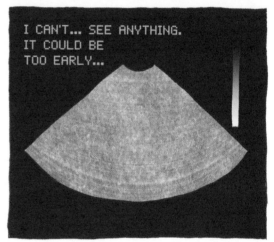

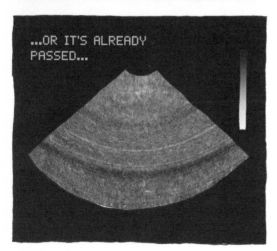

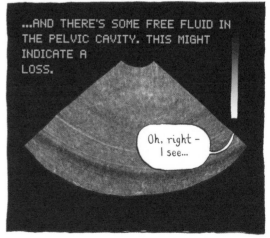

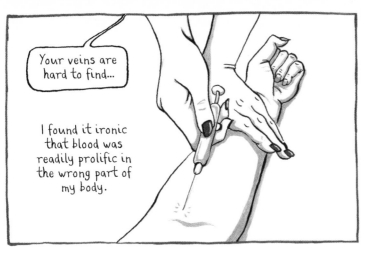

Your veins are hard to find...

I found it ironic that blood was readily prolific in the wrong part of my body.

More weeing...

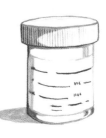

...and waiting in the silent room with the other averted eyes.

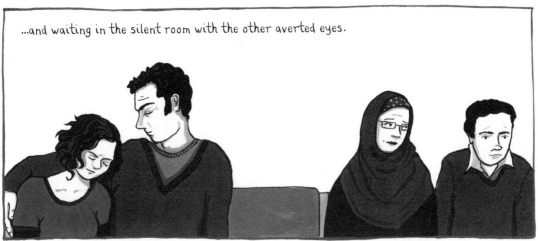

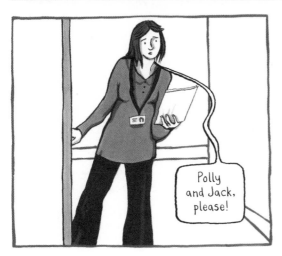

Polly and Jack, please!

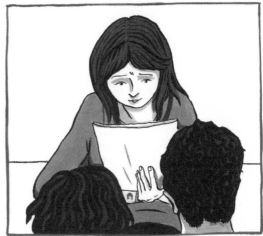

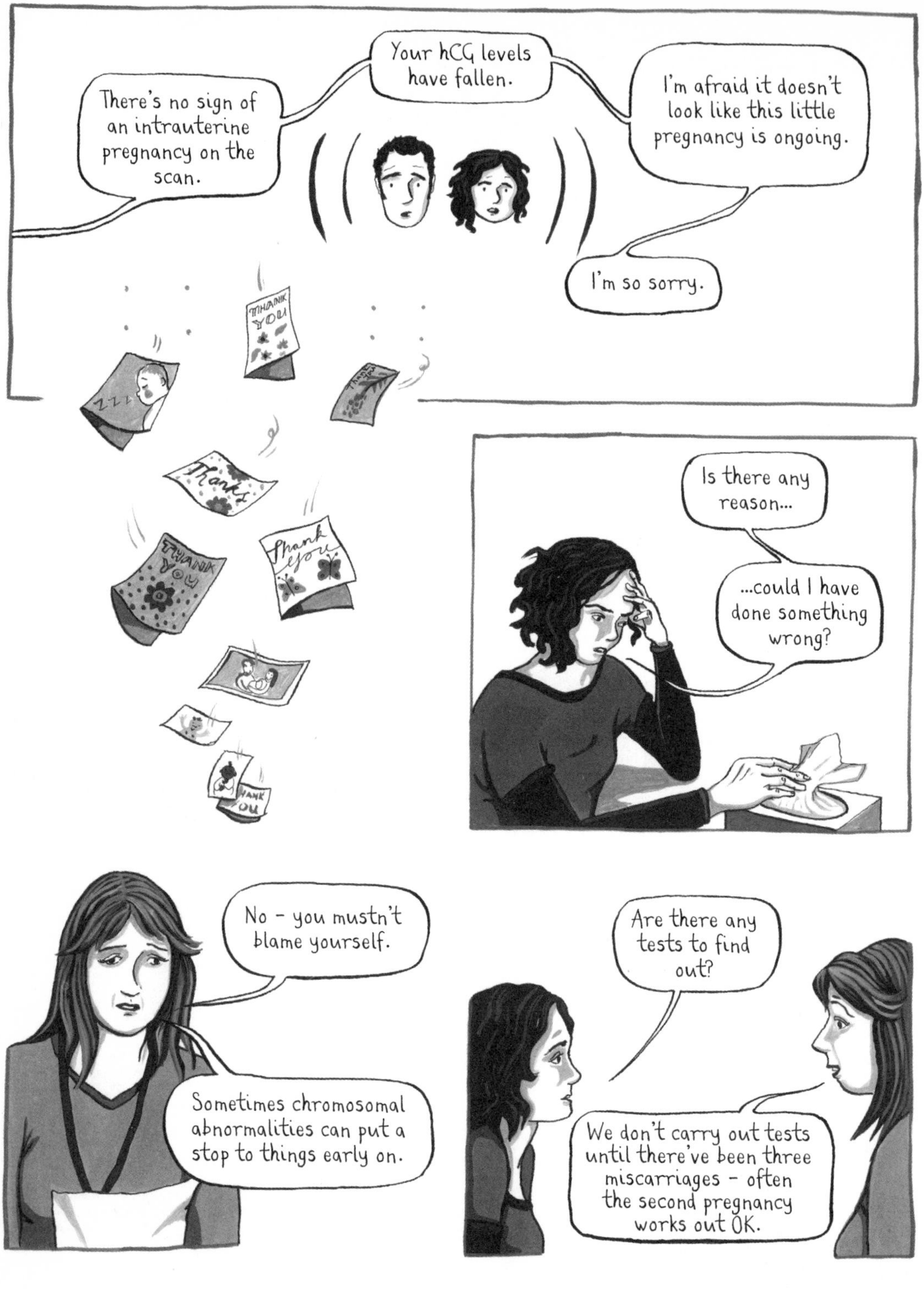
There's no sign of an intrauterine pregnancy on the scan.
Your hCG levels have fallen.
I'm afraid it doesn't look like this little pregnancy is ongoing.
I'm so sorry.
THANK YOU
Thanks
THANK YOU
Thank you
THANK YOU
Is there any reason...
...could I have done something wrong?
No - you mustn't blame yourself.
Sometimes chromosomal abnormalities can put a stop to things early on.
Are there any tests to find out?
We don't carry out tests until there've been three miscarriages - often the second pregnancy works out OK.

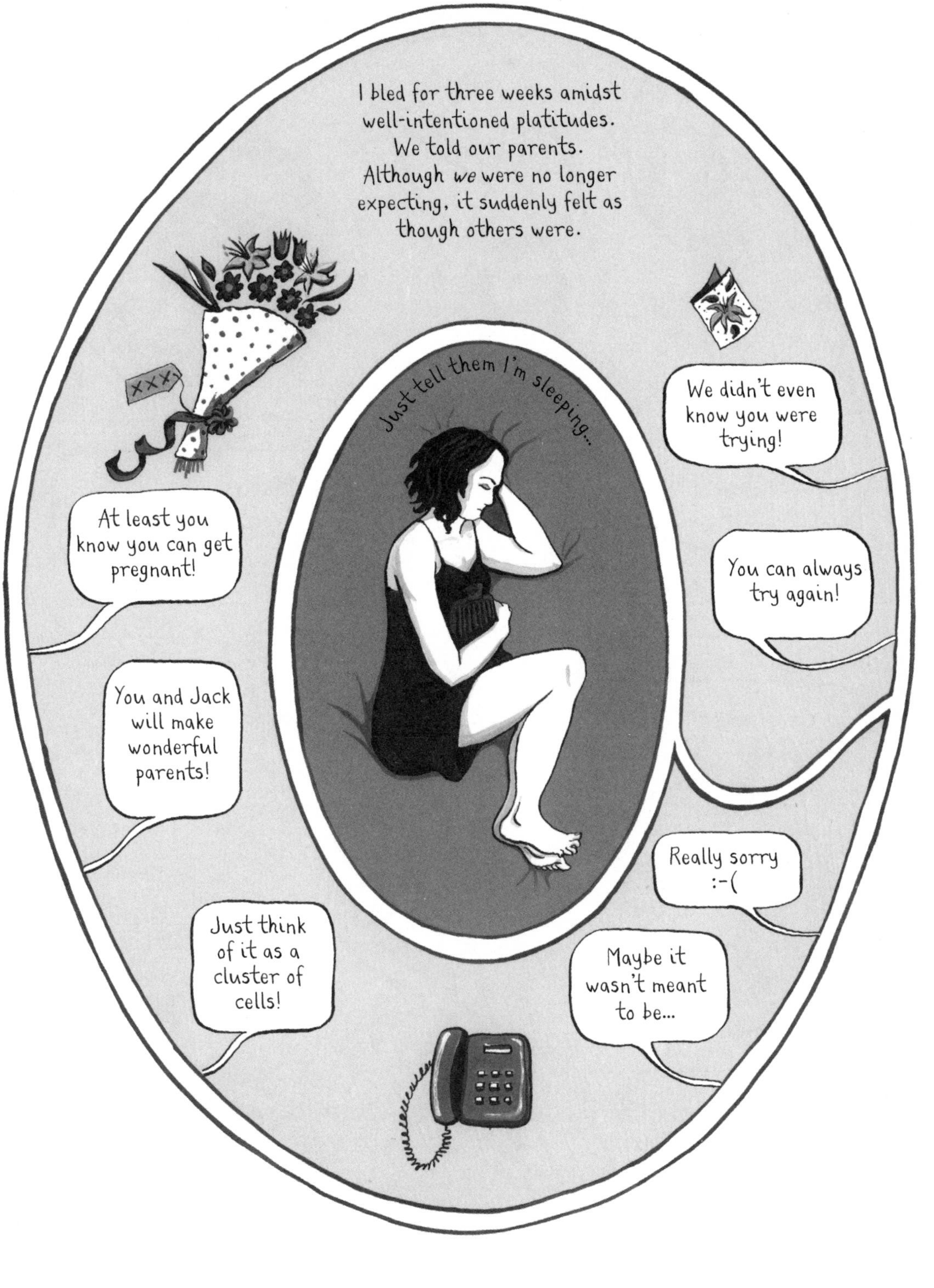
I bled for three weeks amidst well-intentioned platitudes. We told our parents. Although *we* were no longer expecting, it suddenly felt as though others were.
Just tell them I'm sleeping...
We didn't even know you were trying!
At least you know you can get pregnant!
You can always try again!
You and Jack will make wonderful parents!
Really sorry :-(
Just think of it as a cluster of cells!
Maybe it wasn't meant to be...

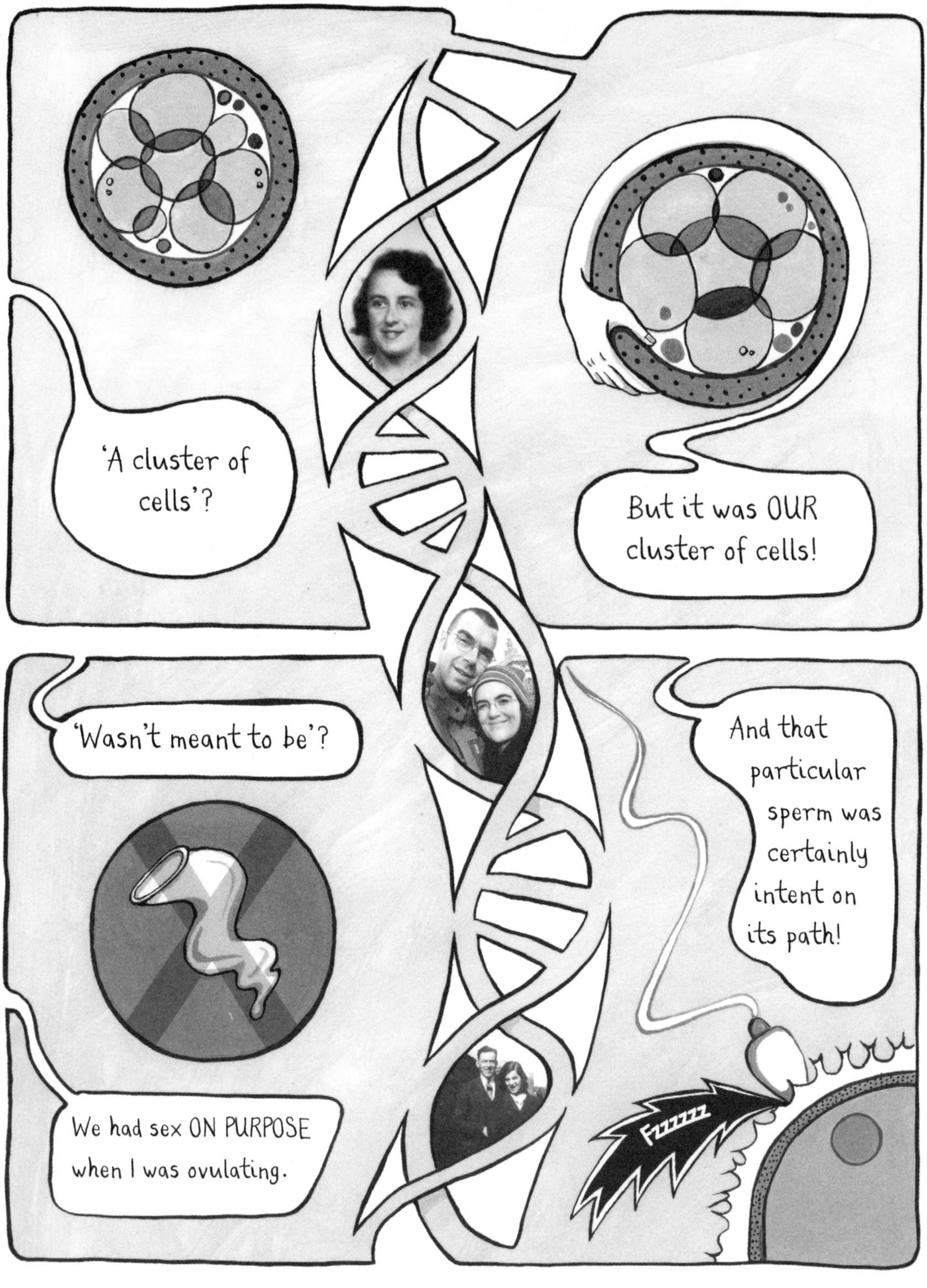
'A cluster of cells'?
But it was OUR cluster of cells!
'Wasn't meant to be'?
And that particular sperm was certainly intent on its path!
We had sex ON PURPOSE when I was ovulating.
Fzzzzzz

It just went wrong, as bodies are prone to do.

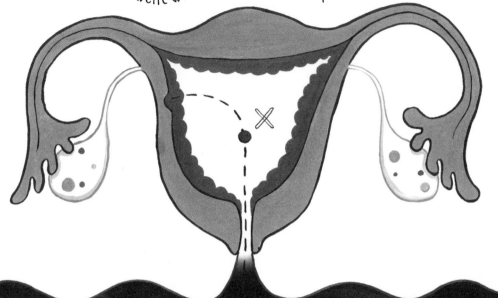

And it was physically and emotionally painful.

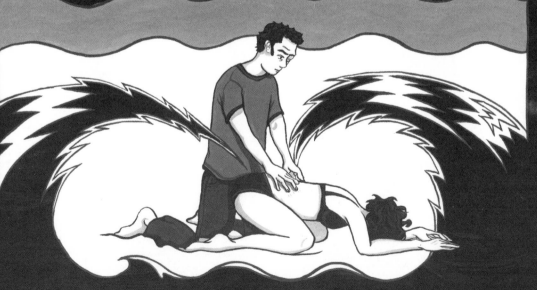

We might never know why, but others would impose their own theories...

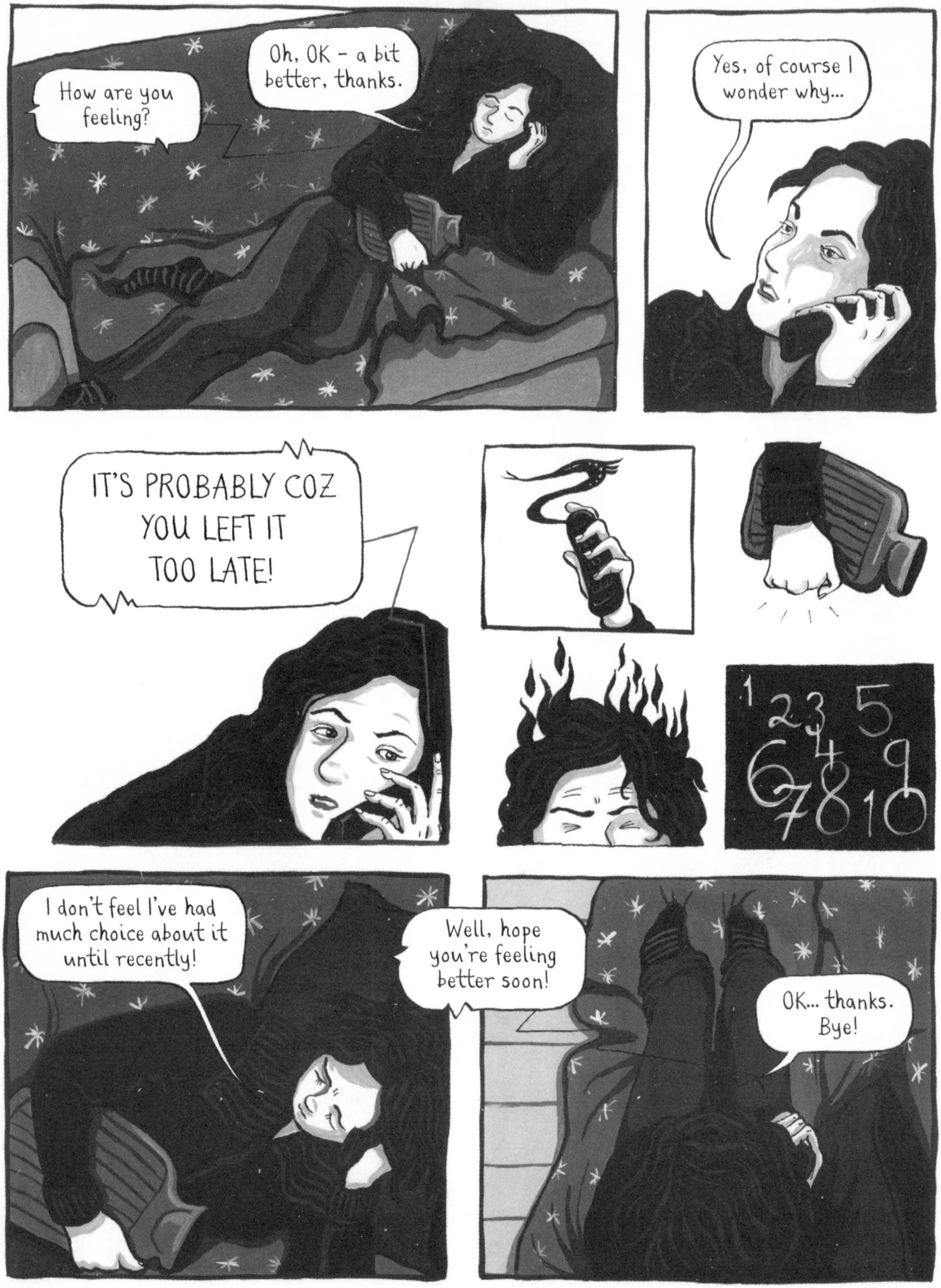
How are you feeling?
Oh, OK - a bit better, thanks.
Yes, of course I wonder why...
IT'S PROBABLY COZ YOU LEFT IT TOO LATE!
1 2 3 4 5 6 7 8 9 10
I don't feel I've had much choice about it until recently!
Well, hope you're feeling better soon!
OK... thanks. Bye!

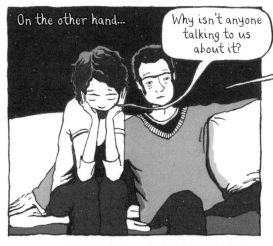

On the other hand...

Why isn't anyone talking to us about it?

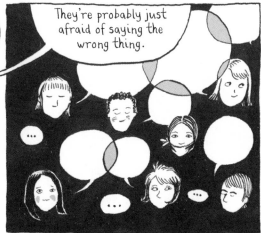

They're probably just afraid of saying the wrong thing.

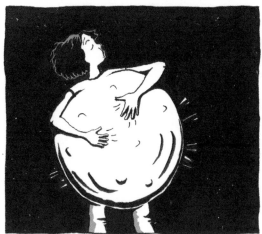

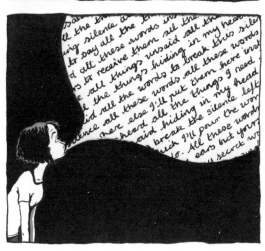

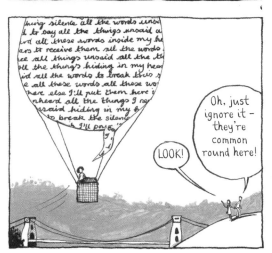

LOOK!

Oh, just ignore it – they're common round here!

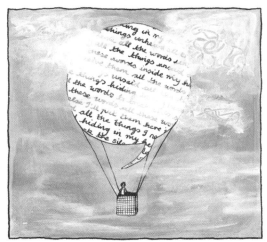

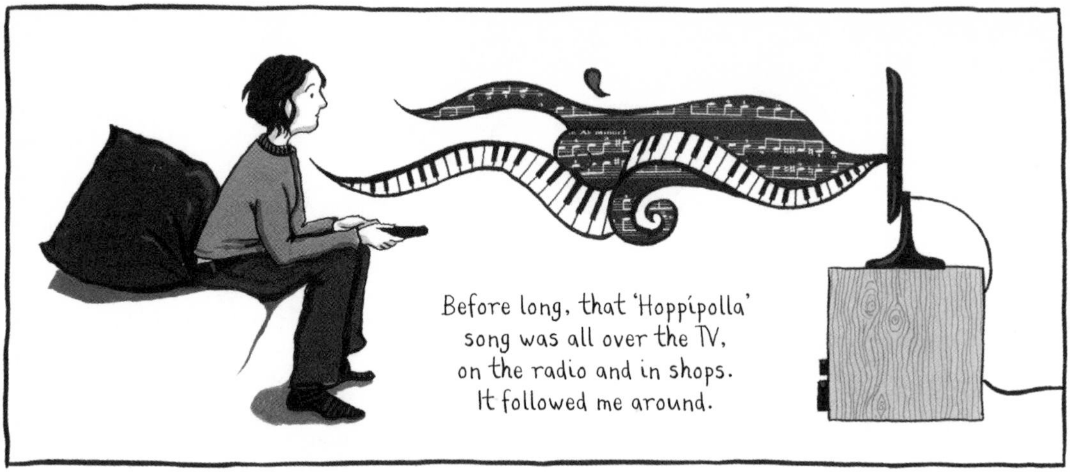
Before long, that 'Hoppípolla' song was all over the TV, on the radio and in shops. It followed me around.

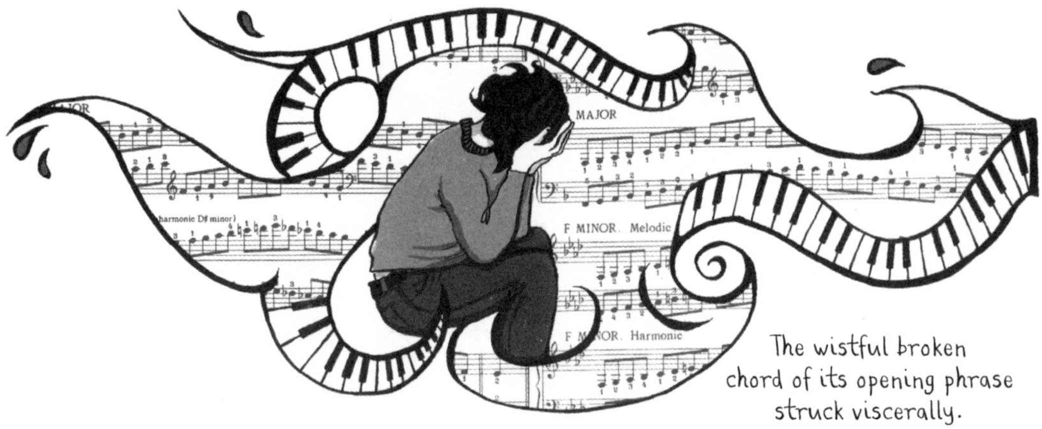
MAJOR
F MINOR. Melodic
F MINOR. Harmonic
The wistful broken chord of its opening phrase struck viscerally.

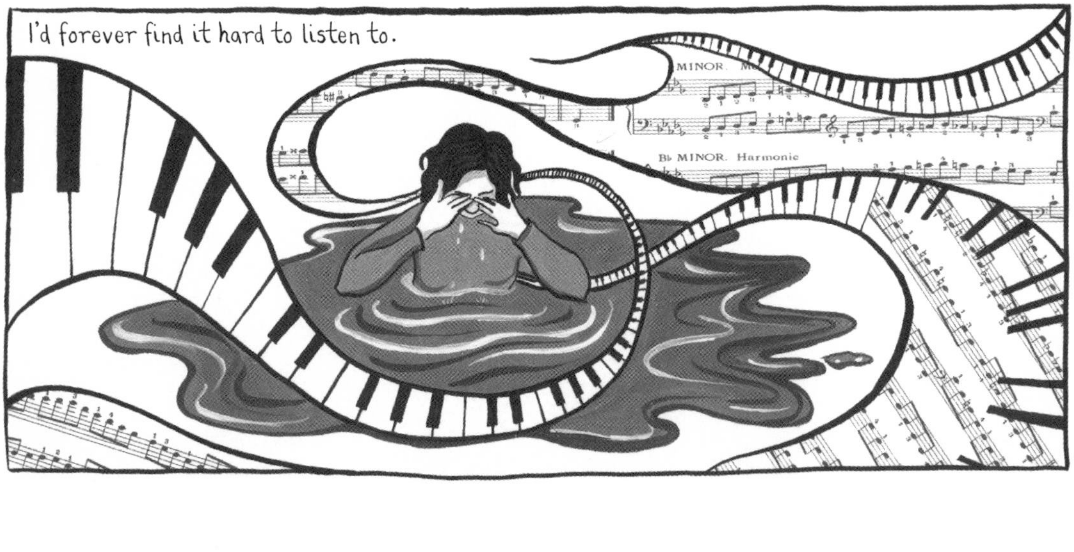
I'd forever find it hard to listen to.
B♭ MINOR. Harmonic

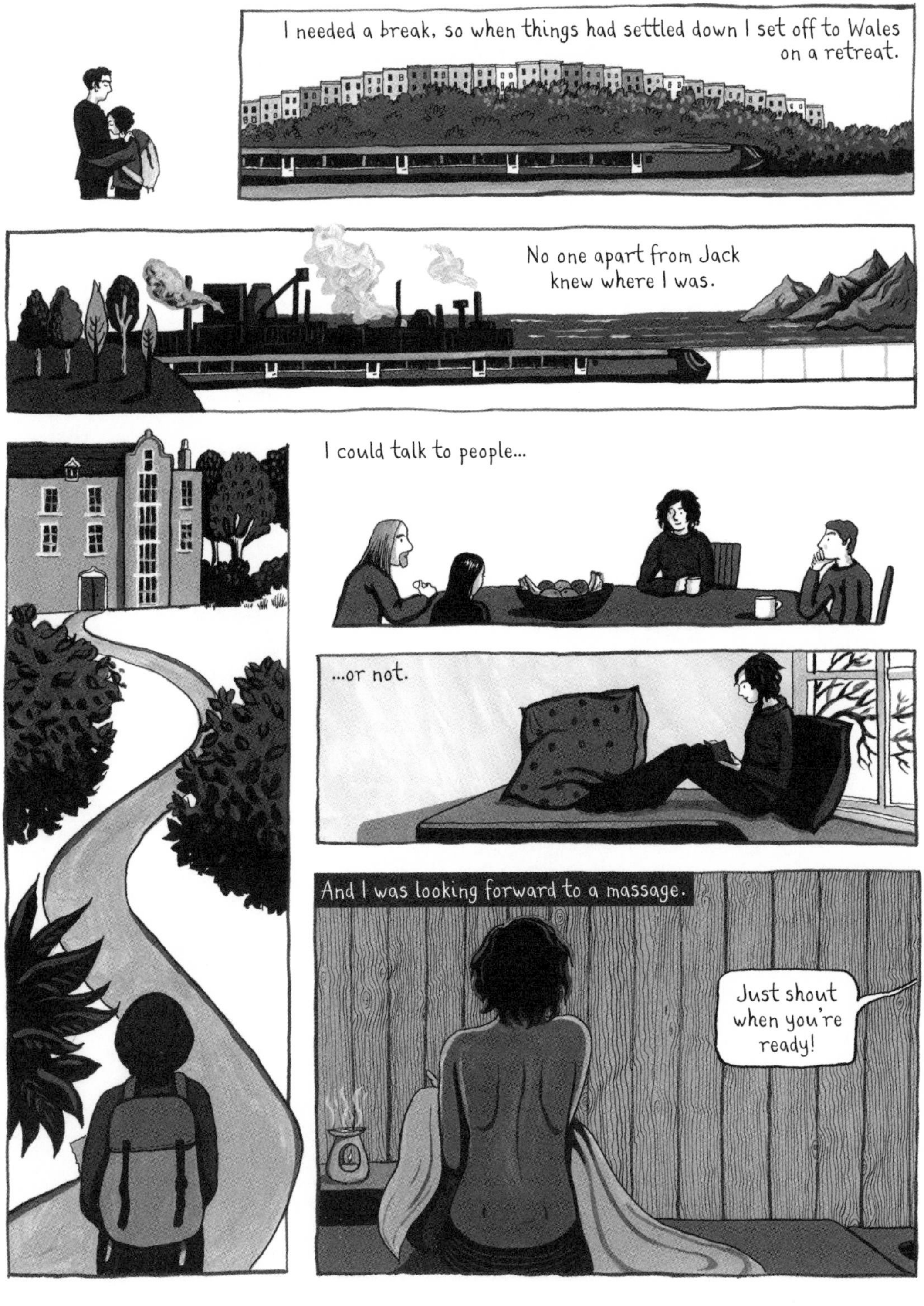
I needed a break, so when things had settled down I set off to Wales on a retreat.
No one apart from Jack knew where I was.
I could talk to people...
...or not.
And I was looking forward to a massage.
Just shout when you're ready!

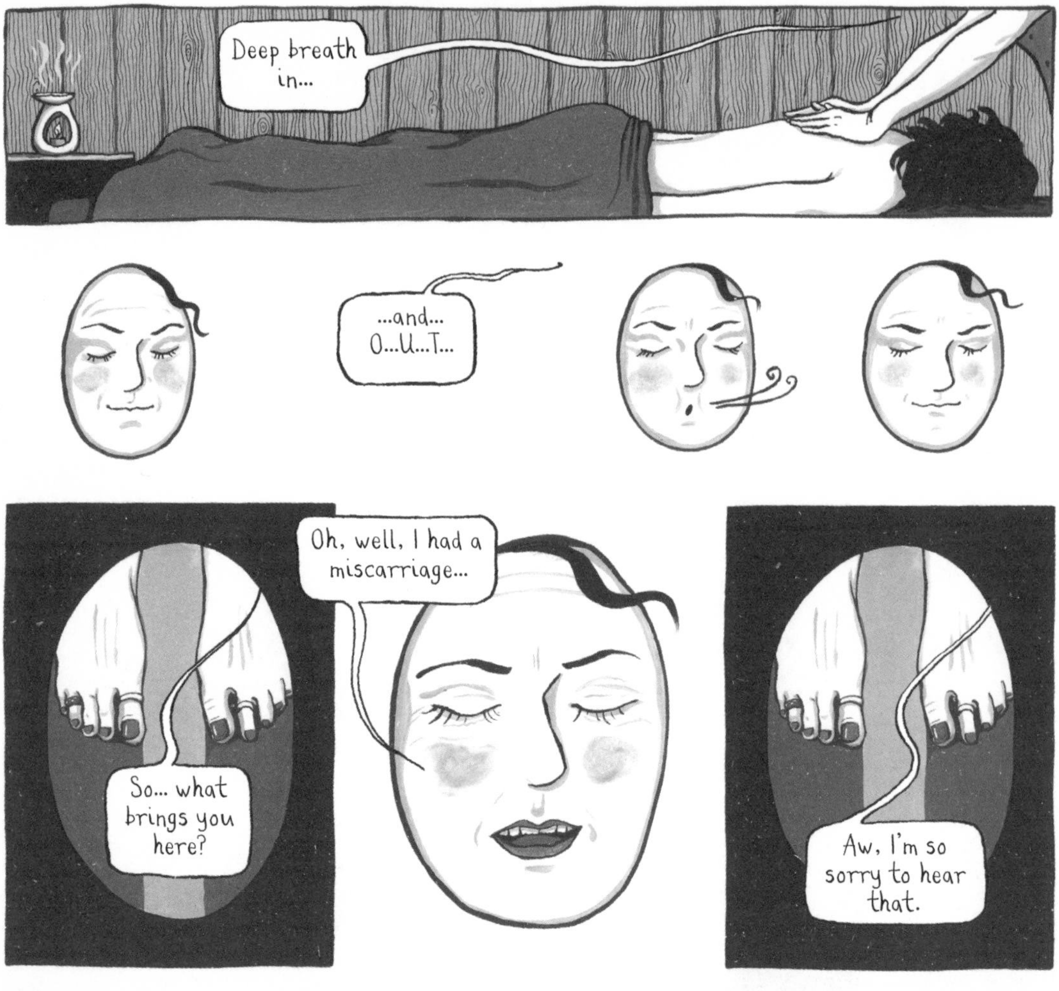
Deep breath in...
...and... O...U...T...
So... what brings you here?
Oh, well, I had a miscarriage...
Aw, I'm so sorry to hear that.
I felt a bit ambivalent about having children, but still wanted to try...
...and I suffered terrible anxiety when I actually did get pregnant.
Ahhh - that's interesting...

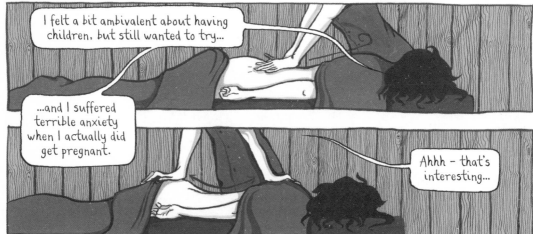

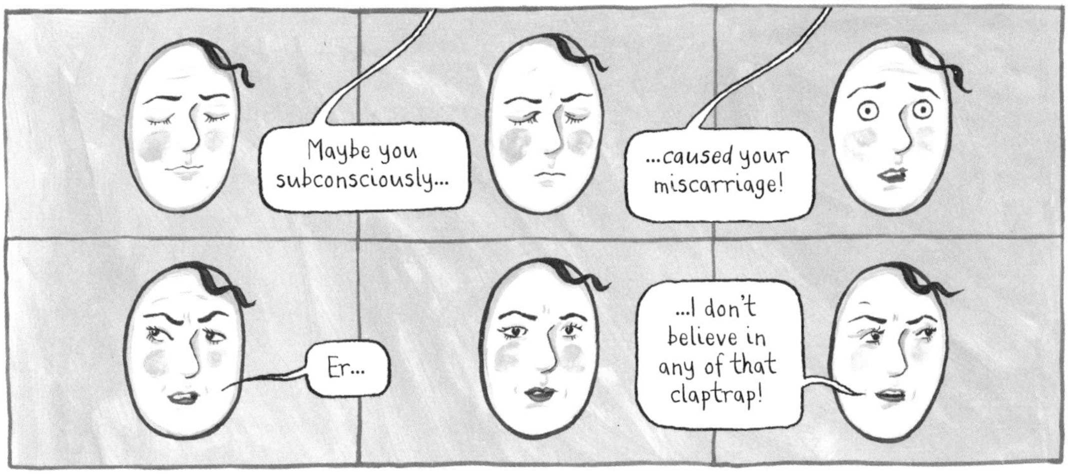
Maybe you subconsciously...
...caused your miscarriage!
Er...
...I don't believe in any of that claptrap!

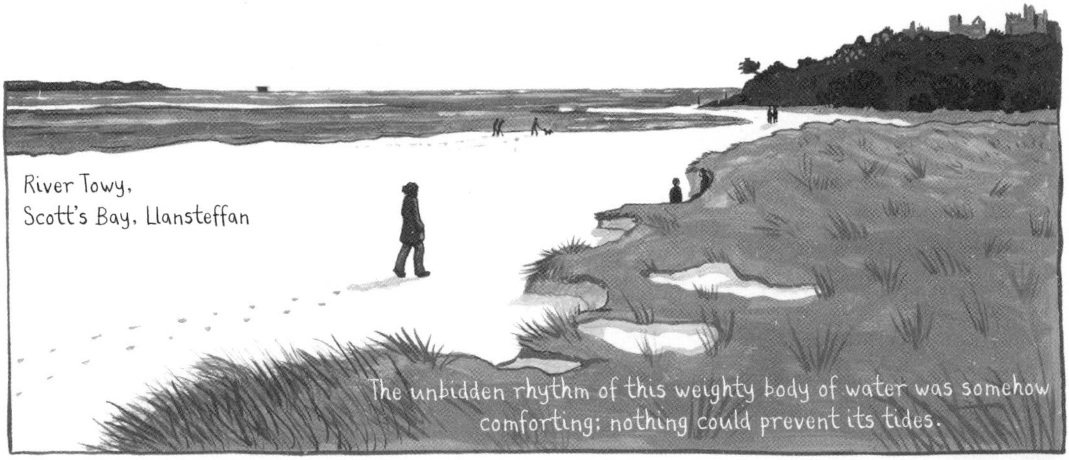
River Towy,
Scott's Bay, Llansteffan
The unbidden rhythm of this weighty body of water was somehow comforting: nothing could prevent its tides.

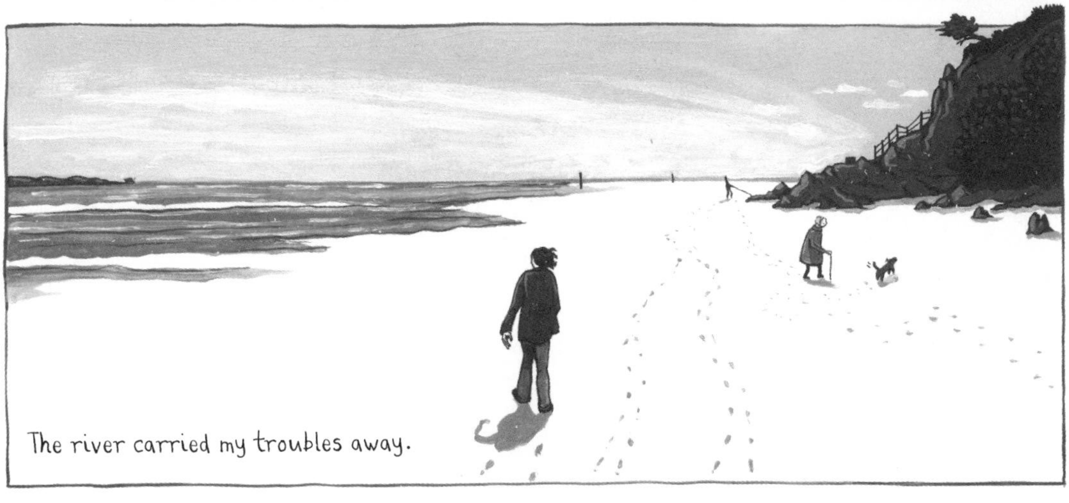
The river carried my troubles away.

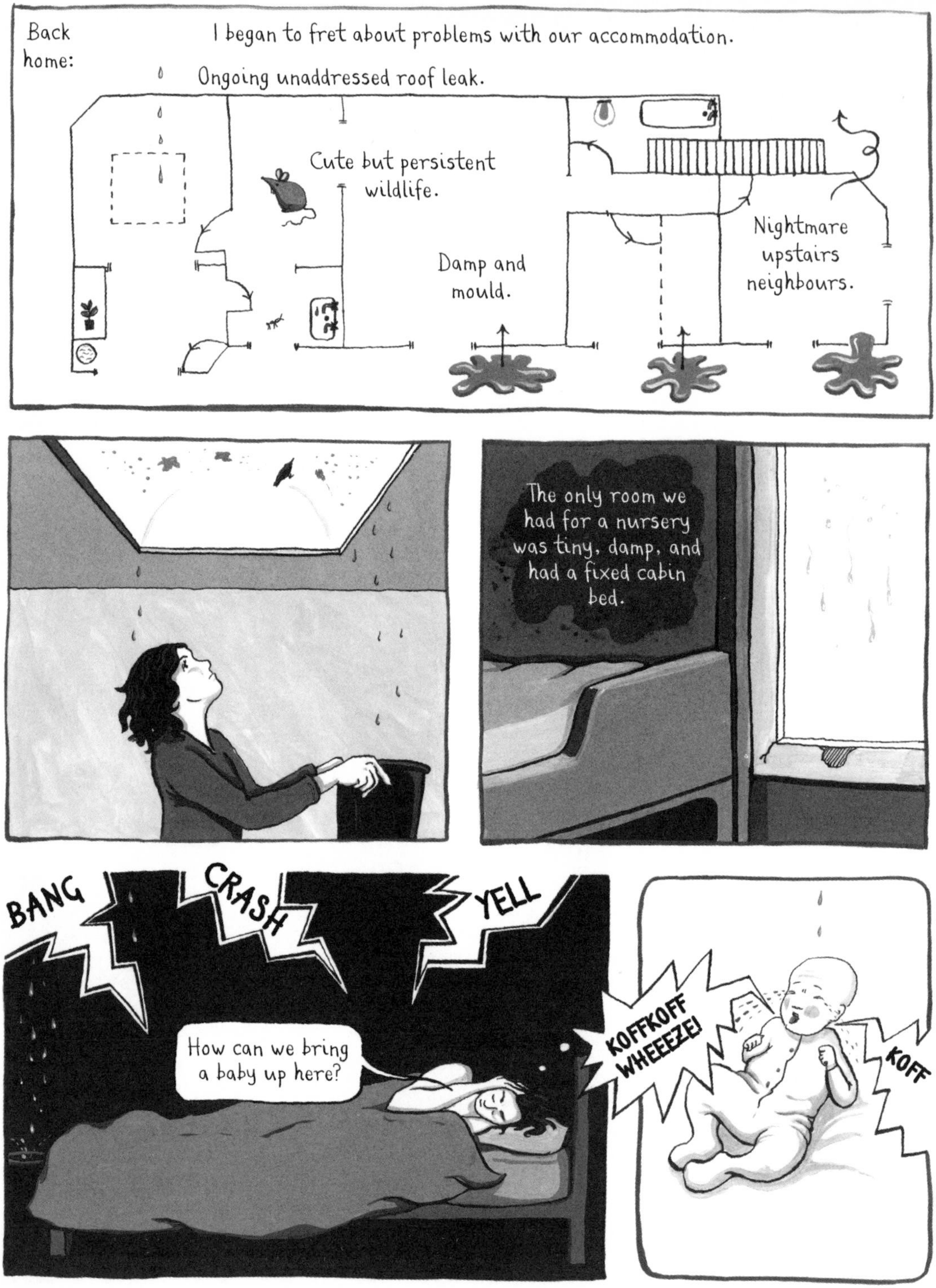
Back home:
I began to fret about problems with our accommodation.
Ongoing unaddressed roof leak.
Cute but persistent wildlife.
Damp and mould.
Nightmare upstairs neighbours.
The only room we had for a nursery was tiny, damp, and had a fixed cabin bed.
BANG
CRASH
YELL
How can we bring a baby up here?
KOFFKOFF WHEEEZE!
KOFF

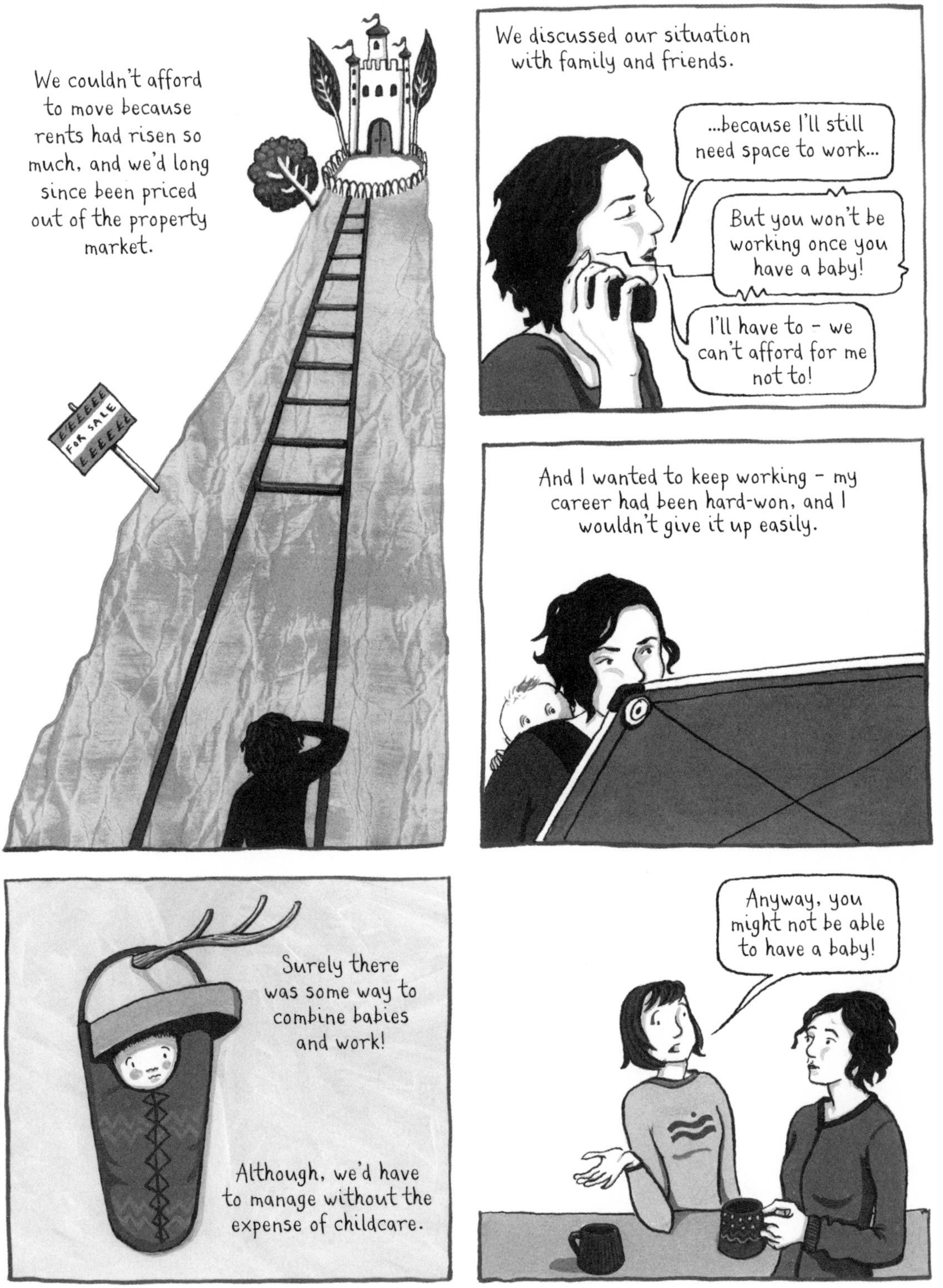
We couldn't afford to move because rents had risen so much, and we'd long since been priced out of the property market.
FOR SALE
We discussed our situation with family and friends.
...because I'll still need space to work...
But you won't be working once you have a baby!
I'll have to – we can't afford for me not to!
And I wanted to keep working – my career had been hard-won, and I wouldn't give it up easily.
Surely there was some way to combine babies and work!
Although, we'd have to manage without the expense of childcare.
Anyway, you might not be able to have a baby!

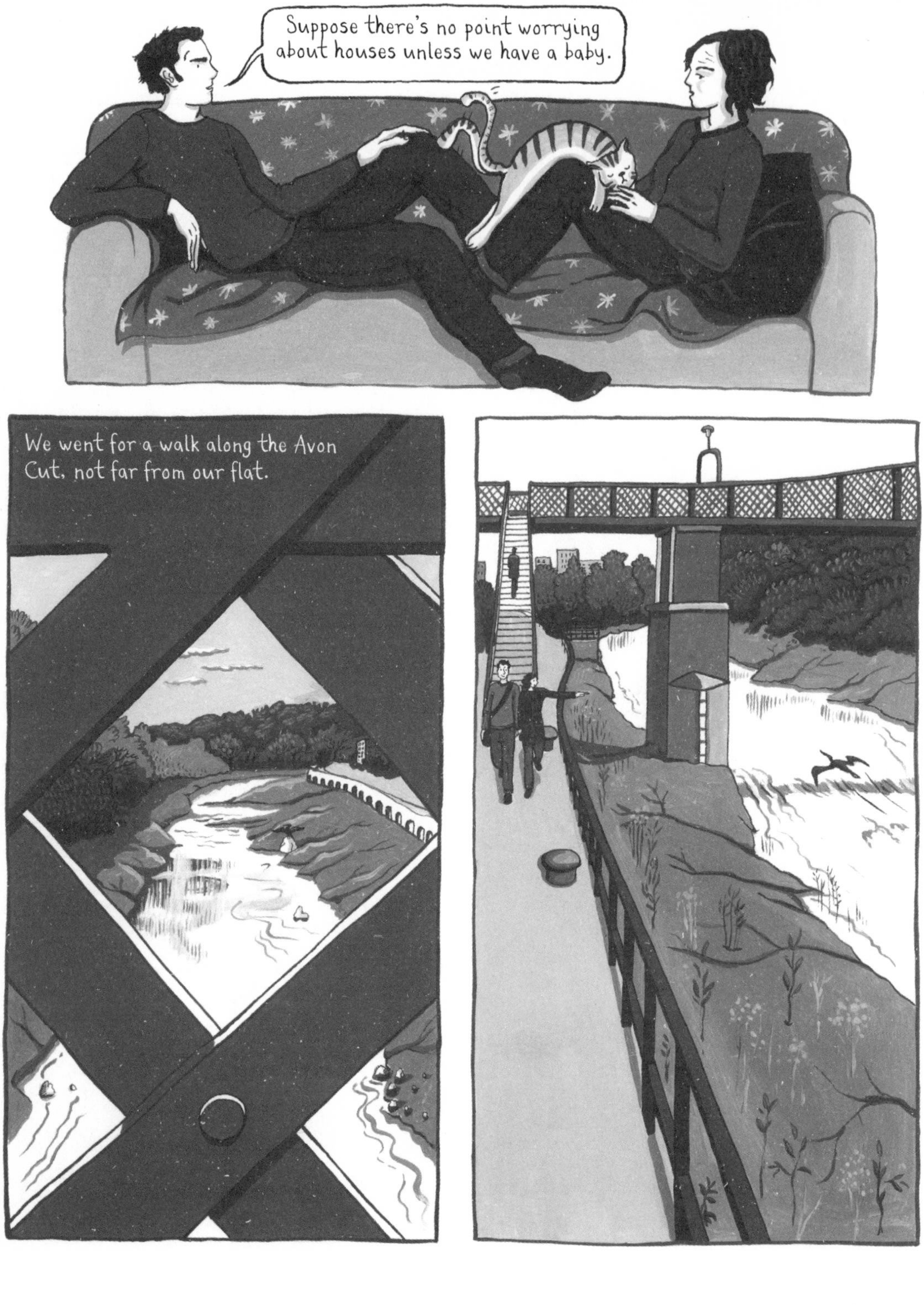
Suppose there's no point worrying about houses unless we have a baby.
We went for a walk along the Avon Cut, not far from our flat.

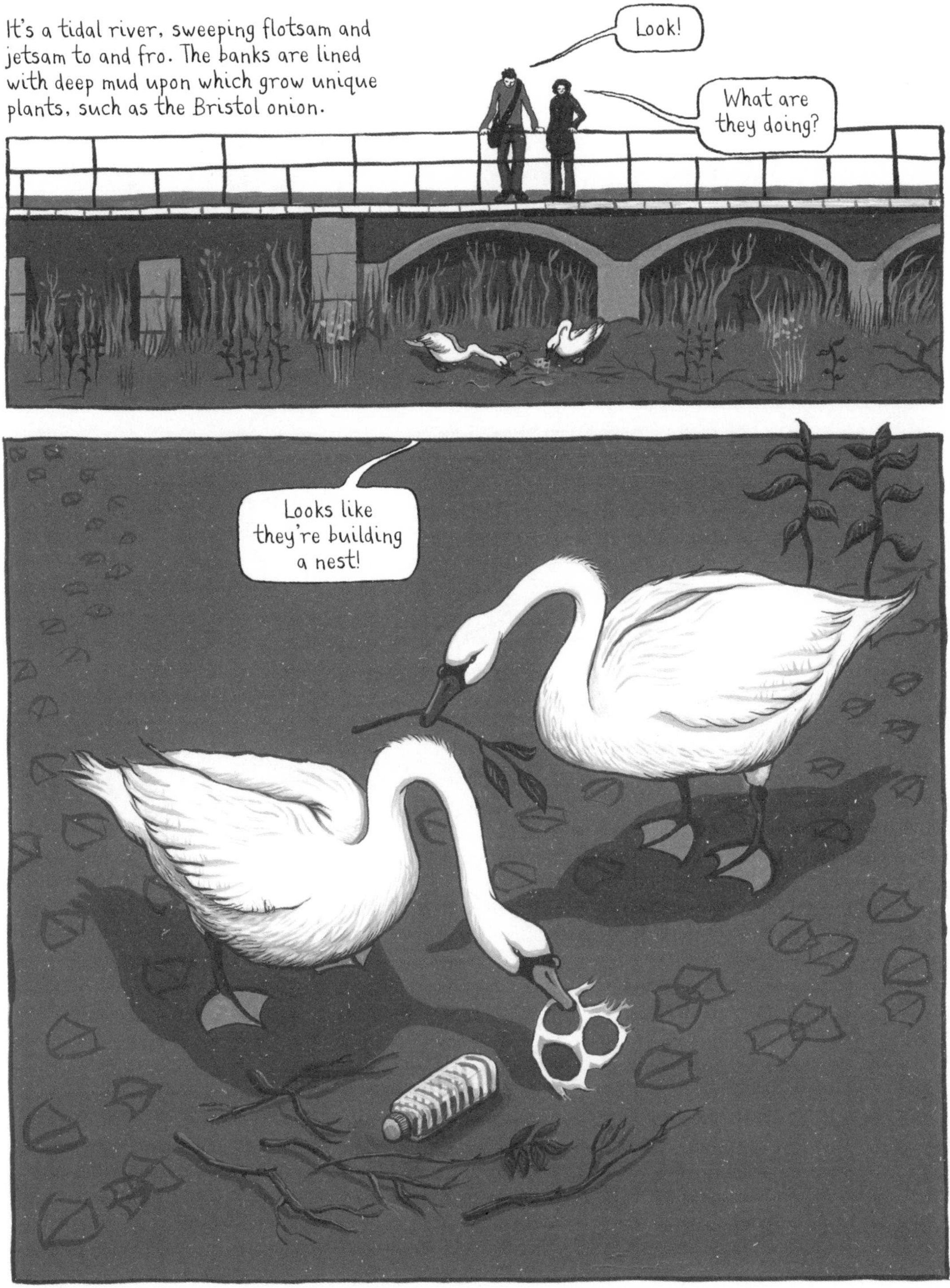
It's a tidal river, sweeping flotsam and jetsam to and fro. The banks are lined with deep mud upon which grow unique plants, such as the Bristol onion.
Look!
What are they doing?
Looks like they're building a nest!

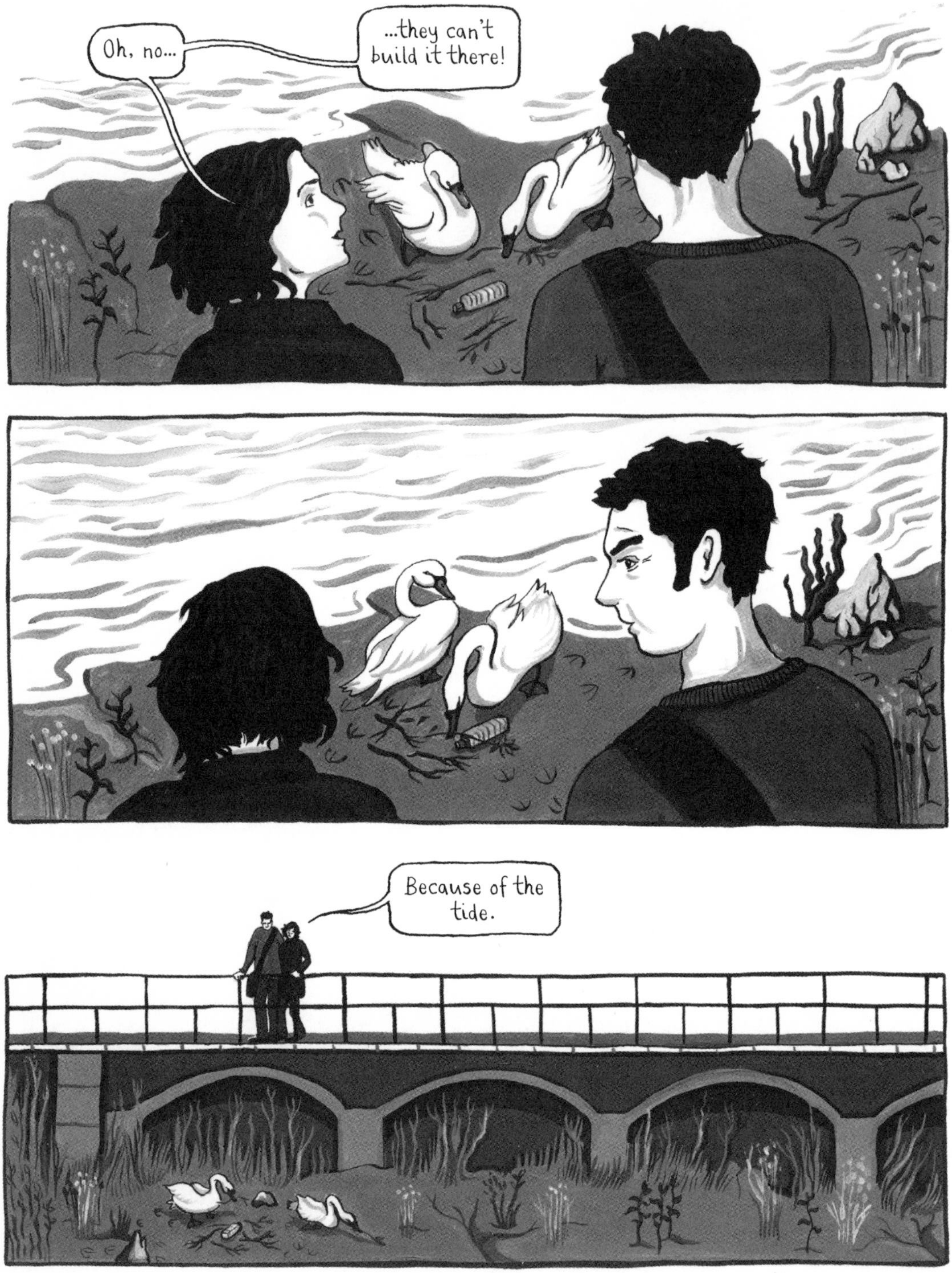
Oh, no...
...they can't build it there!
Because of the tide.

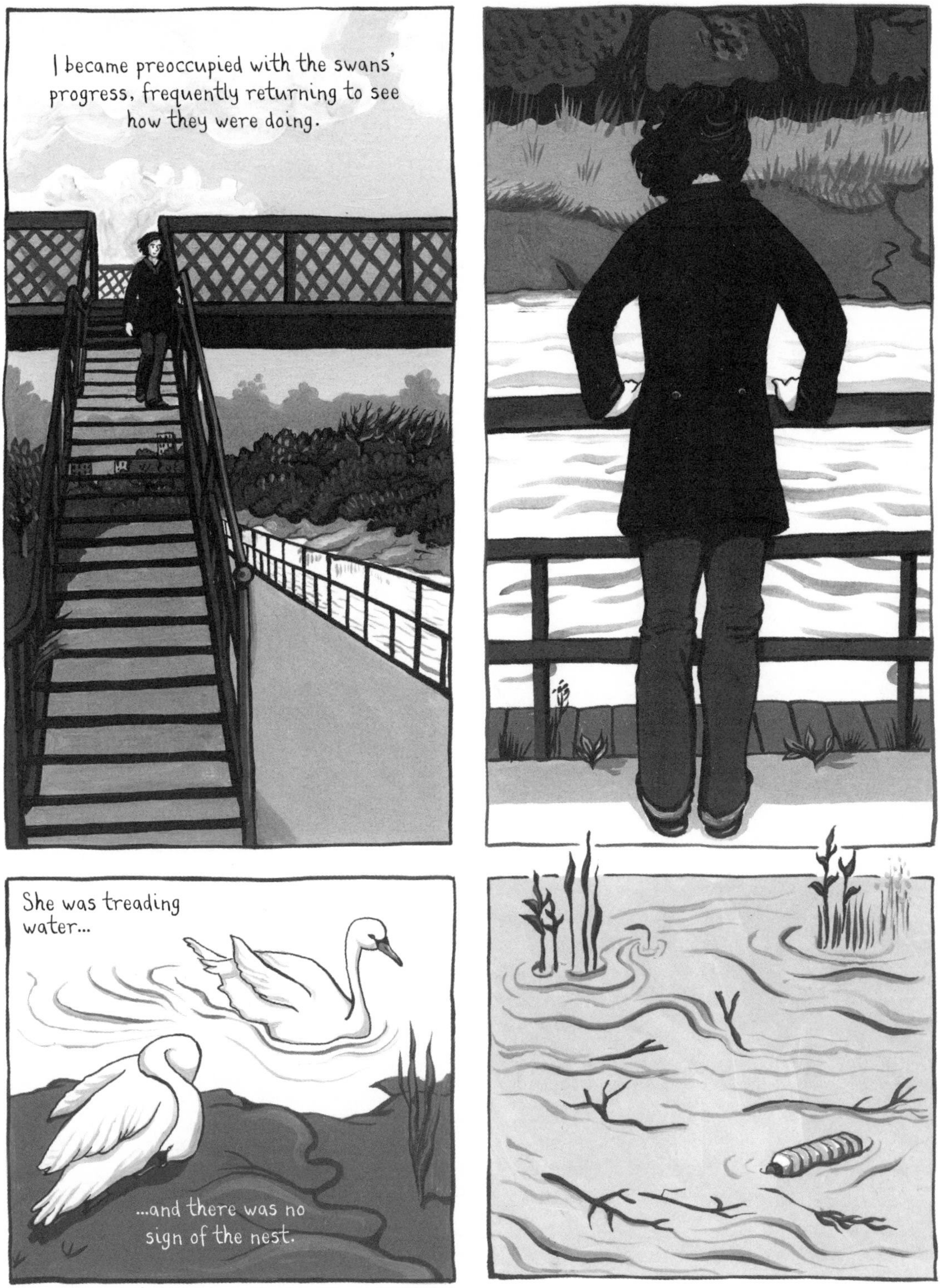
I became preoccupied with the swans' progress, frequently returning to see how they were doing.
She was treading water...
...and there was no sign of the nest.

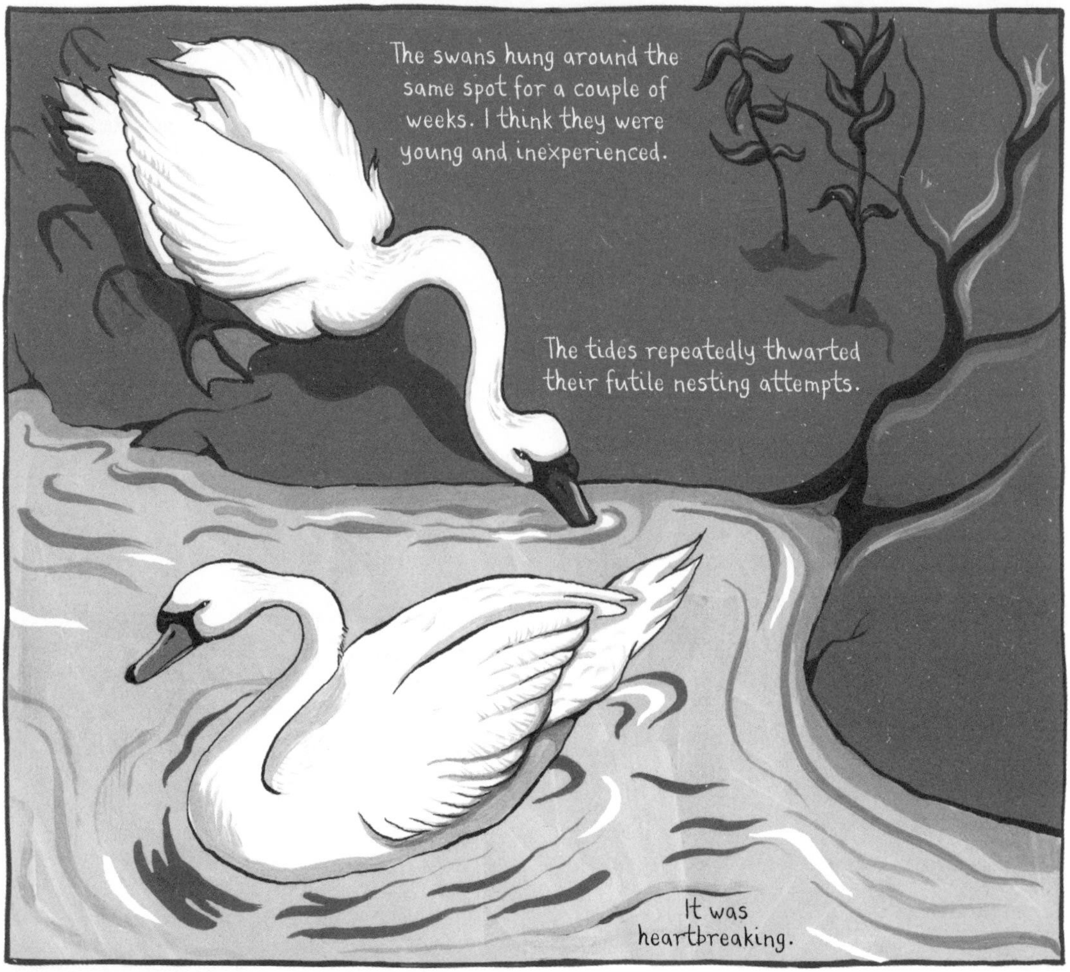
The swans hung around the same spot for a couple of weeks. I think they were young and inexperienced.
The tides repeatedly thwarted their futile nesting attempts.
It was heartbreaking.

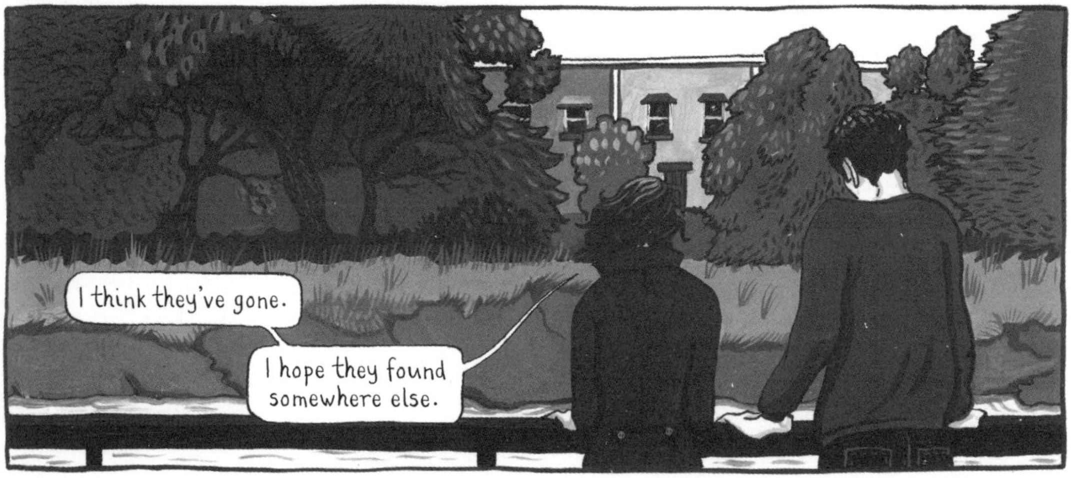
I think they've gone.
I hope they found somewhere else.

Later that year:

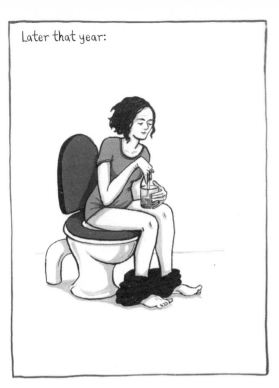

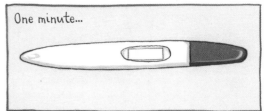

One minute...

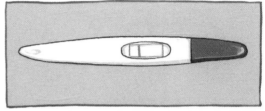

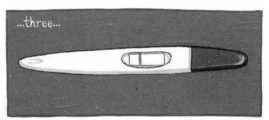

...three...

WHAT'S...

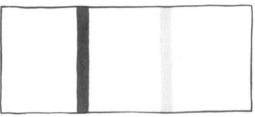

...THAT?

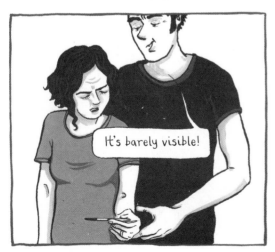

It's barely visible!

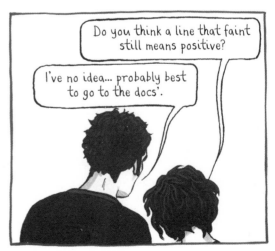

Do you think a line that faint still means positive?

I've no idea... probably best to go to the docs'.

All the signs seemed to be the same:

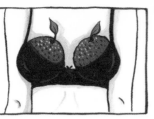

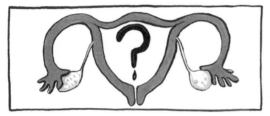

I was feeling tired, but also experiencing...

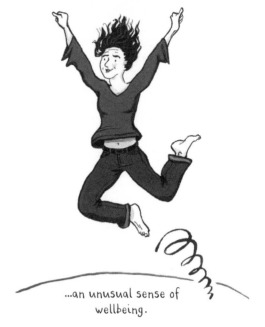

...an unusual sense of wellbeing.

The next day, me and the ever-so-faint line took ourselves...

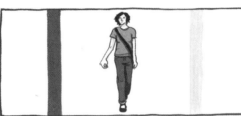

...to the doctors' to see what was occurring.

Polly Woods to room four please!

Hello!

What can I do for you today?

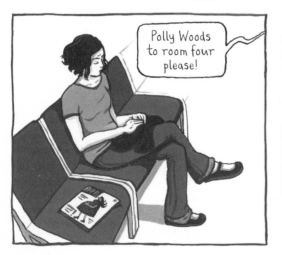

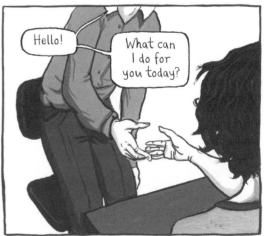

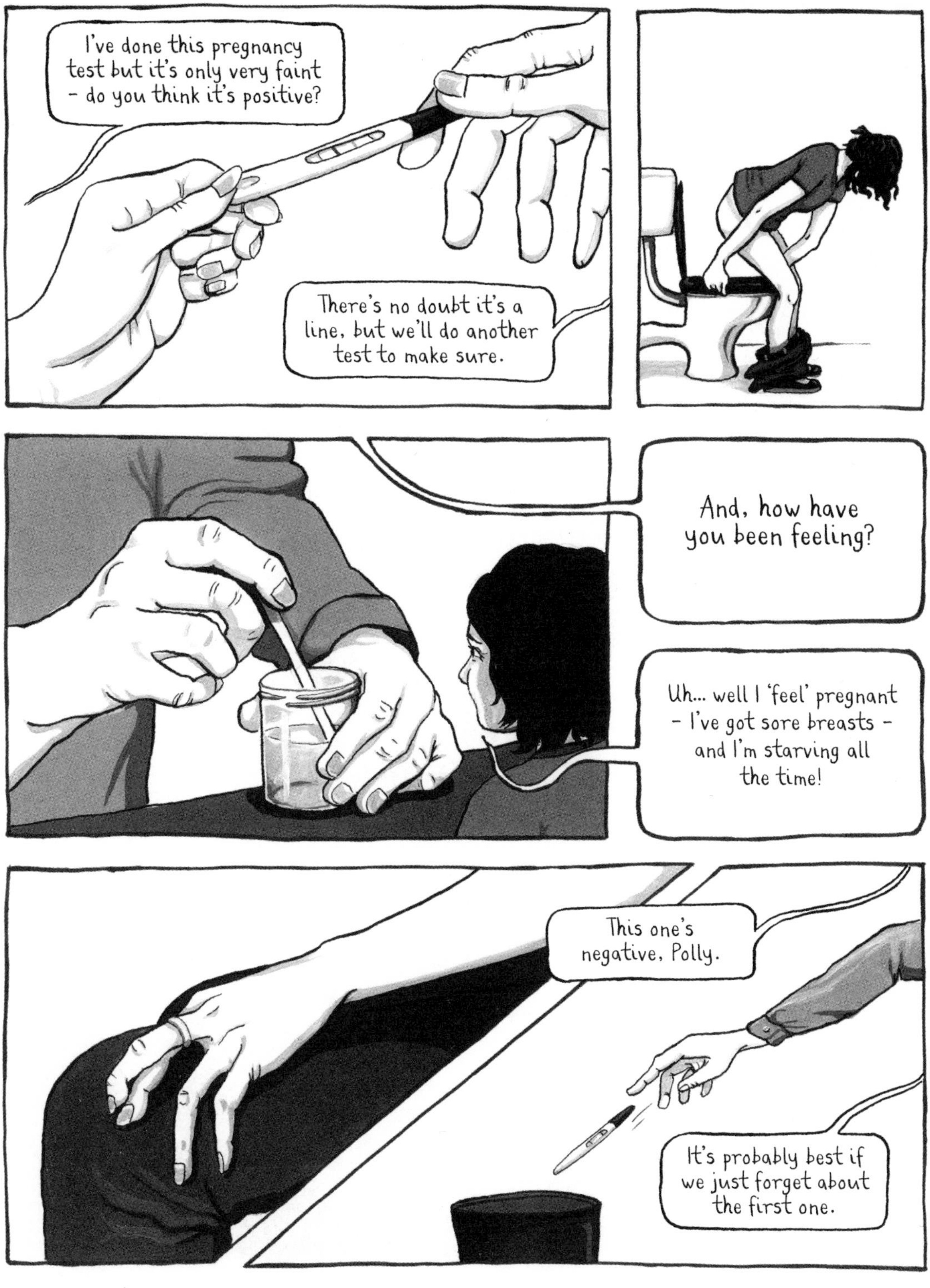
I've done this pregnancy test but it's only very faint - do you think it's positive?
There's no doubt it's a line, but we'll do another test to make sure.
And, how have you been feeling?
Uh... well I 'feel' pregnant - I've got sore breasts - and I'm starving all the time!
This one's negative, Polly.
It's probably best if we just forget about the first one.

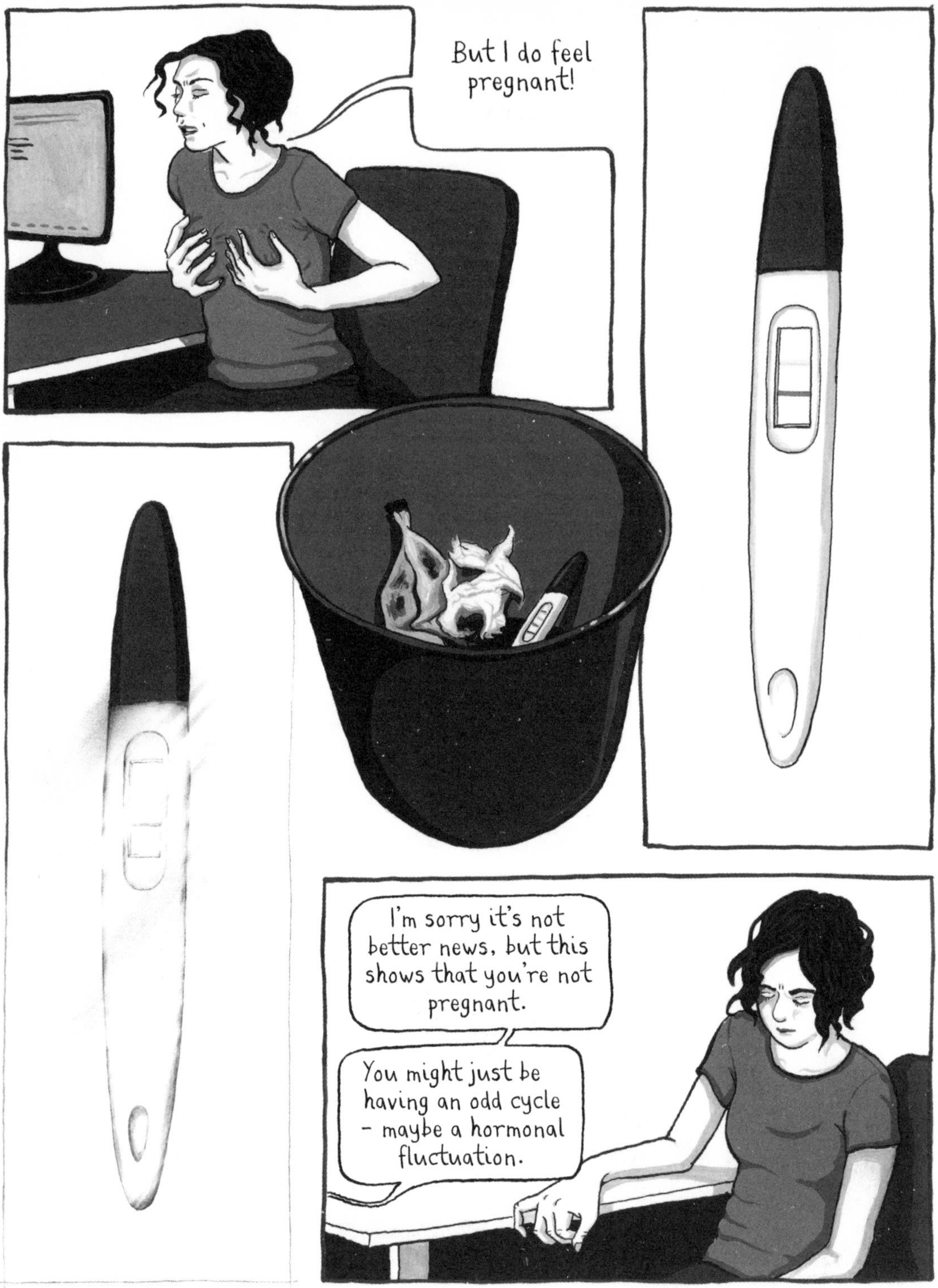
But I do feel pregnant!
I'm sorry it's not better news, but this shows that you're not pregnant.
You might just be having an odd cycle - maybe a hormonal fluctuation.

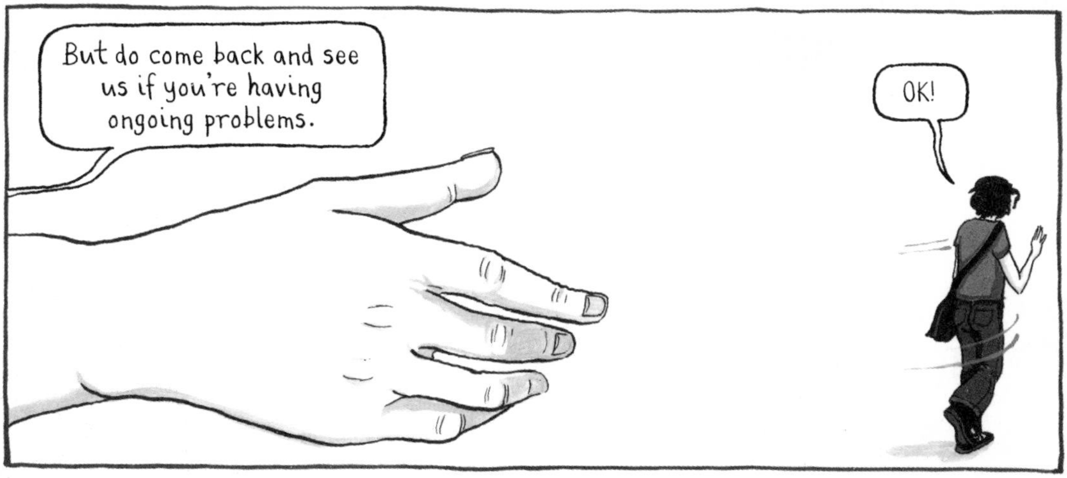
But do come back and see us if you're having ongoing problems.
OK!

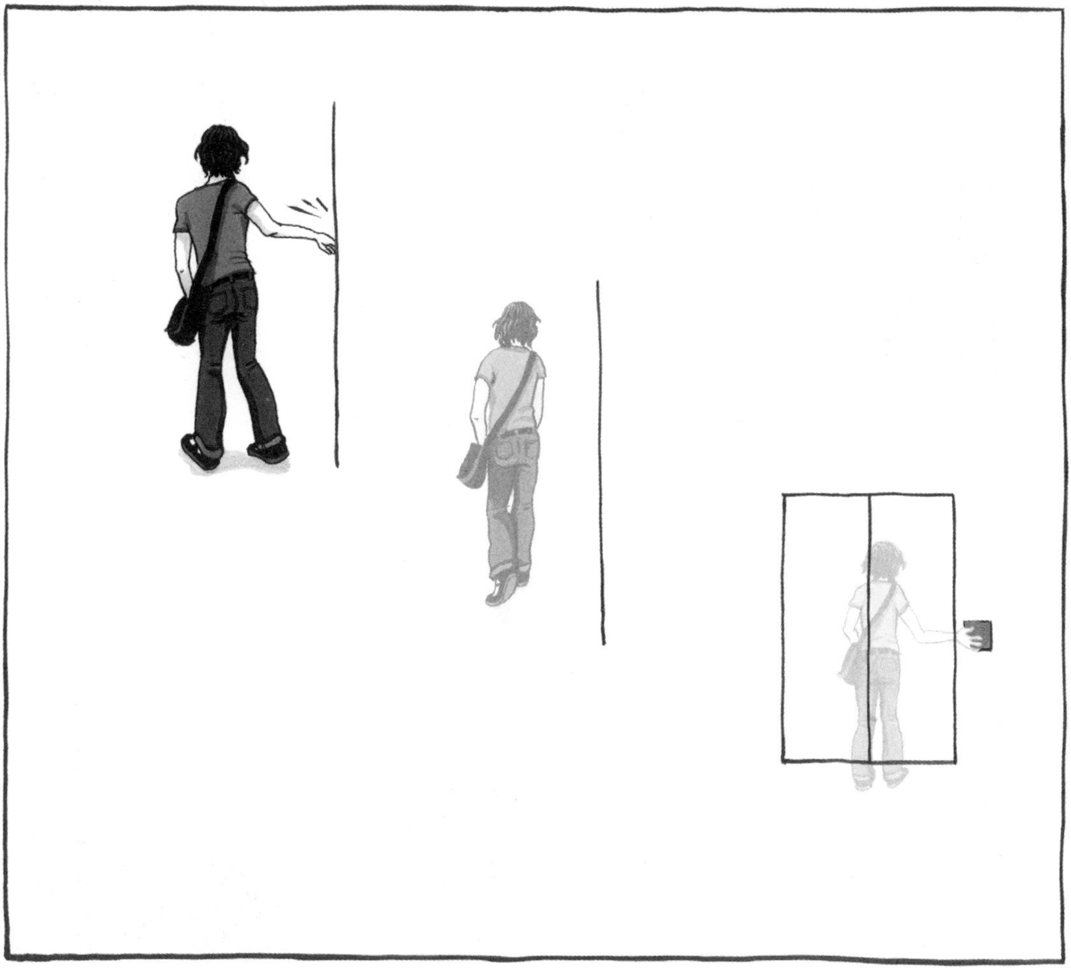

Within a week, we were at the top of Sheffield Pike overlooking Ullswater. We hadn't wanted to disappoint my parents by cancelling plans to meet up.

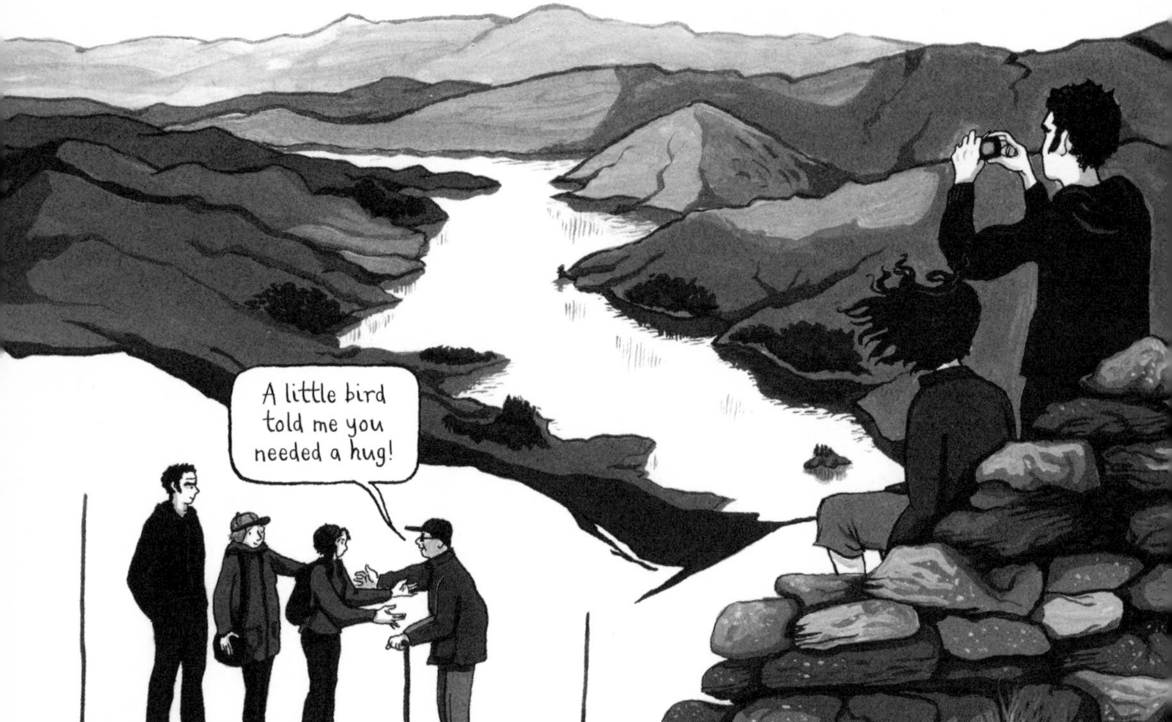
A little bird told me you needed a hug!

I bled for ten days – longer than any period I'd ever had. I had to have had three miscarriages before any tests could be carried out, and, due to the faint line, I felt that this bleeding was a very early miscarriage, or biochemical pregnancy.

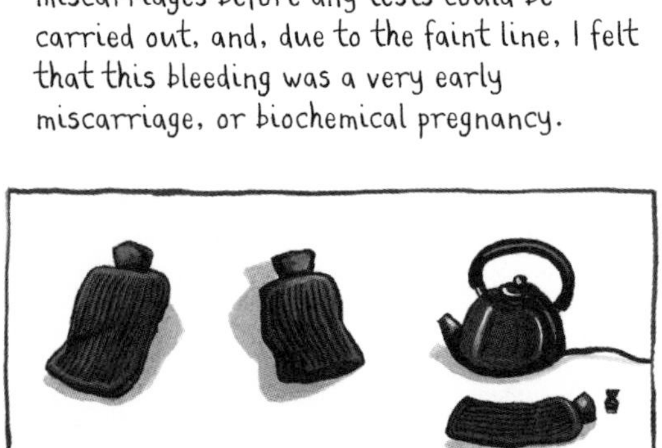

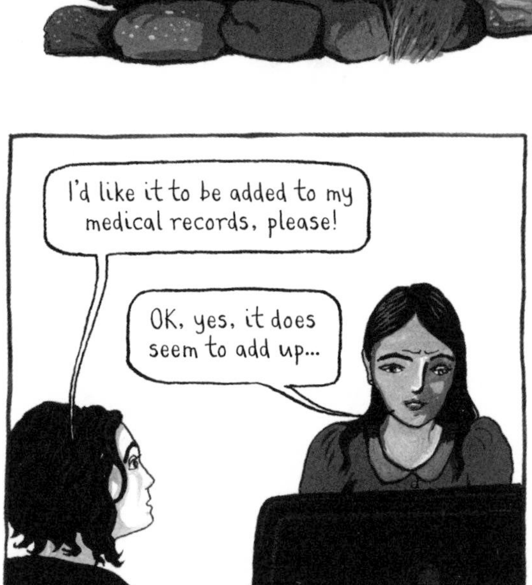
I'd like it to be added to my medical records, please!
OK, yes, it does seem to add up...

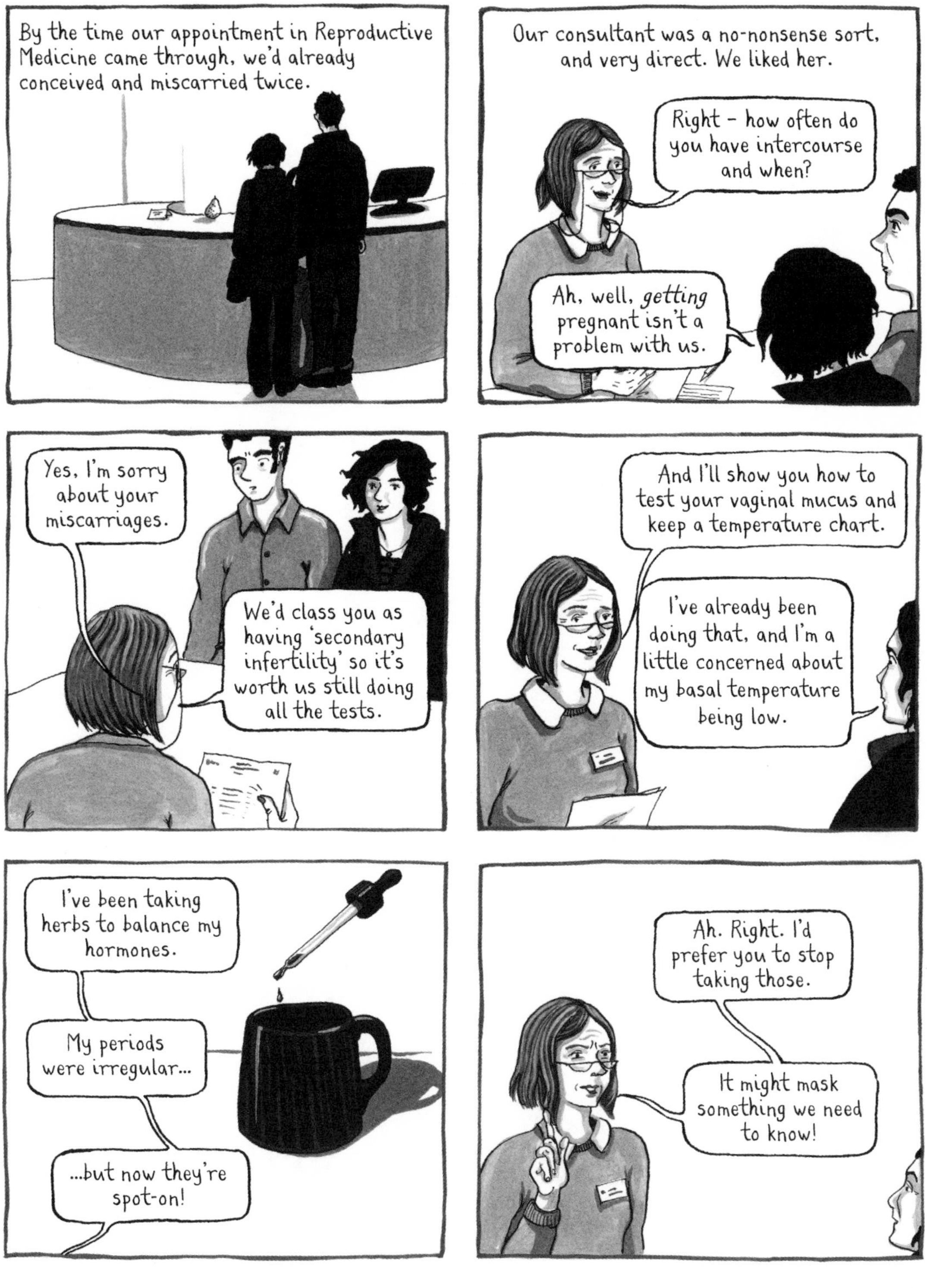
By the time our appointment in Reproductive Medicine came through, we'd already conceived and miscarried twice.
Our consultant was a no-nonsense sort, and very direct. We liked her.
Right – how often do you have intercourse and when?
Ah, well, *getting* pregnant isn't a problem with us.
Yes, I'm sorry about your miscarriages.
We'd class you as having 'secondary infertility' so it's worth us still doing all the tests.
And I'll show you how to test your vaginal mucus and keep a temperature chart.
I've already been doing that, and I'm a little concerned about my basal temperature being low.
I've been taking herbs to balance my hormones.
My periods were irregular...
...but now they're spot-on!
Ah. Right. I'd prefer you to stop taking those.
It might mask something we need to know!

My tests involved repeated trips to St Michael's Hospital over three months.

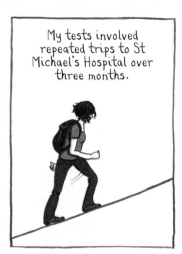

The hospital is located at the top of one of Bristol's steepest hills (depending on one's direction of travel).

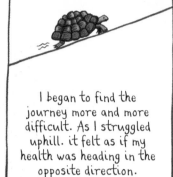

I began to find the journey more and more difficult. As I struggled uphill, it felt as if my health was heading in the opposite direction.

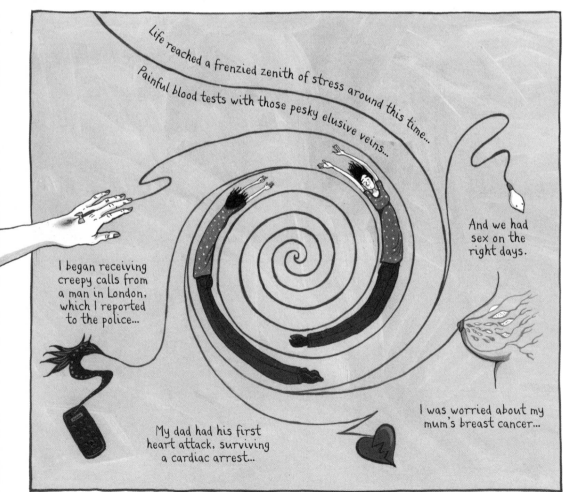

Life reached a frenzied zenith of stress around this time...

Painful blood tests with those pesky elusive veins...

I began receiving creepy calls from a man in London, which I reported to the police...

My dad had his first heart attack, surviving a cardiac arrest...

And we had sex on the right days.

I was worried about my mum's breast cancer...

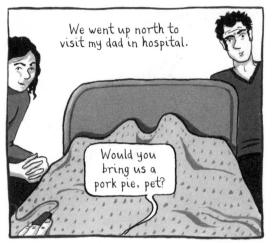

We went up north to visit my dad in hospital.

Would you bring us a pork pie, pet?

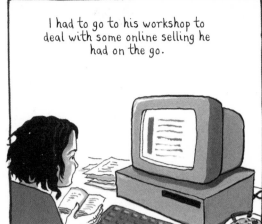

I had to go to his workshop to deal with some online selling he had on the go.

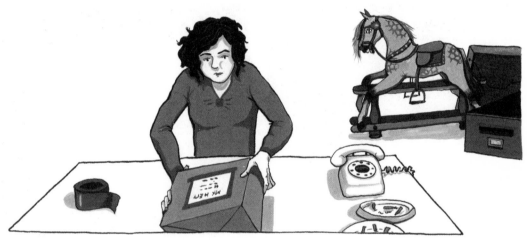

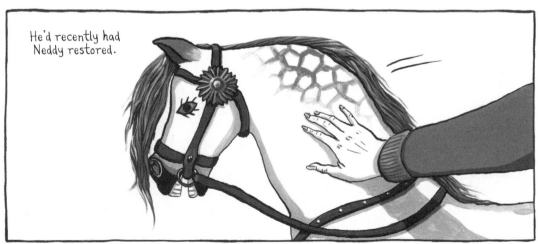

He'd recently had Neddy restored.

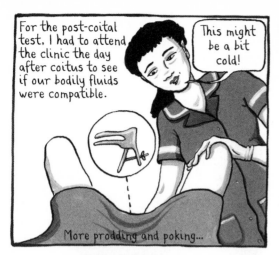

For the post-coital test, I had to attend the clinic the day after coitus to see if our bodily fluids were compatible.

This might be a bit cold!

More prodding and poking...

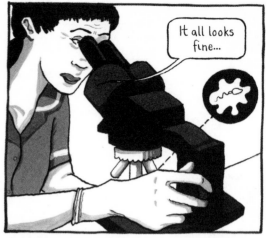

It all looks fine...

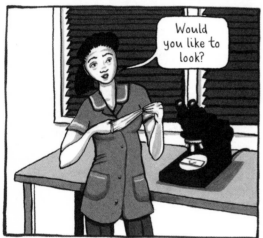

Would you like to look?

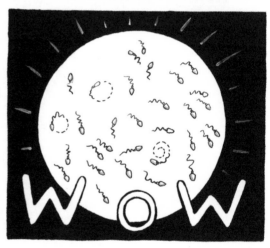

W O W

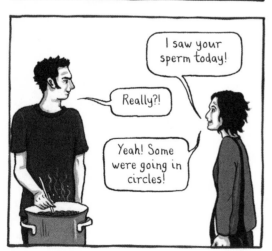

I saw your sperm today!

Really?!

Yeah! Some were going in circles!

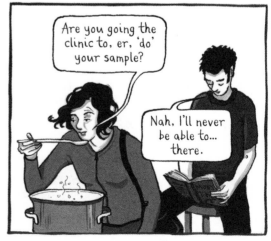

Are you going the clinic to, er, 'do' your sample?

Nah, I'll never be able to... there.

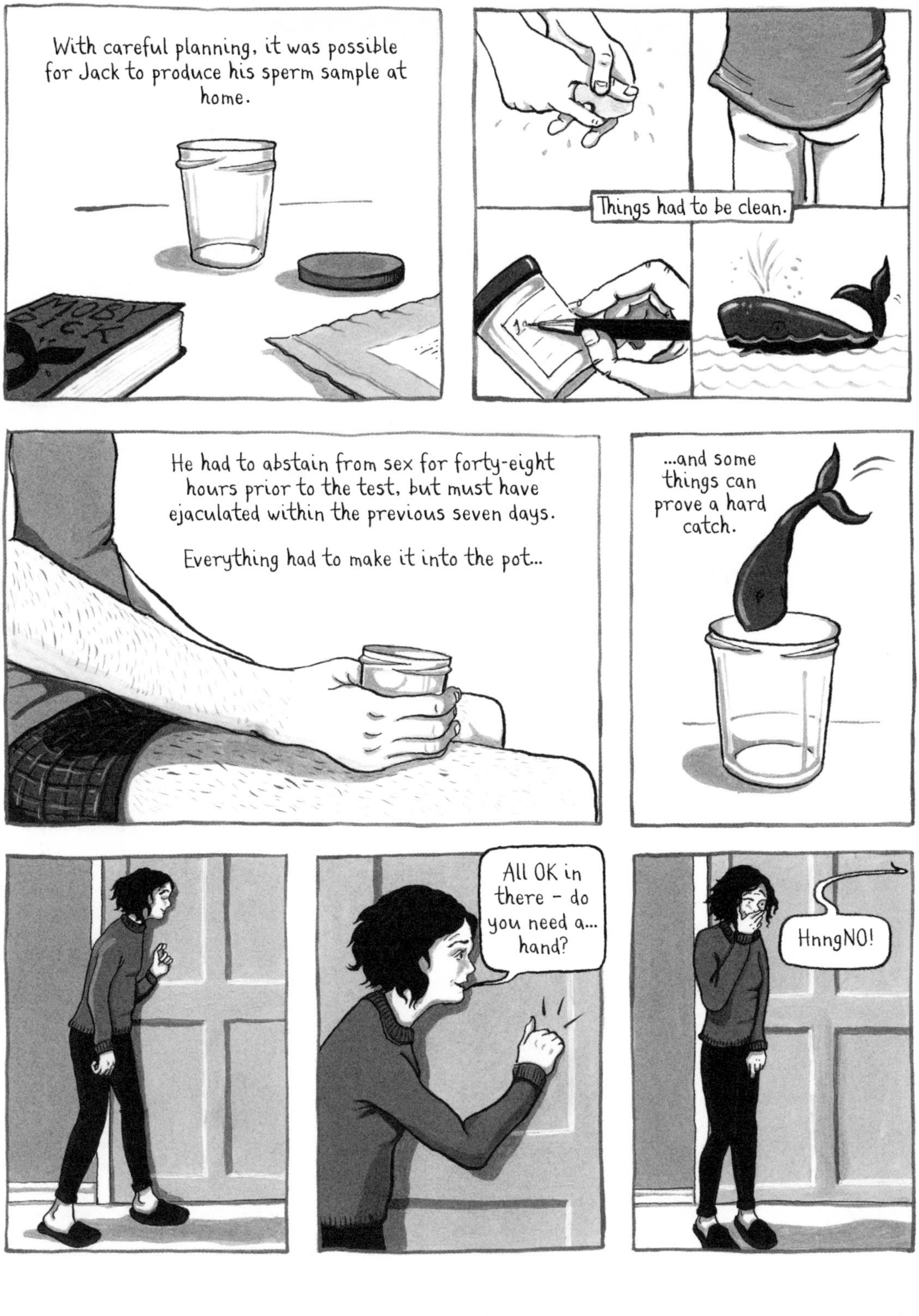
With careful planning, it was possible for Jack to produce his sperm sample at home.
MOBY DICK
Things had to be clean.
He had to abstain from sex for forty-eight hours prior to the test, but must have ejaculated within the previous seven days.
Everything had to make it into the pot...
...and some things can prove a hard catch.
All OK in there - do you need a... hand?
HnngNO!

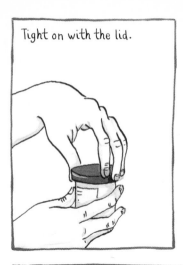

Tight on with the lid.

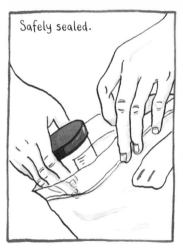

Safely sealed.

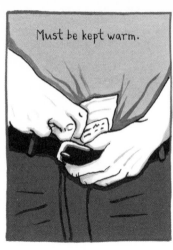

Must be kept warm.

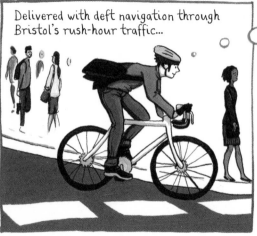

Delivered with deft navigation through Bristol's rush-hour traffic...

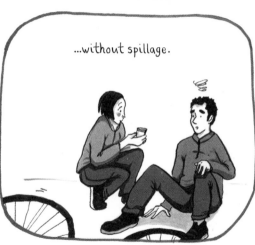

...without spillage.

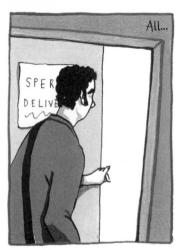

All...

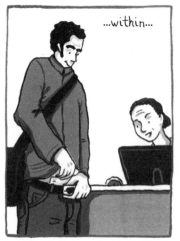

...within...

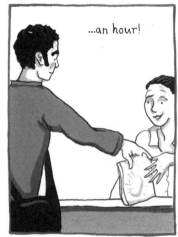

...an hour!

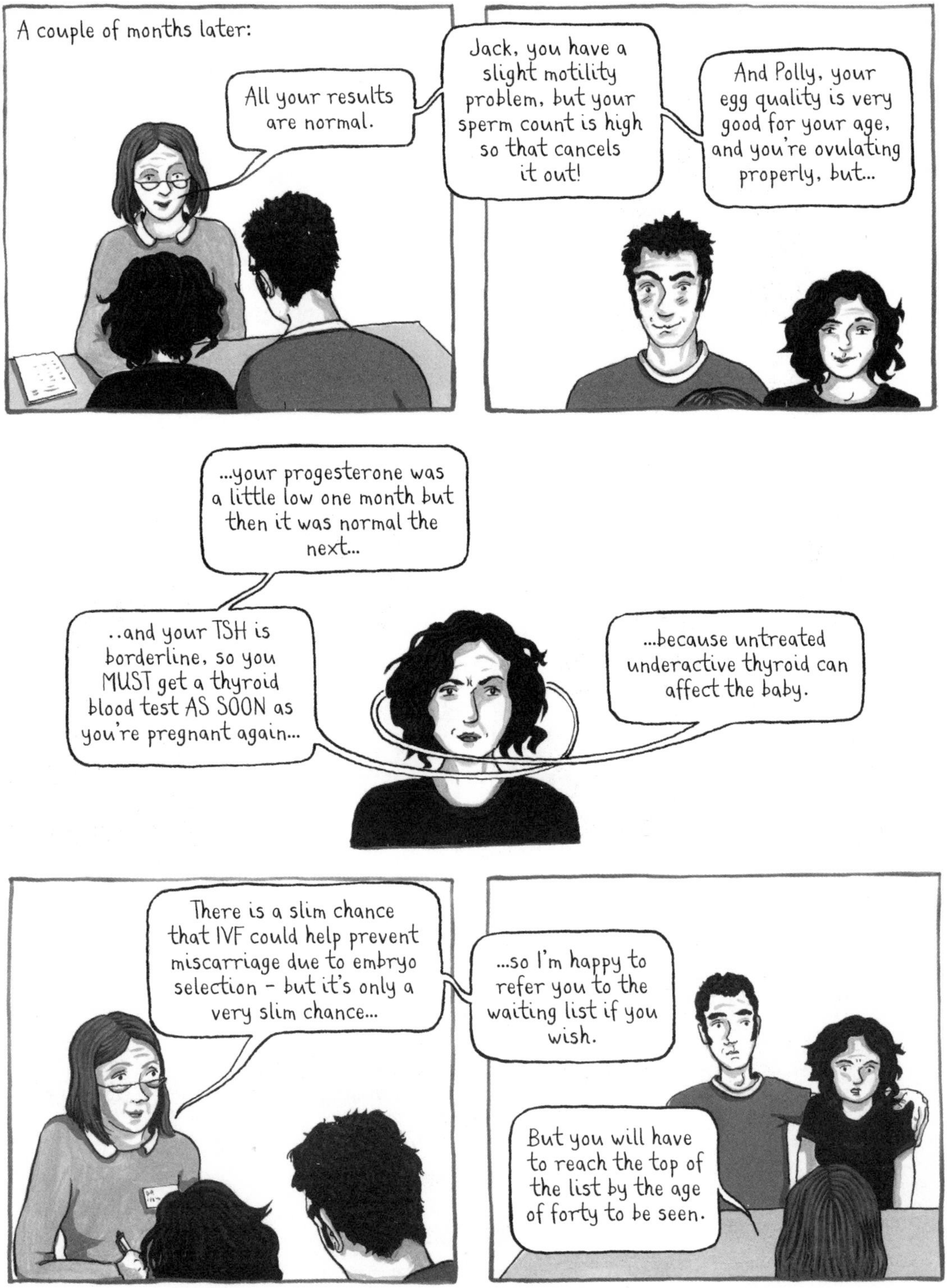
A couple of months later:
All your results are normal.
Jack, you have a slight motility problem, but your sperm count is high so that cancels it out!
And Polly, your egg quality is very good for your age, and you're ovulating properly, but...
...your progesterone was a little low one month but then it was normal the next...
..and your TSH is borderline, so you MUST get a thyroid blood test AS SOON as you're pregnant again...
...because untreated underactive thyroid can affect the baby.
There is a slim chance that IVF could help prevent miscarriage due to embryo selection - but it's only a very slim chance...
...so I'm happy to refer you to the waiting list if you wish.
But you will have to reach the top of the list by the age of forty to be seen.

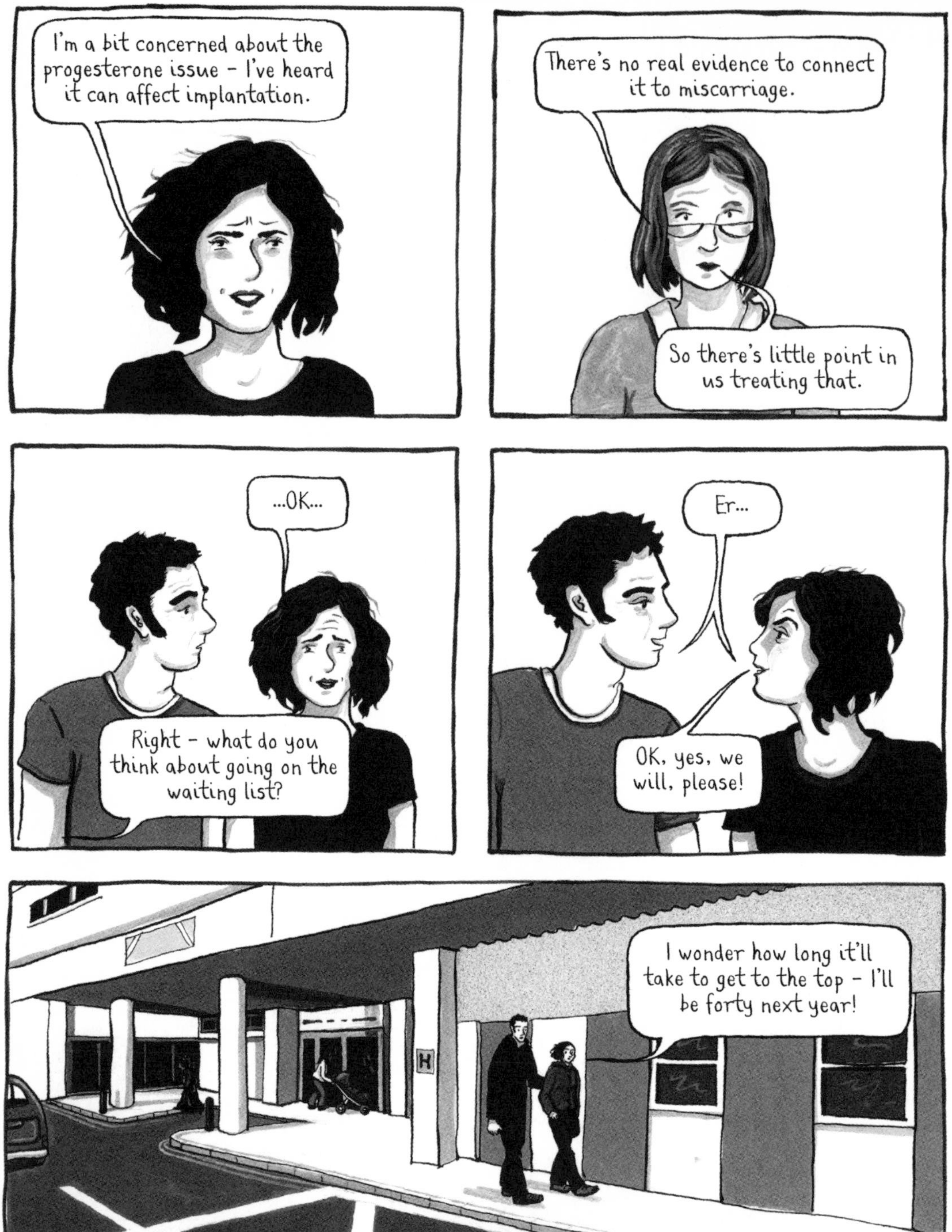
I'm a bit concerned about the progesterone issue - I've heard it can affect implantation.
There's no real evidence to connect it to miscarriage.
So there's little point in us treating that.
...OK...
Right - what do you think about going on the waiting list?
Er...
OK, yes, we will, please!
I wonder how long it'll take to get to the top - I'll be forty next year!

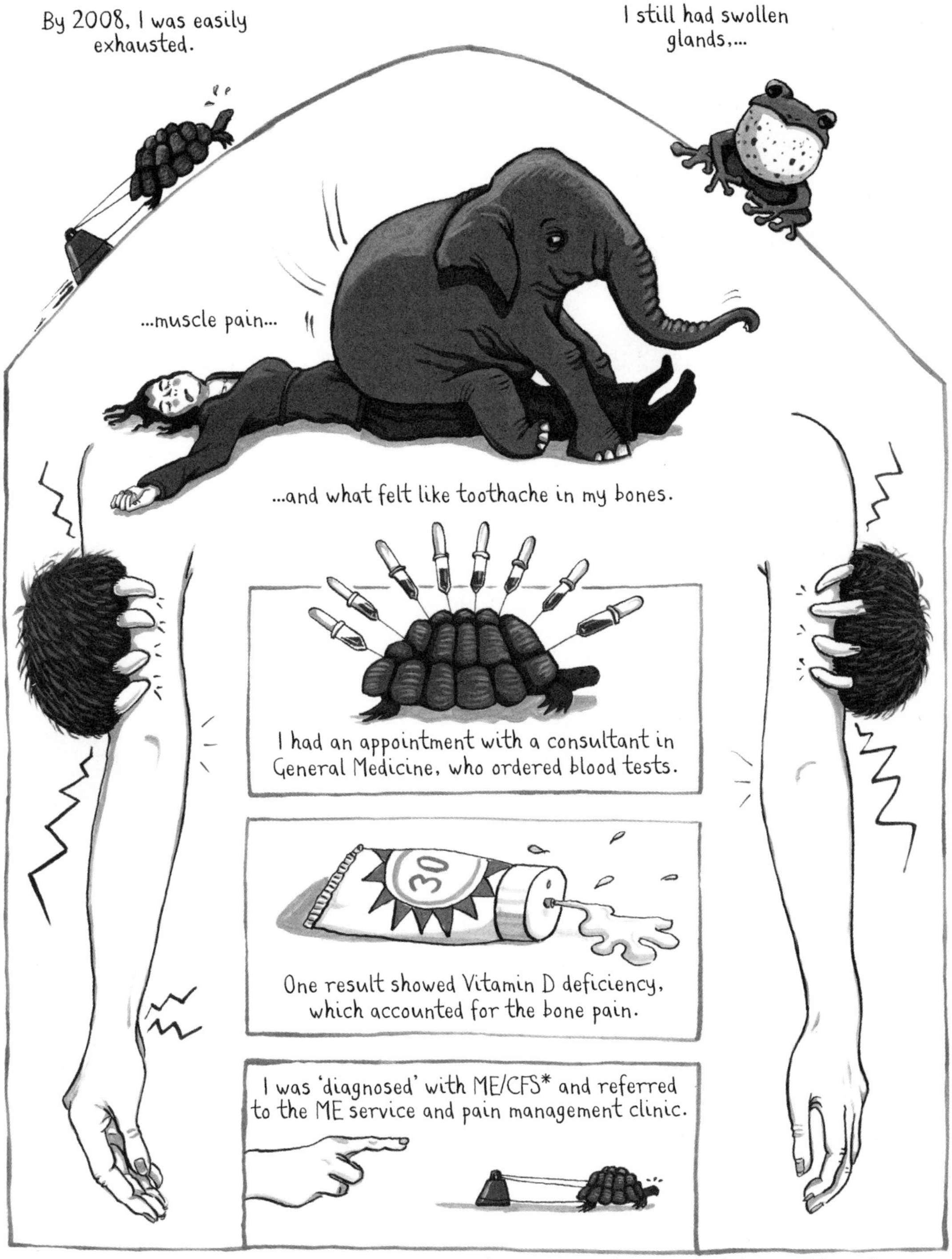

By 2008, I was easily exhausted.
I still had swollen glands,...
...muscle pain...
...and what felt like toothache in my bones.
I had an appointment with a consultant in General Medicine, who ordered blood tests.
30
One result showed Vitamin D deficiency, which accounted for the bone pain.
I was 'diagnosed' with ME/CFS* and referred to the ME service and pain management clinic.

* Myalgic Encephalomyelitis/ Chronic Fatigue Syndrome

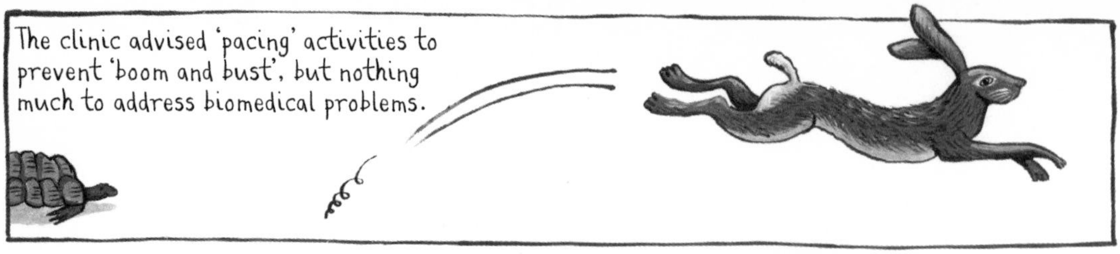
The clinic advised 'pacing' activities to prevent 'boom and bust', but nothing much to address biomedical problems.

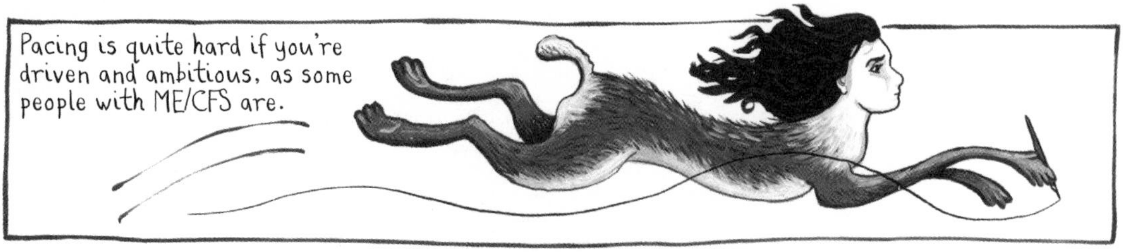
Pacing is quite hard if you're driven and ambitious, as some people with ME/CFS are.

Some ME sufferers refer to relapses as being in 'The Pit'. But they are the ones, like me, who are lucky enough to have some energy, and not be house- or bed-bound.

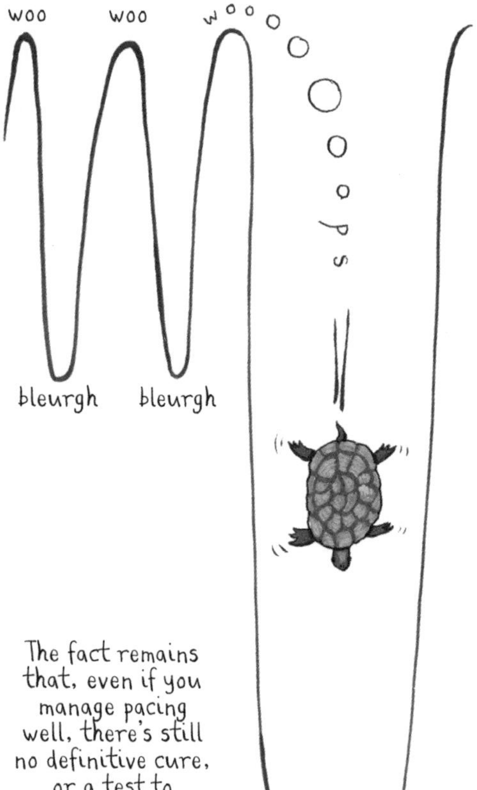
woo
woo
woooooooops
bleurgh
bleurgh
The fact remains that, even if you manage pacing well, there's still no definitive cure, or a test to diagnose ME.

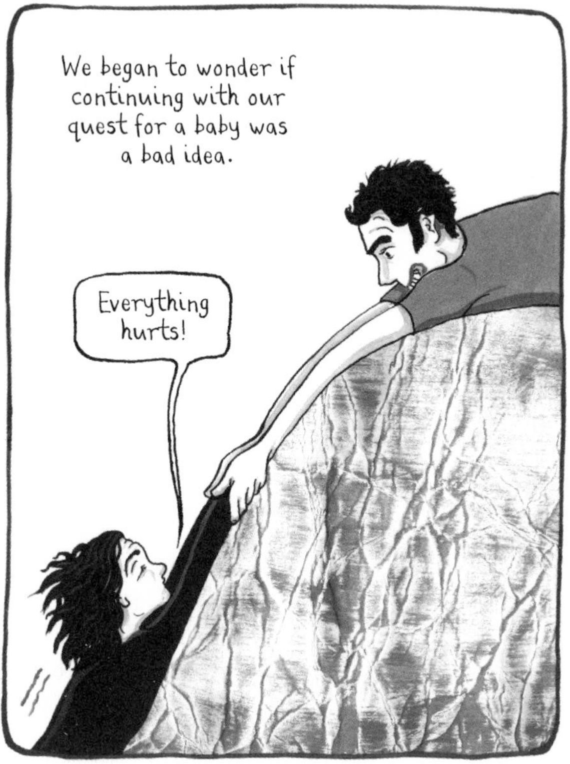
We began to wonder if continuing with our quest for a baby was a bad idea.
Everything hurts!

At certain times of the month, I became obsessed with checking my breasts for signs. June 2008 showed some promise.

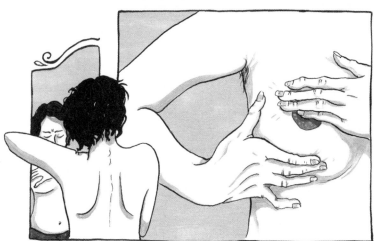

The first test was negative.

But the next day...

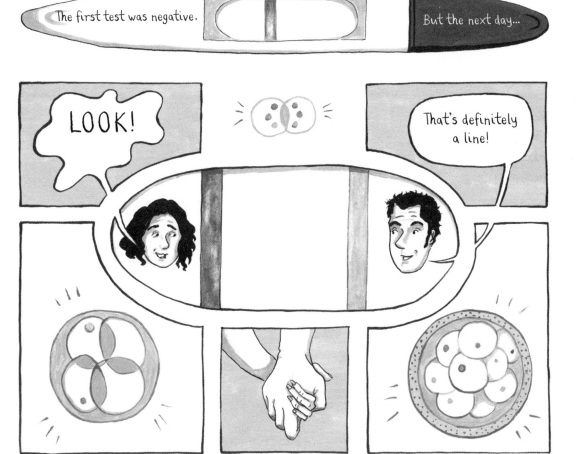

LOOK!

That's definitely a line!

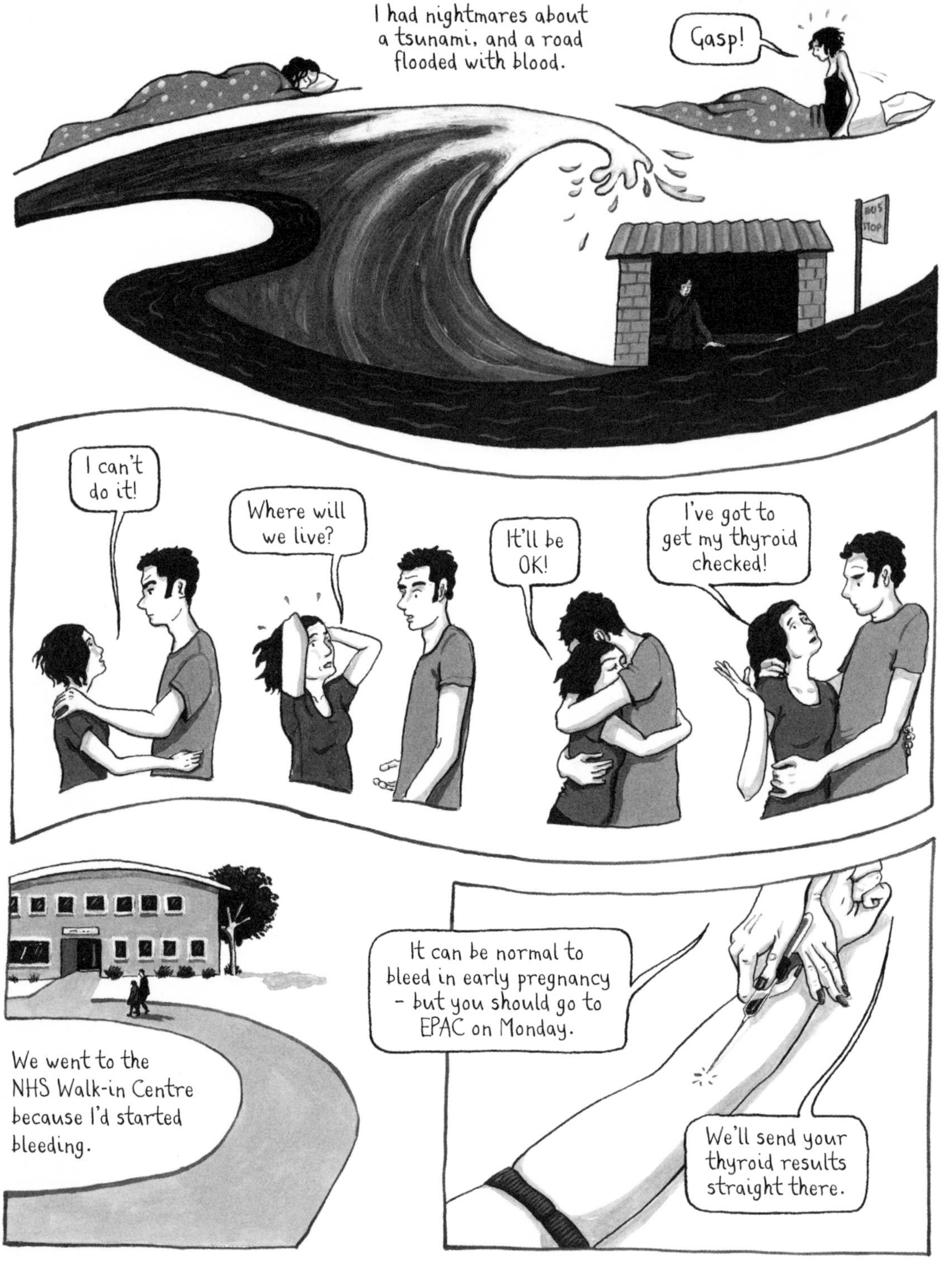
I had nightmares about a tsunami, and a road flooded with blood.
Gasp!
BUS STOP
I can't do it!
Where will we live?
It'll be OK!
I've got to get my thyroid checked!
We went to the NHS Walk-in Centre because I'd started bleeding.
It can be normal to bleed in early pregnancy - but you should go to EPAC on Monday.
We'll send your thyroid results straight there.

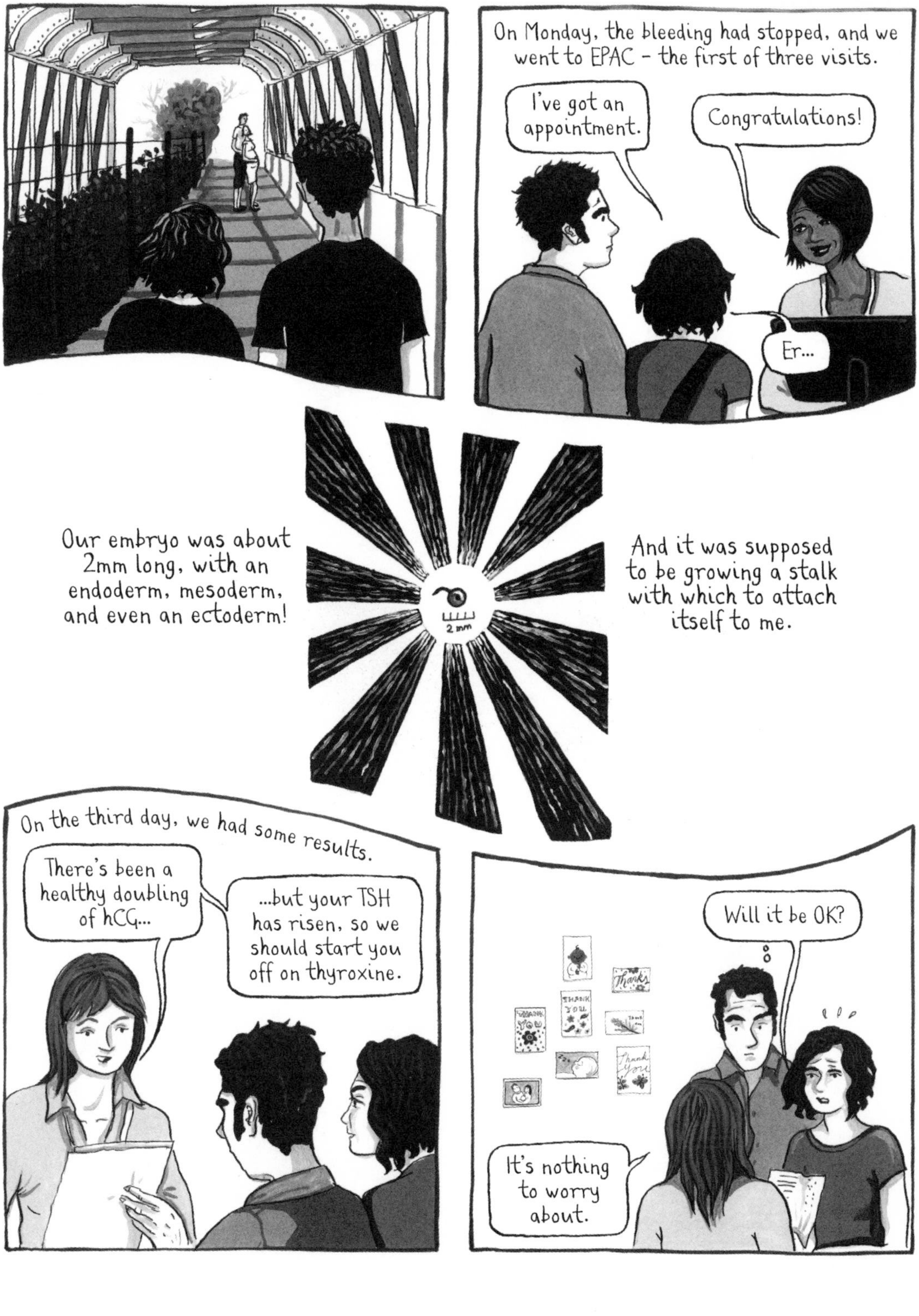
On Monday, the bleeding had stopped, and we went to EPAC – the first of three visits.
I've got an appointment.
Congratulations!
Er...
Our embryo was about 2mm long, with an endoderm, mesoderm, and even an ectoderm!
2 mm
And it was supposed to be growing a stalk with which to attach itself to me.
On the third day, we had some results.
There's been a healthy doubling of hCG...
...but your TSH has risen, so we should start you off on thyroxine.
Will it be OK?
It's nothing to worry about.

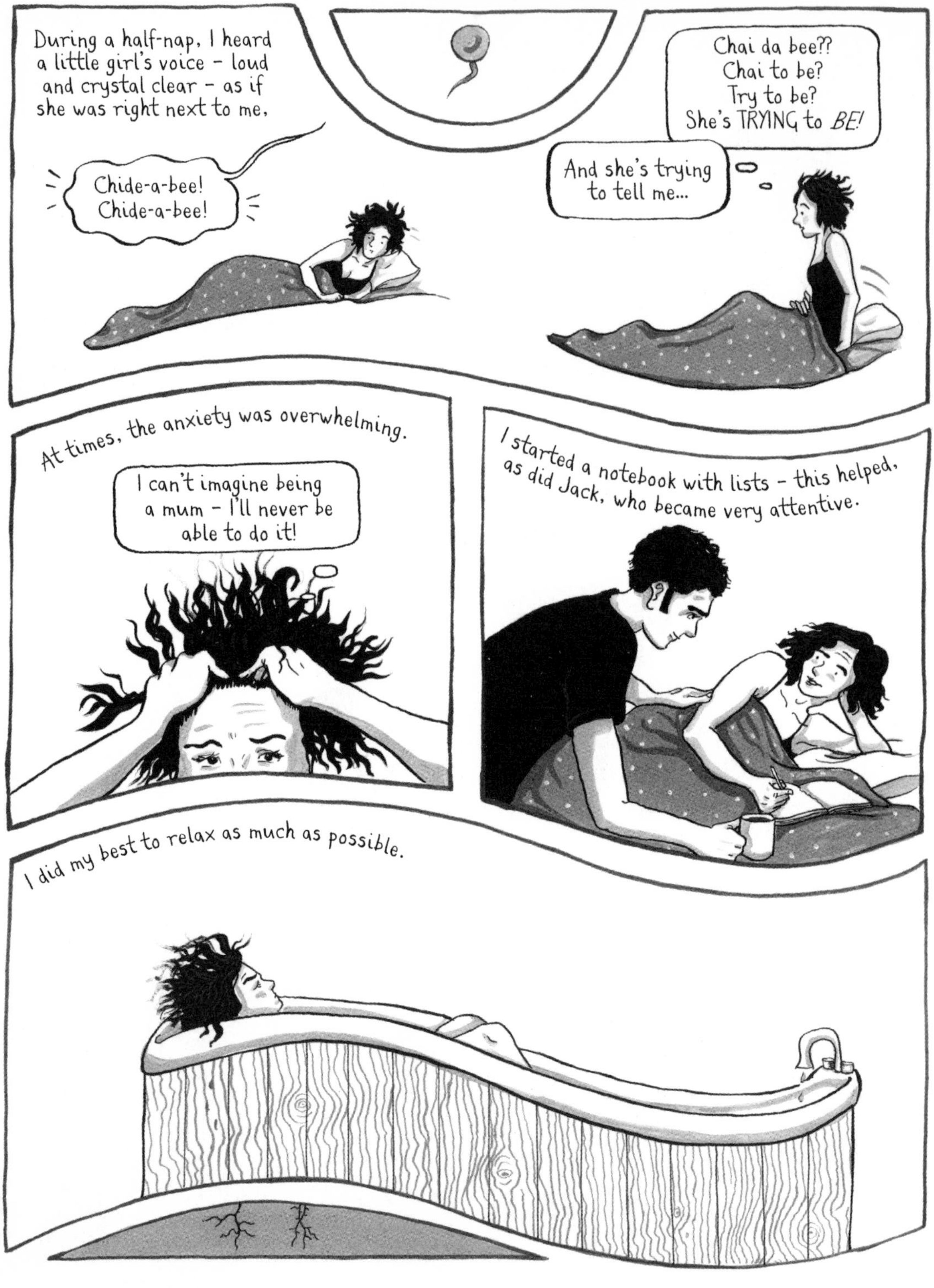

During a half-nap, I heard a little girl's voice - loud and crystal clear - as if she was right next to me,
Chide-a-bee! Chide-a-bee!
Chai da bee?? Chai to be? Try to be? She's TRYING to BE!
And she's trying to tell me...
At times, the anxiety was overwhelming.
I can't imagine being a mum - I'll never be able to do it!
I started a notebook with lists - this helped, as did Jack, who became very attentive.
I did my best to relax as much as possible.

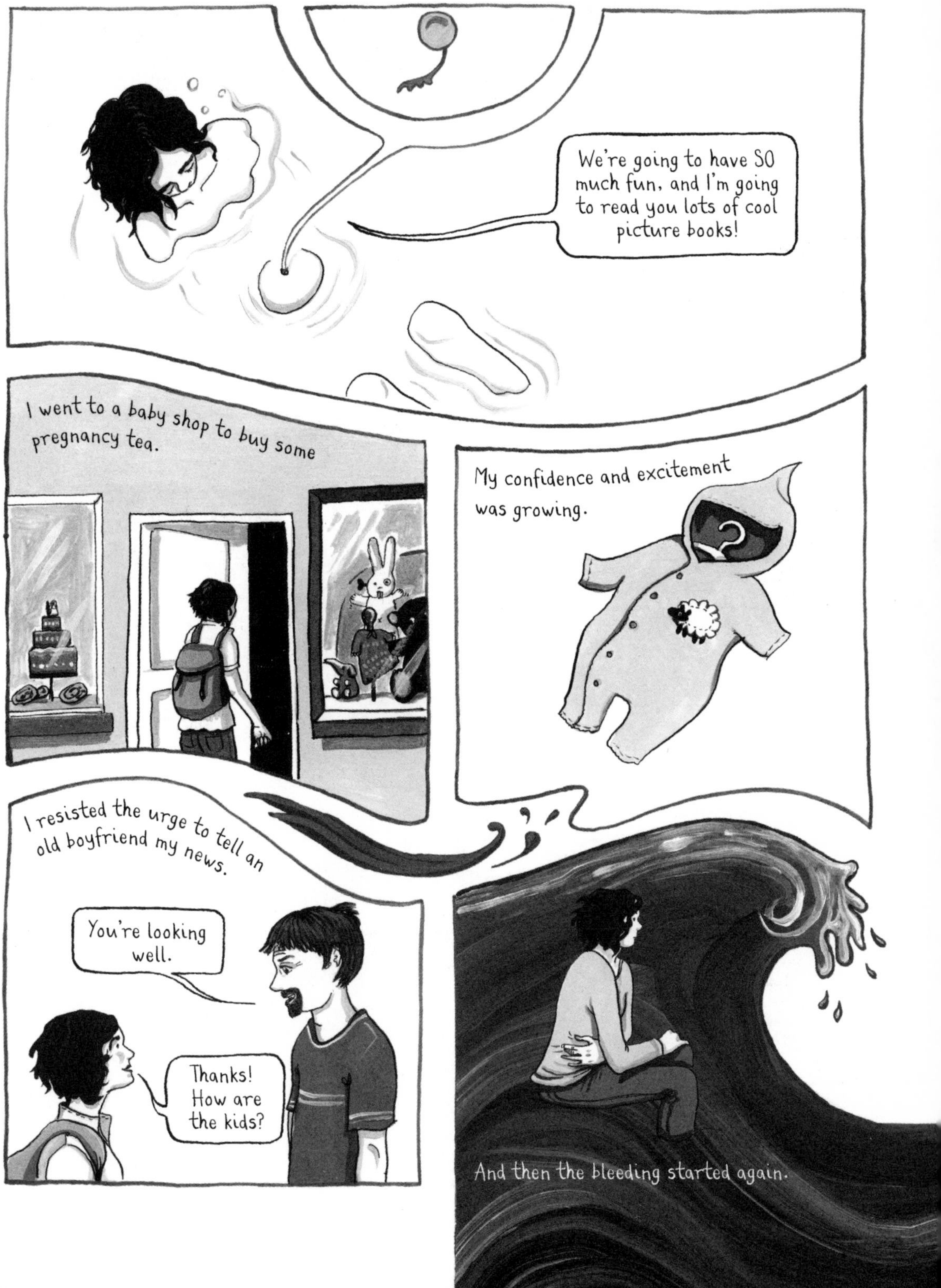
We're going to have SO much fun, and I'm going to read you lots of cool picture books!
I went to a baby shop to buy some pregnancy tea.
My confidence and excitement was growing.
I resisted the urge to tell an old boyfriend my news.
You're looking well.
Thanks! How are the kids?
And then the bleeding started again.

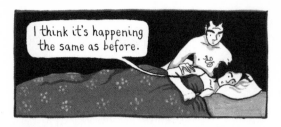

I think it's happening the same as before.

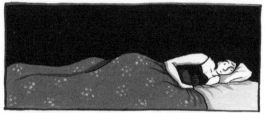

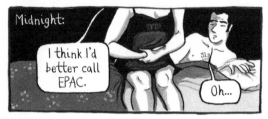

Midnight:

I think I'd better call EPAC.

Oh...

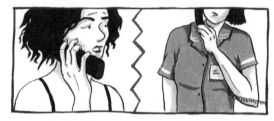

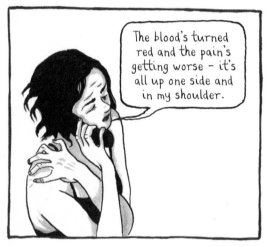

The blood's turned red and the pain's getting worse – it's all up one side and in my shoulder.

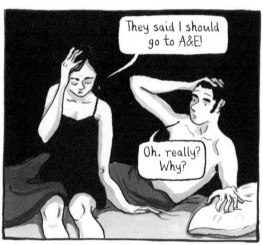

They said I should go to A&E!

Oh, really? Why?

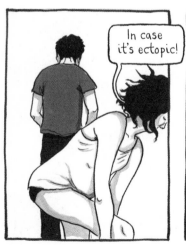

In case it's ectopic!

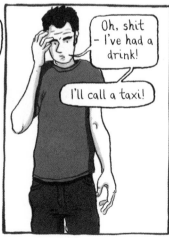

Oh, shit – I've had a drink!

I'll call a taxi!

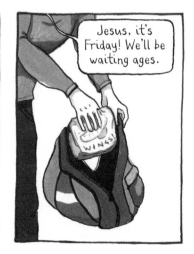

Jesus, it's Friday! We'll be waiting ages.

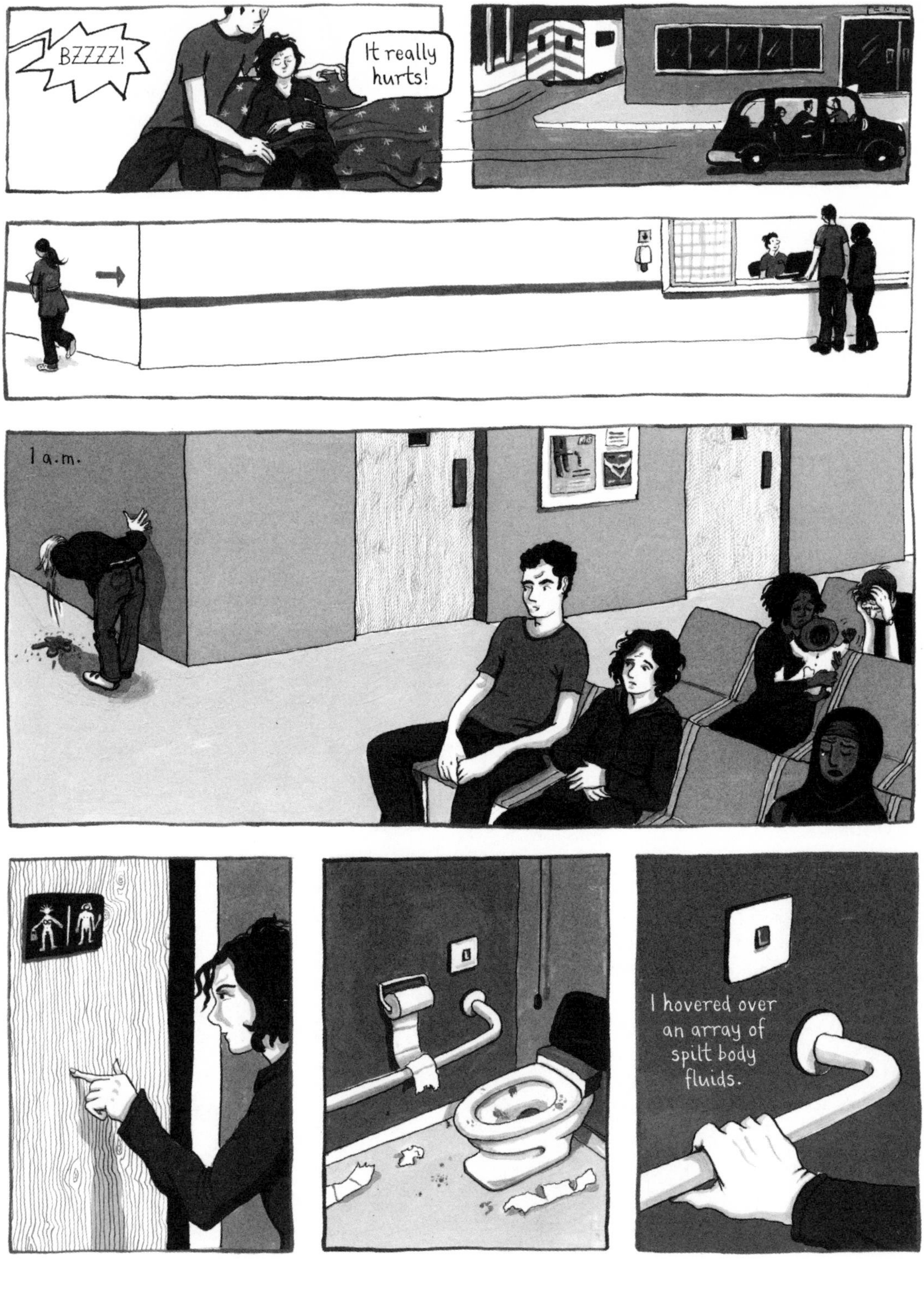
BZZZZ!
It really hurts!
1 a.m.
I hovered over an array of spilt body fluids.

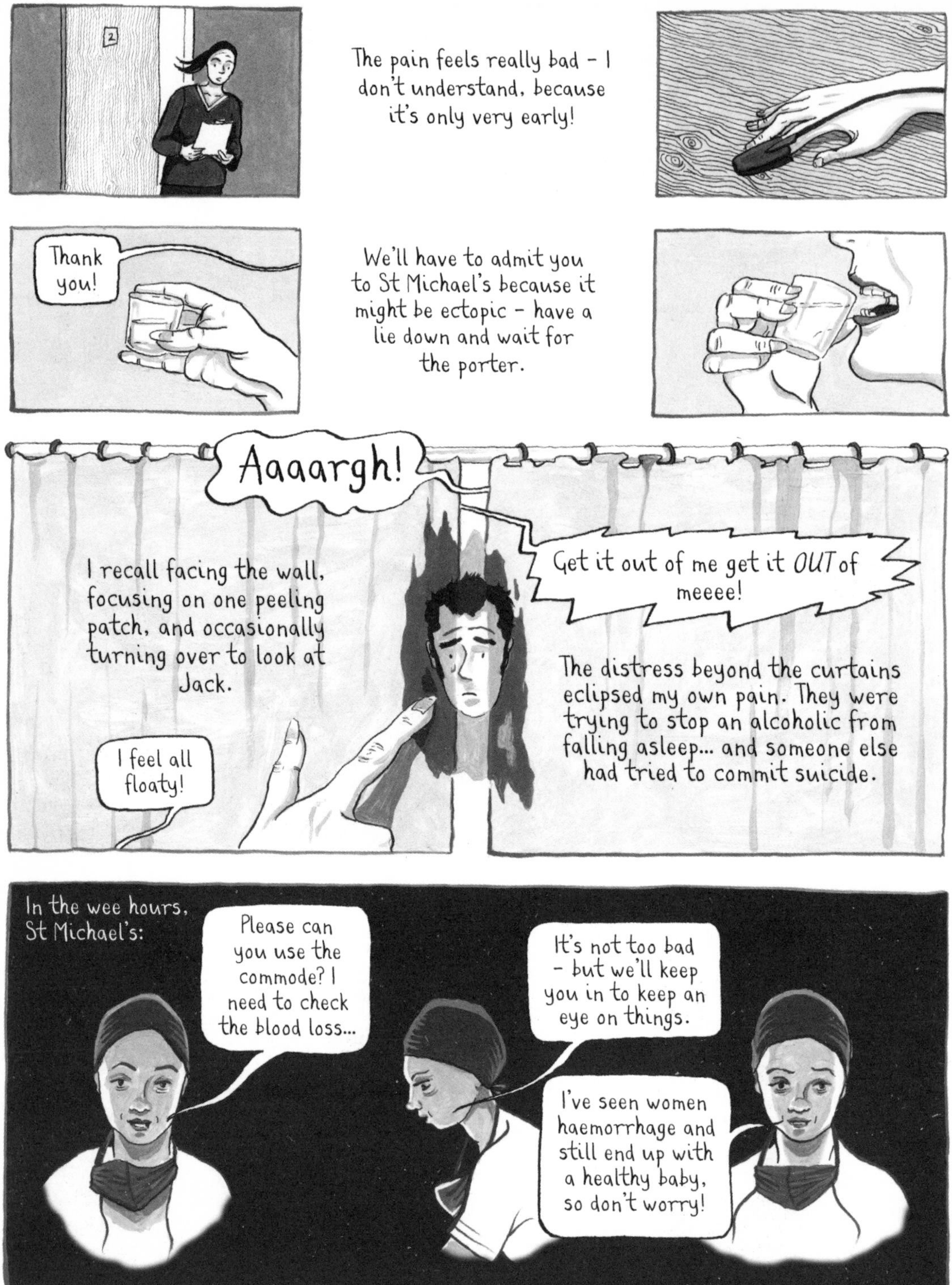

The pain feels really bad - I don't understand, because it's only very early!
Thank you!
We'll have to admit you to St Michael's because it might be ectopic - have a lie down and wait for the porter.
Aaaargh!
I recall facing the wall, focusing on one peeling patch, and occasionally turning over to look at Jack.
Get it out of me get it OUT of meeee!
The distress beyond the curtains eclipsed my own pain. They were trying to stop an alcoholic from falling asleep... and someone else had tried to commit suicide.
I feel all floaty!
In the wee hours, St Michael's:
Please can you use the commode? I need to check the blood loss...
It's not too bad - but we'll keep you in to keep an eye on things.
I've seen women haemorrhage and still end up with a healthy baby, so don't worry!

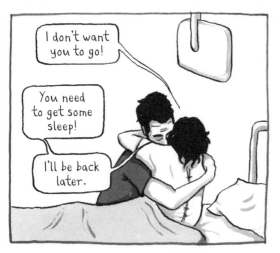

I don't want you to go!

You need to get some sleep!

I'll be back later.

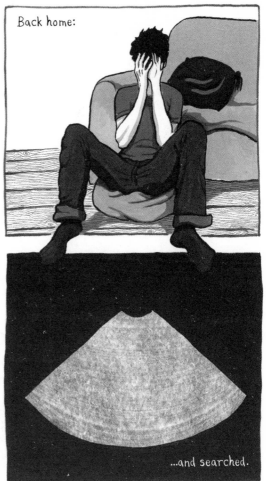

Back home:

The next day, the radiographer searched...

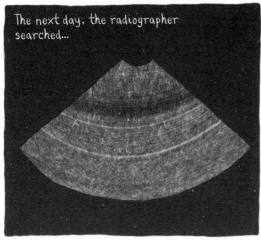

...and searched.

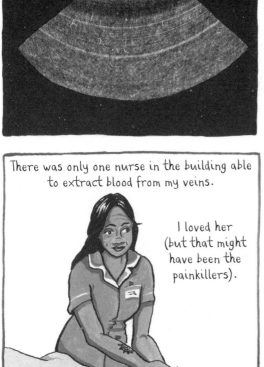

There was only one nurse in the building able to extract blood from my veins.

I loved her (but that might have been the painkillers).

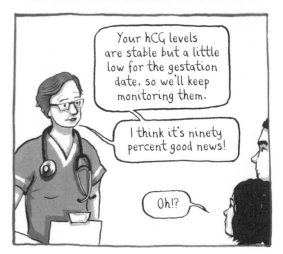

Your hCG levels are stable but a little low for the gestation date, so we'll keep monitoring them.

I think it's ninety percent good news!

Oh!?

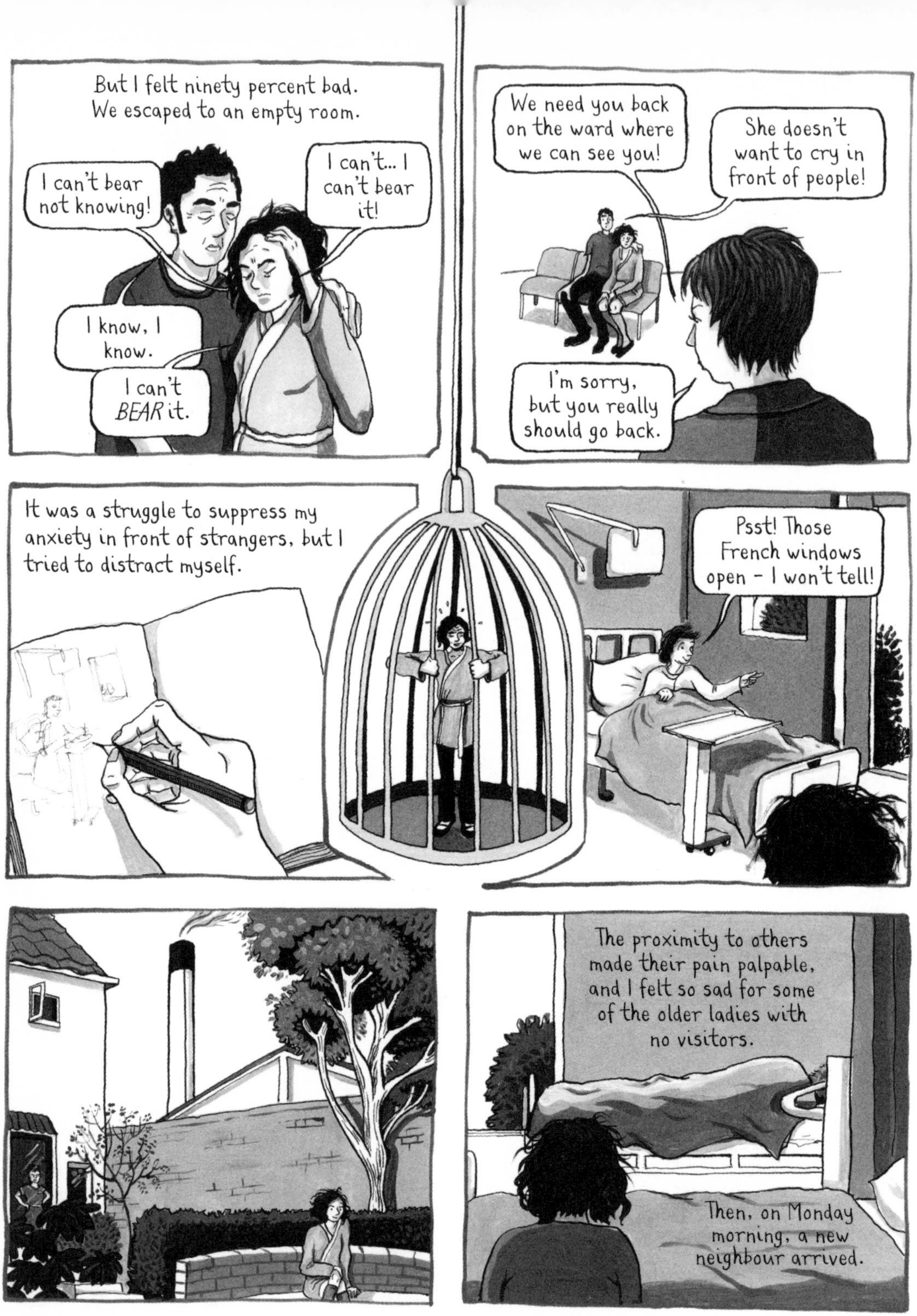

But I felt ninety percent bad. We escaped to an empty room.
I can't bear not knowing!
I can't... I can't bear it!
I know, I know.
I can't *BEAR* it.
We need you back on the ward where we can see you!
She doesn't want to cry in front of people!
I'm sorry, but you really should go back.
It was a struggle to suppress my anxiety in front of strangers, but I tried to distract myself.
Psst! Those French windows open - I won't tell!
The proximity to others made their pain palpable, and I felt so sad for some of the older ladies with no visitors.
Then, on Monday morning, a new neighbour arrived.

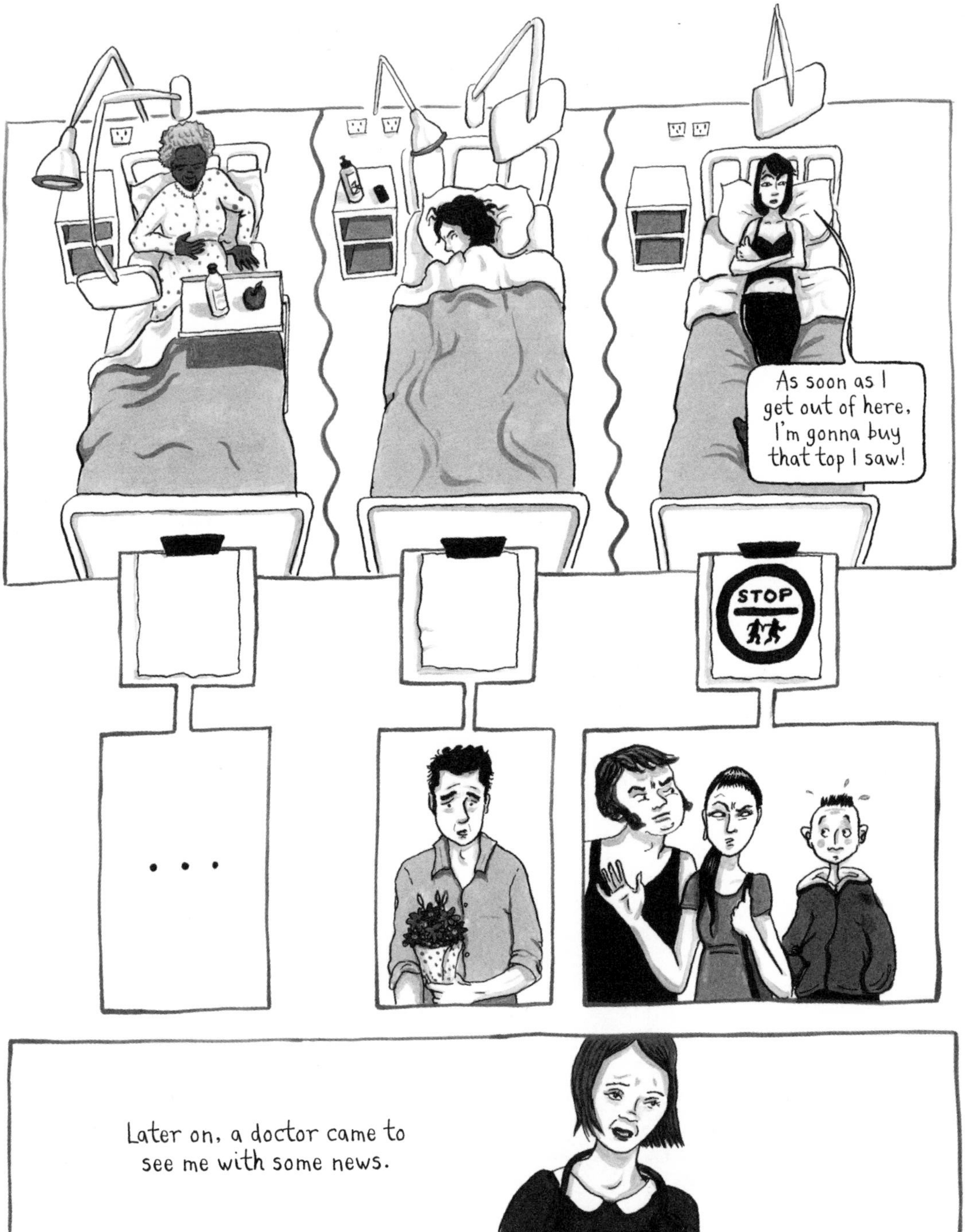
As soon as I get out of here, I'm gonna buy that top I saw!
STOP
...
Later on, a doctor came to see me with some news.

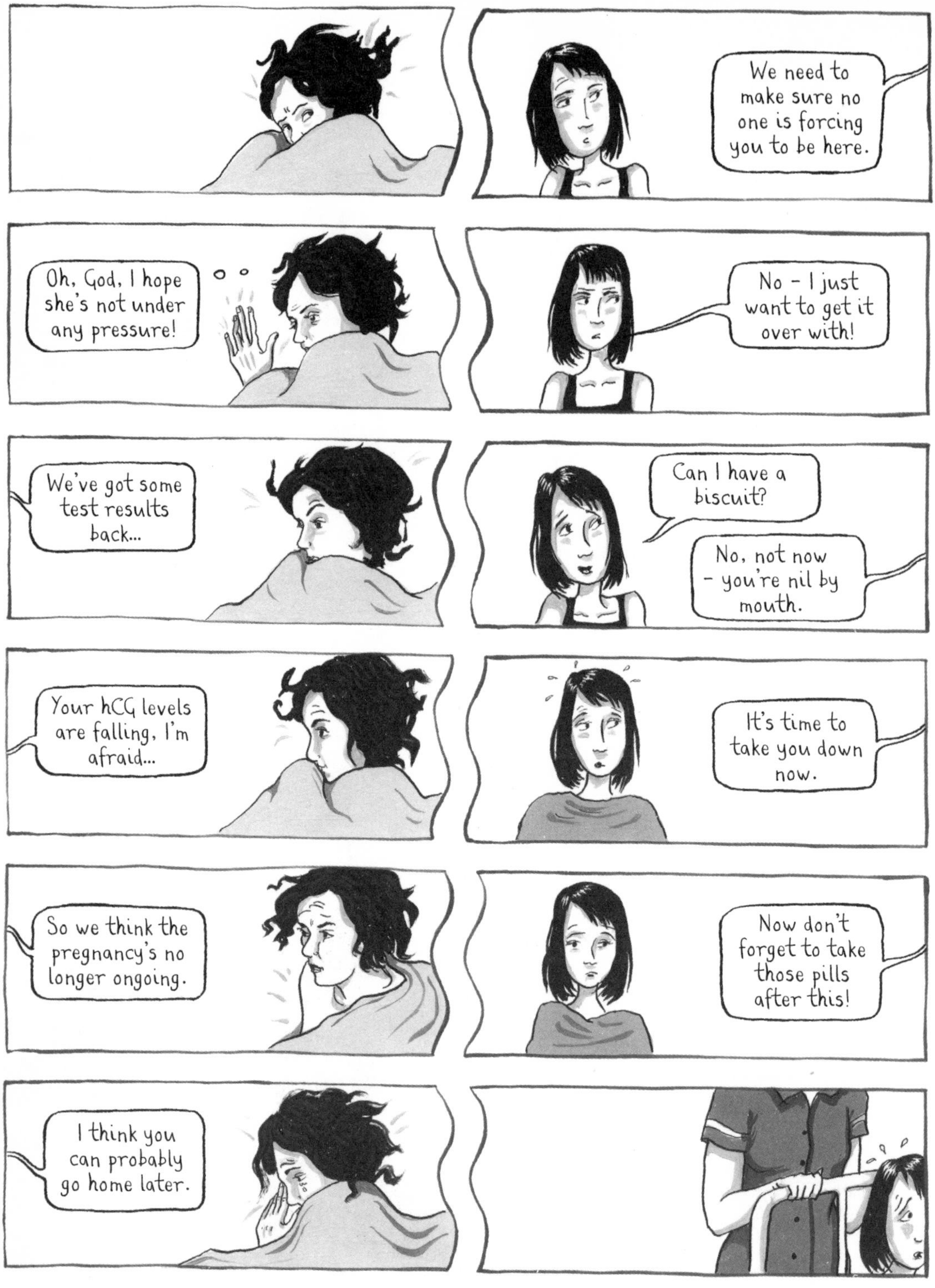
We need to make sure no one is forcing you to be here.
Oh, God, I hope she's not under any pressure!
No - I just want to get it over with!
We've got some test results back...
Can I have a biscuit?
No, not now - you're nil by mouth.
Your hCG levels are falling, I'm afraid...
It's time to take you down now.
So we think the pregnancy's no longer ongoing.
Now don't forget to take those pills after this!
I think you can probably go home later.

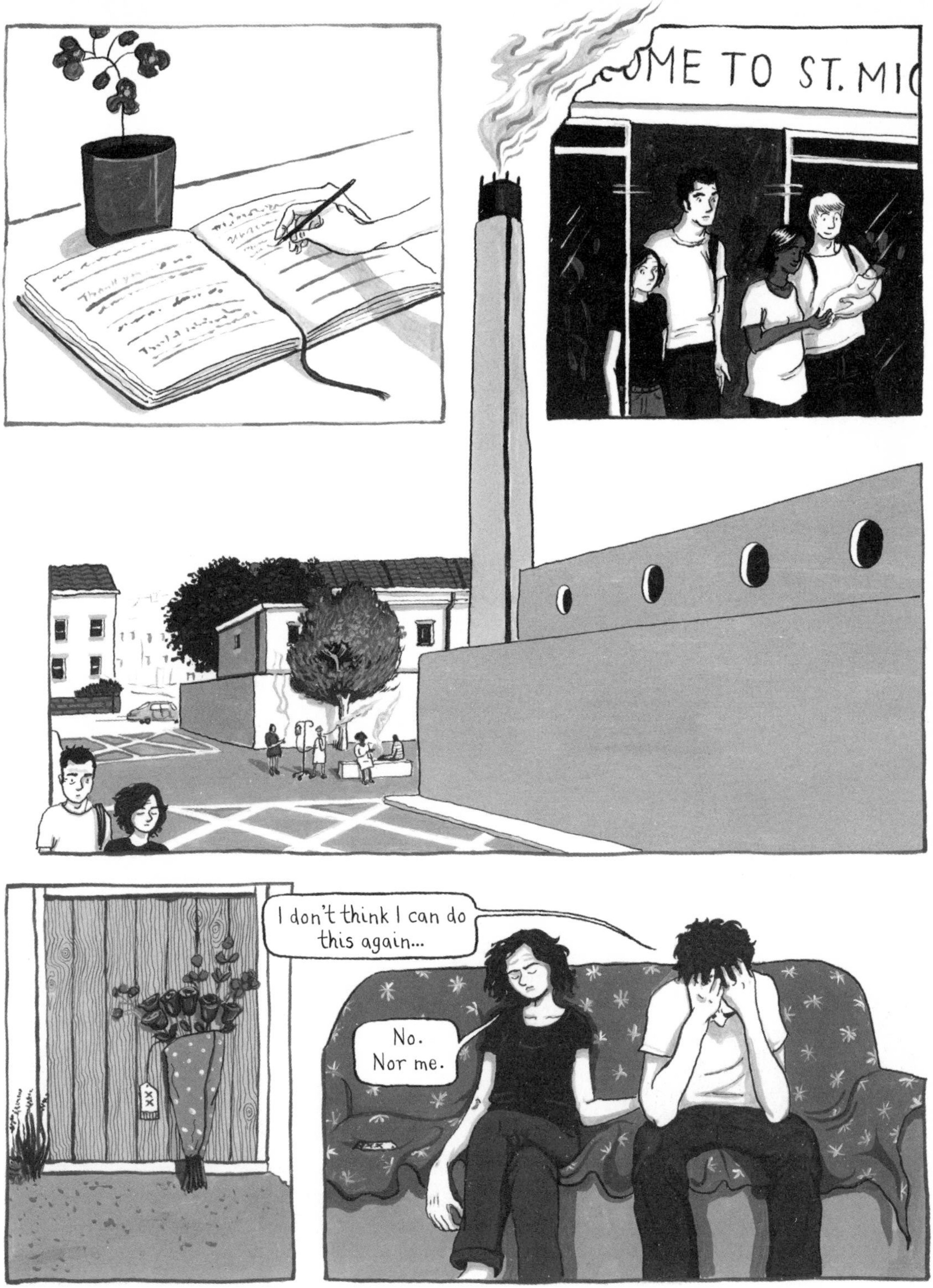
COME TO ST. MIC
I don't think I can do this again...
No. Nor me.

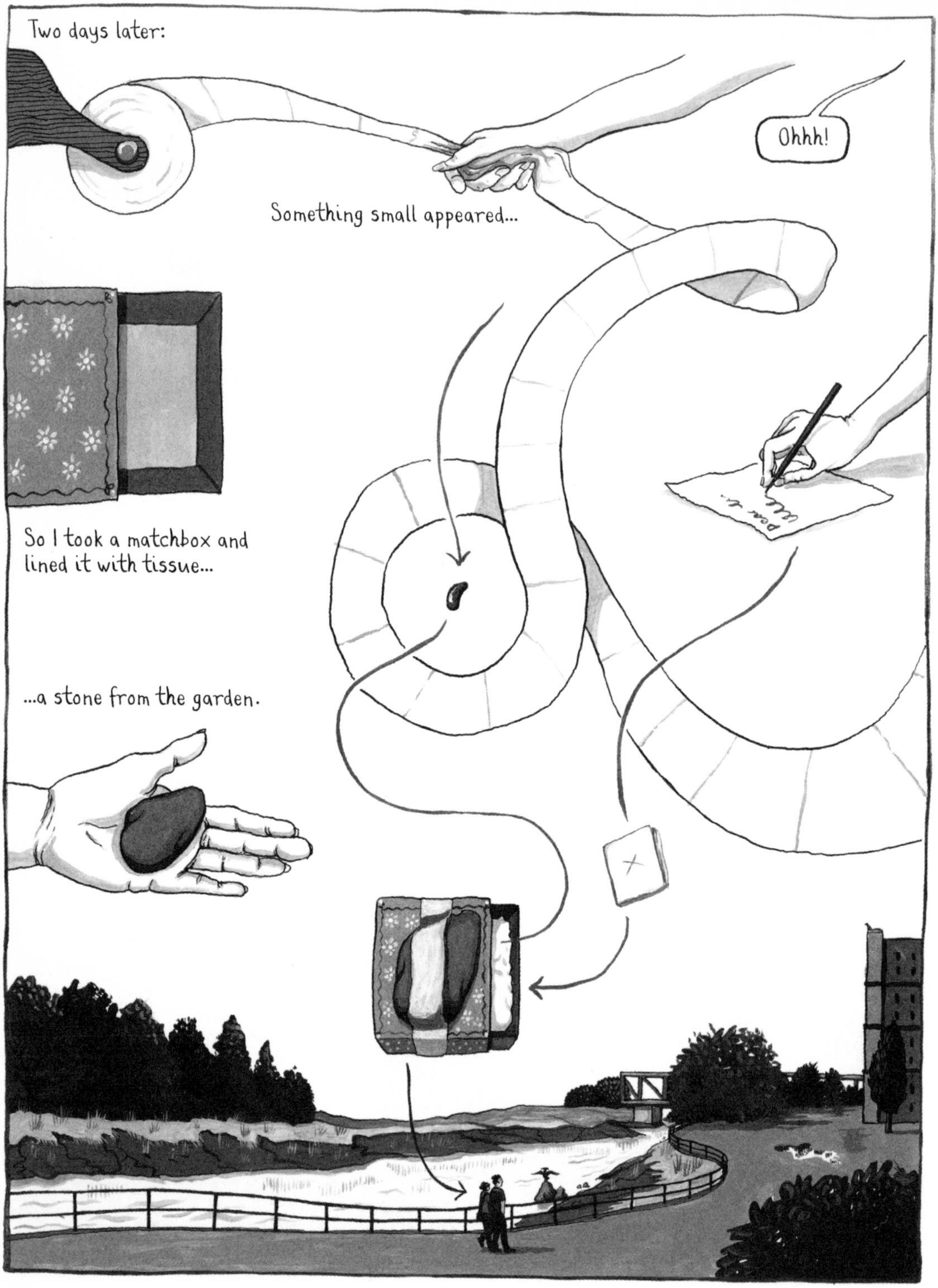
Two days later:
Ohhh!
Something small appeared...
So I took a matchbox and
lined it with tissue...
...a stone from the garden.

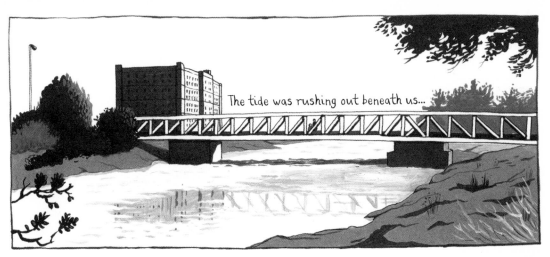

The tide was rushing out beneath us...

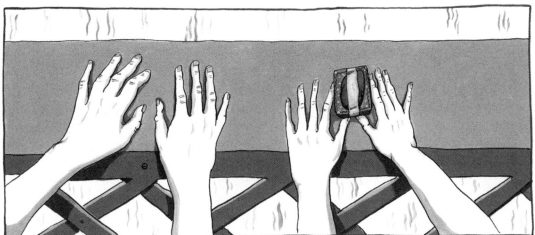

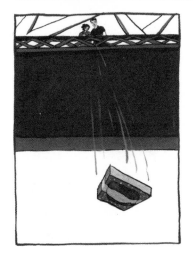

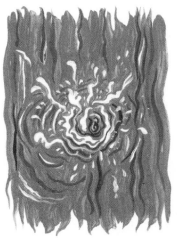

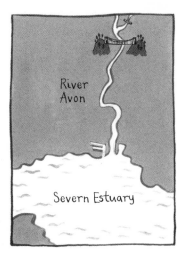

River
Avon

Severn Estuary

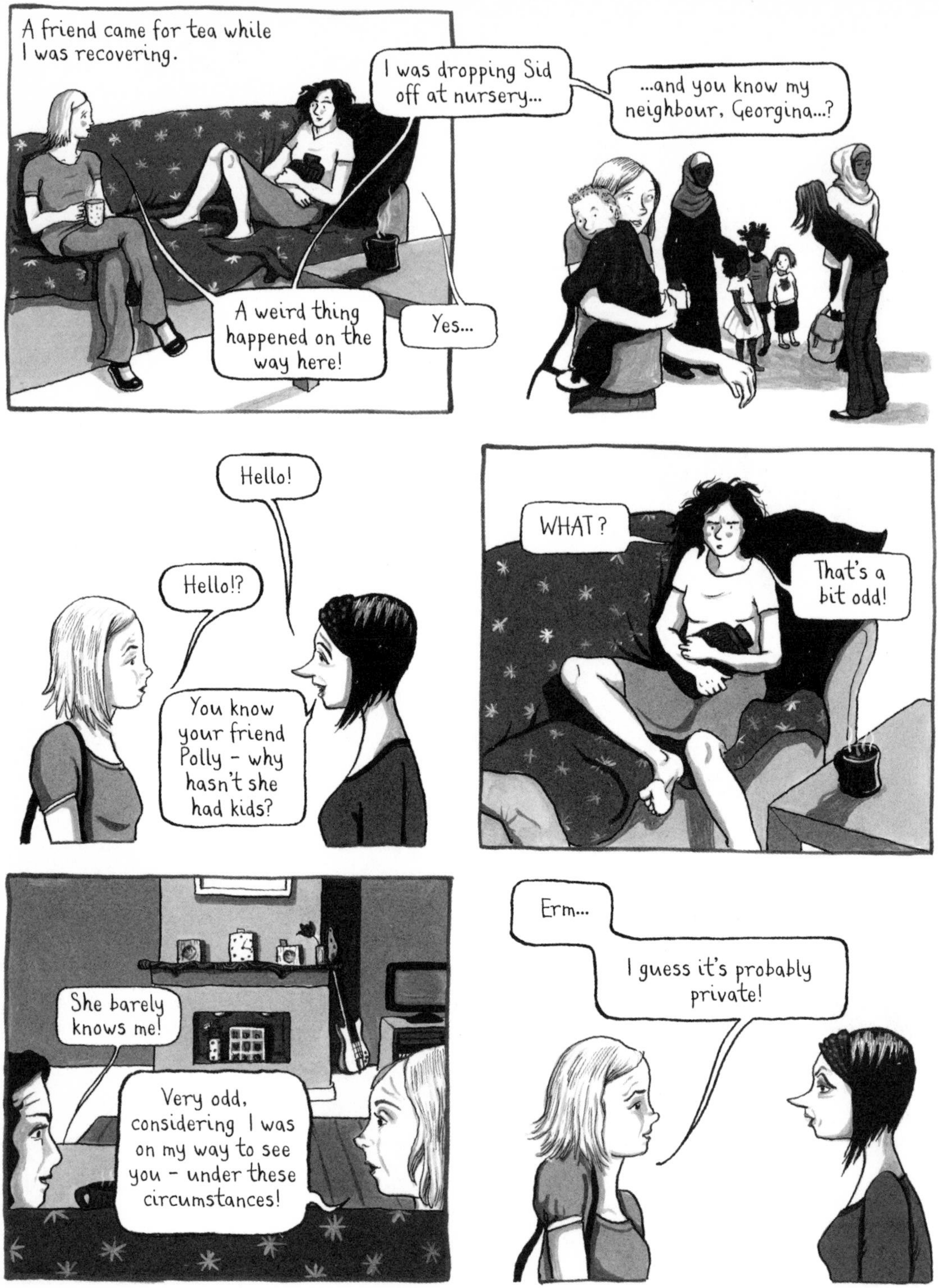
A friend came for tea while I was recovering.
A weird thing happened on the way here!
Yes...
I was dropping Sid off at nursery...
...and you know my neighbour, Georgina...?
Hello!
Hello!?
You know your friend Polly - why hasn't she had kids?
WHAT?
That's a bit odd!
She barely knows me!
Very odd, considering I was on my way to see you - under these circumstances!
Erm...
I guess it's probably private!

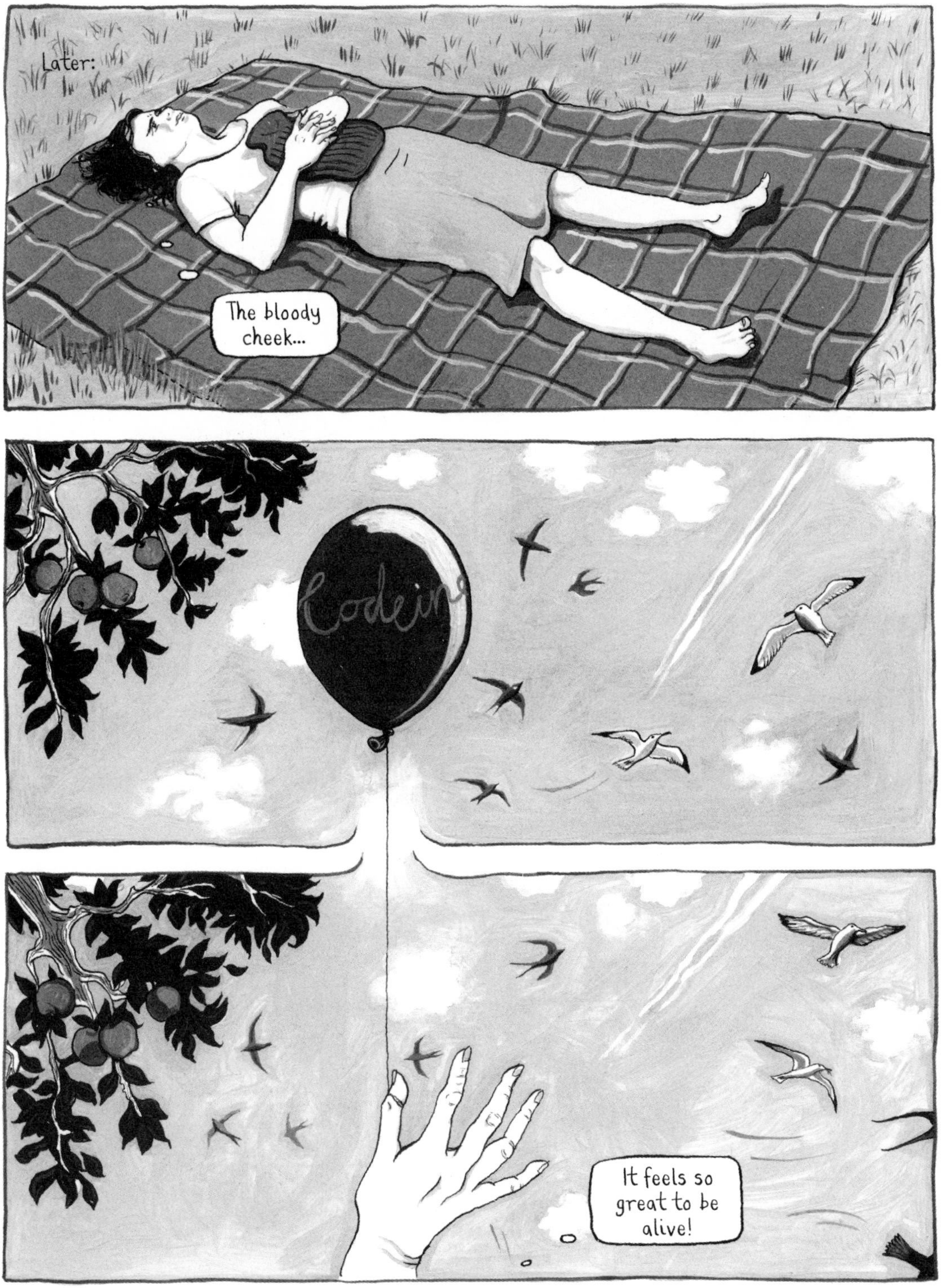
Later:
The bloody cheek...
Codeine
It feels so great to be alive!

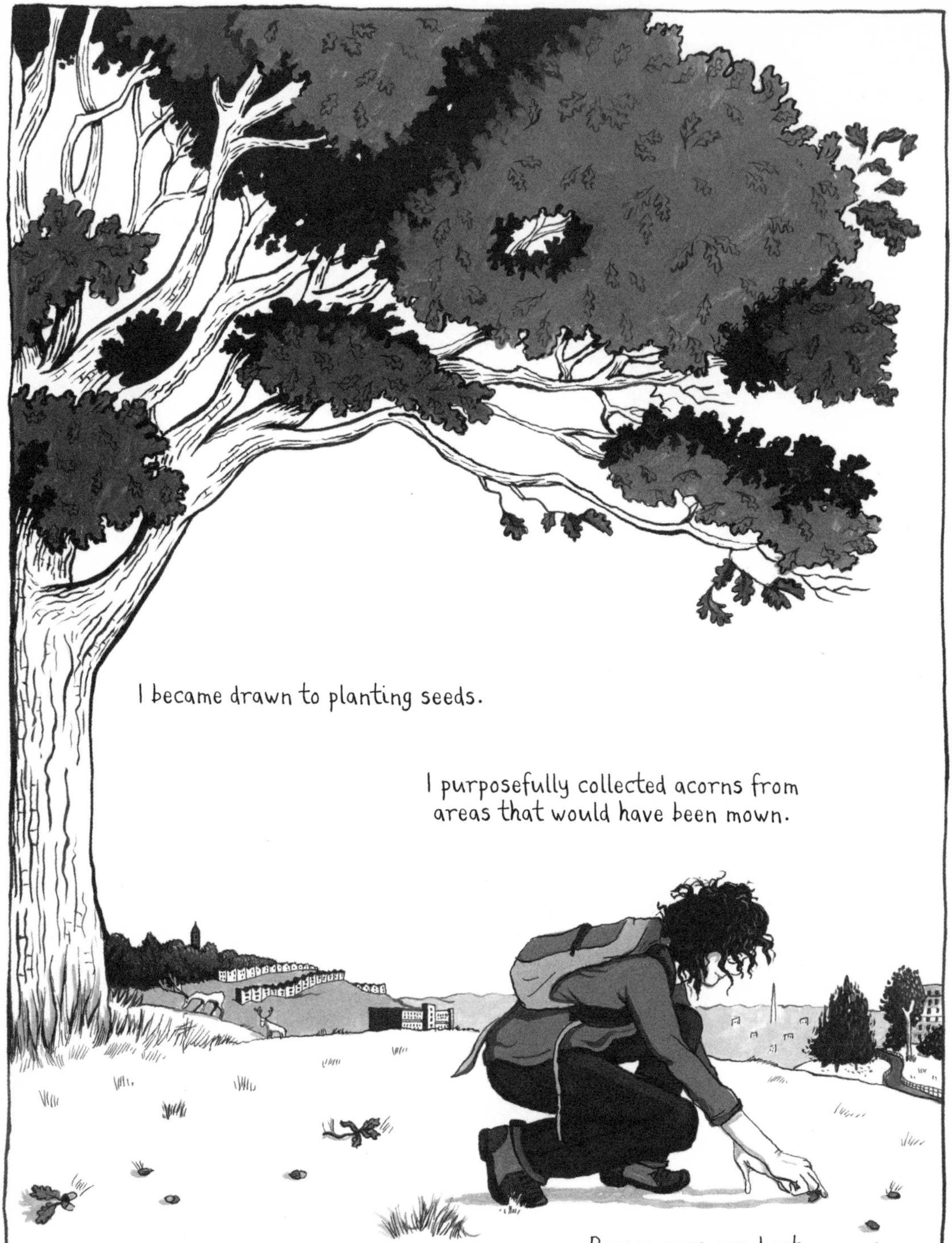
I became drawn to planting seeds.
I purposefully collected acorns from areas that would have been mown.
Brown ones are best.

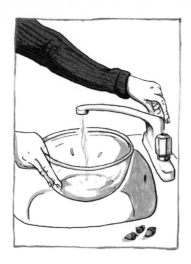

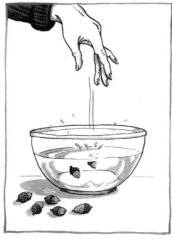

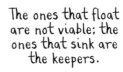

The ones that float are not viable; the ones that sink are the keepers.

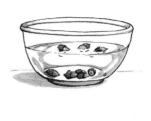

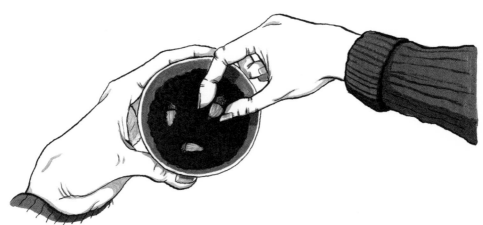

I pledged three of them to a tree-planting scheme in the National Forest. I'd be invited to plant them in the third season, if they grew strong enough.

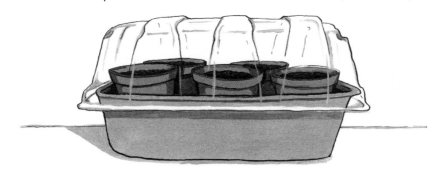

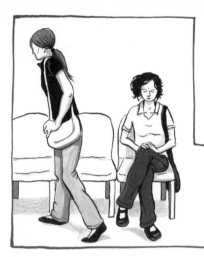

Now I'd had three miscarriages, I was able to have tests to investigate possible causes.

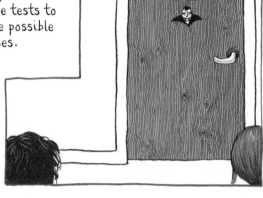

Owww!

Meanwhile...

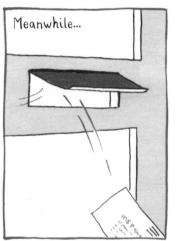

Jack!

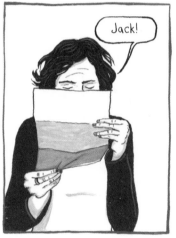

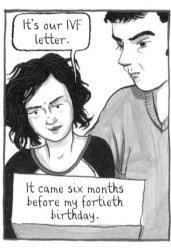

It's our IVF letter.

It came six months before my fortieth birthday.

Thing is...

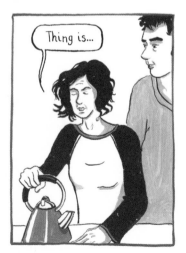

...it's more a matter of staying pregnant, not getting pregnant...

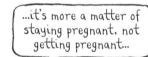

...and IVF's no guarantee of that.

It'd be an awful lot to put ourselves through.

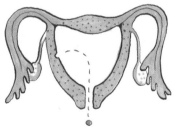

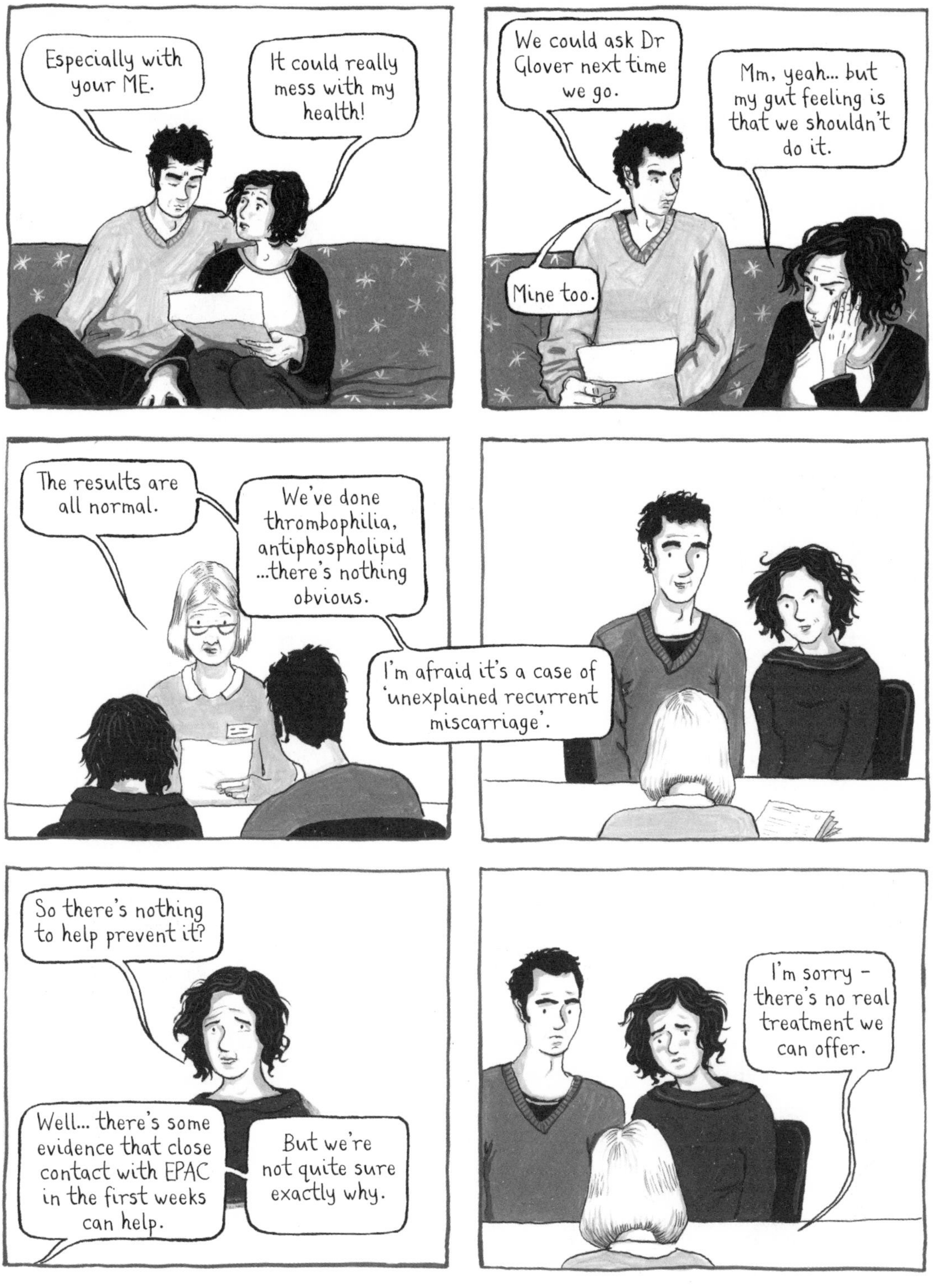
Especially with your ME.
It could really mess with my health!
We could ask Dr Glover next time we go.
Mm, yeah... but my gut feeling is that we shouldn't do it.
Mine too.
The results are all normal.
We've done thrombophilia, antiphospholipid ...there's nothing obvious.
I'm afraid it's a case of 'unexplained recurrent miscarriage'.
So there's nothing to help prevent it?
Well... there's some evidence that close contact with EPAC in the first weeks can help.
But we're not quite sure exactly why.
I'm sorry - there's no real treatment we can offer.

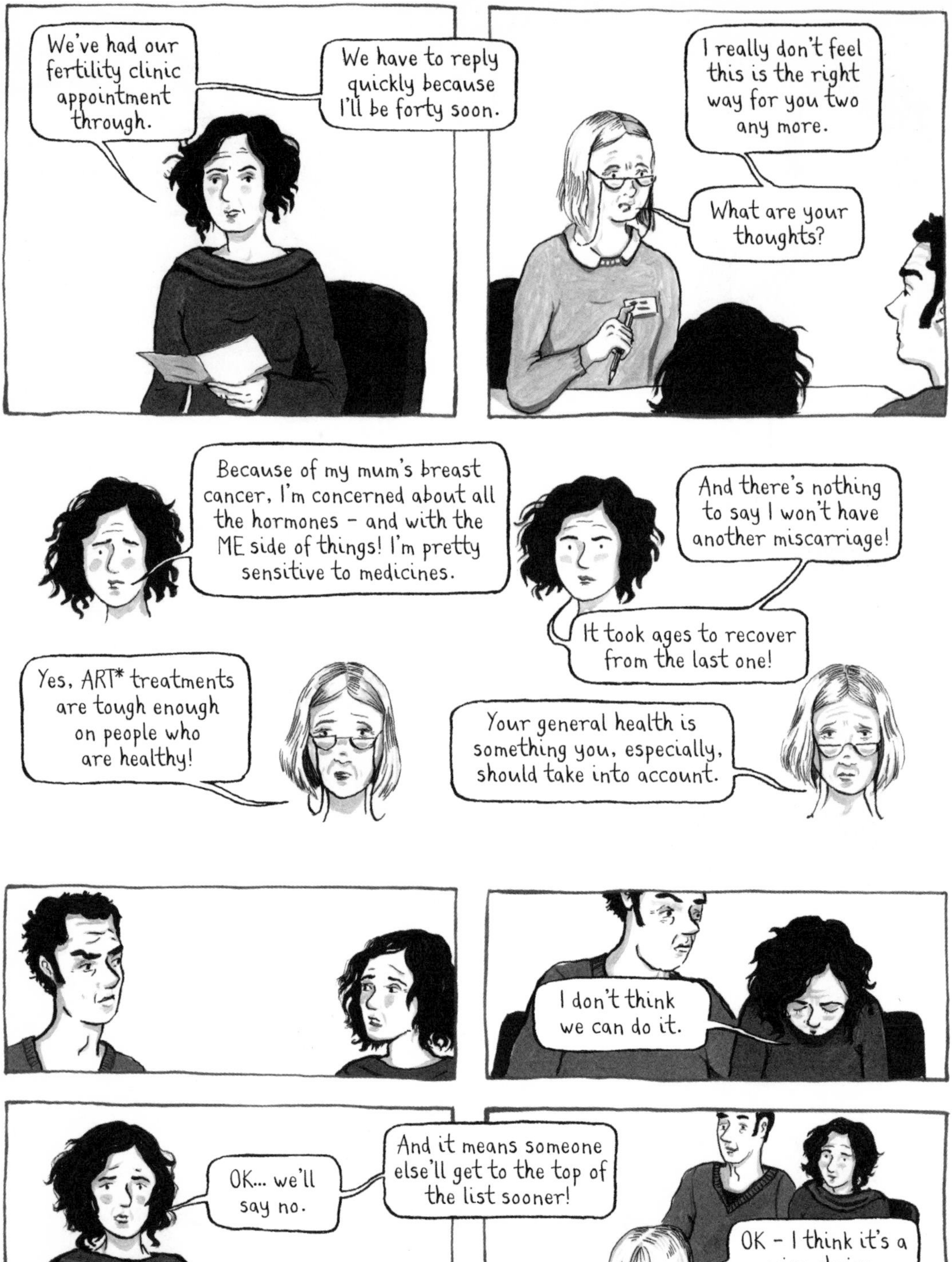
We've had our fertility clinic appointment through.
We have to reply quickly because I'll be forty soon.
I really don't feel this is the right way for you two any more.
What are your thoughts?
Because of my mum's breast cancer, I'm concerned about all the hormones - and with the ME side of things! I'm pretty sensitive to medicines.
And there's nothing to say I won't have another miscarriage!
It took ages to recover from the last one!
Yes, ART* treatments are tough enough on people who are healthy!
Your general health is something you, especially, should take into account.
I don't think we can do it.
OK... we'll say no.
And it means someone else'll get to the top of the list sooner!
OK - I think it's a wise choice.

*Assisted Reproductive Technology

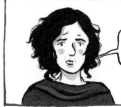

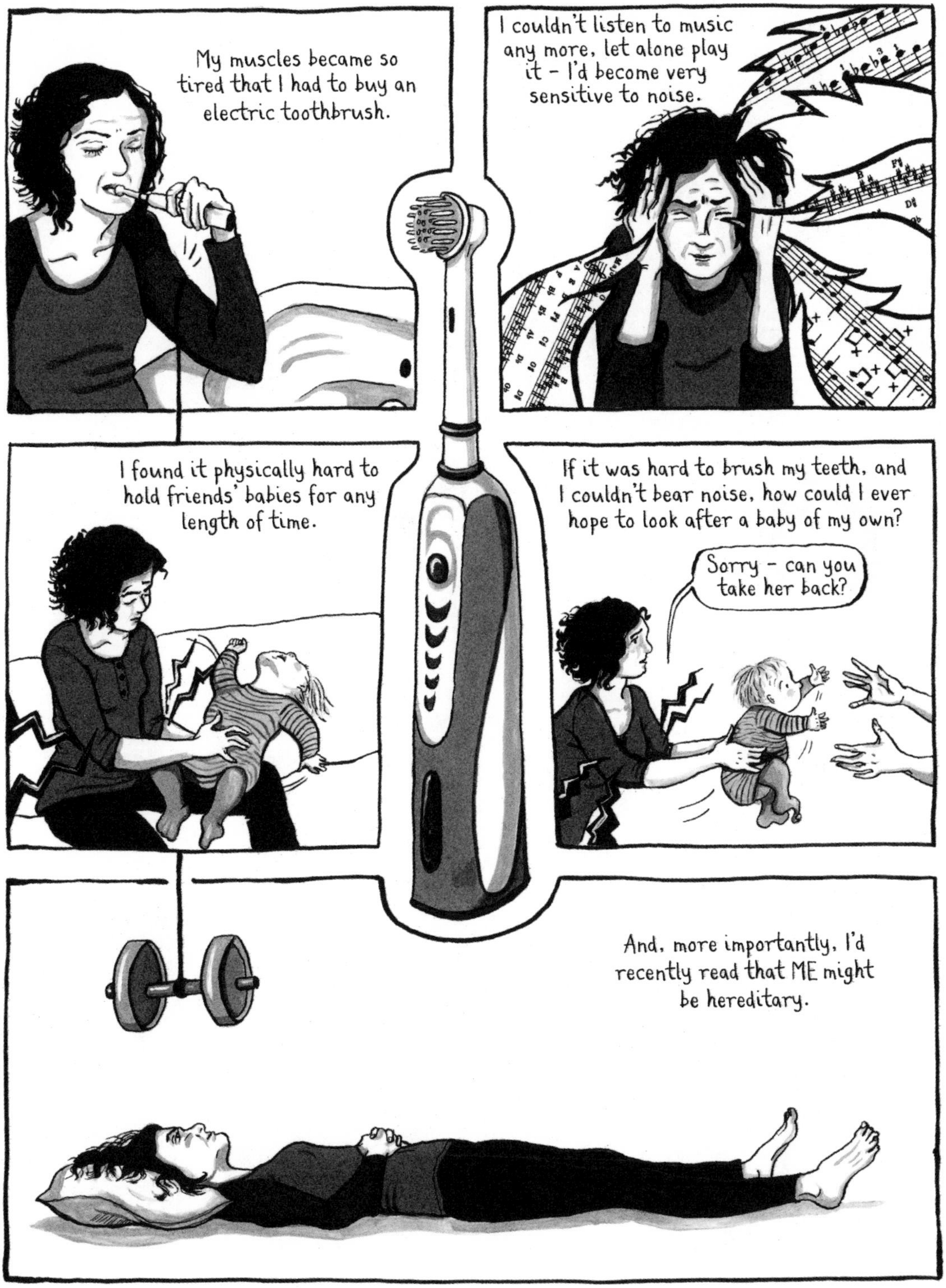
My muscles became so tired that I had to buy an electric toothbrush.
I couldn't listen to music any more, let alone play it – I'd become very sensitive to noise.
I found it physically hard to hold friends' babies for any length of time.
If it was hard to brush my teeth, and I couldn't bear noise, how could I ever hope to look after a baby of my own?
Sorry – can you take her back?
And, more importantly, I'd recently read that ME might be hereditary.

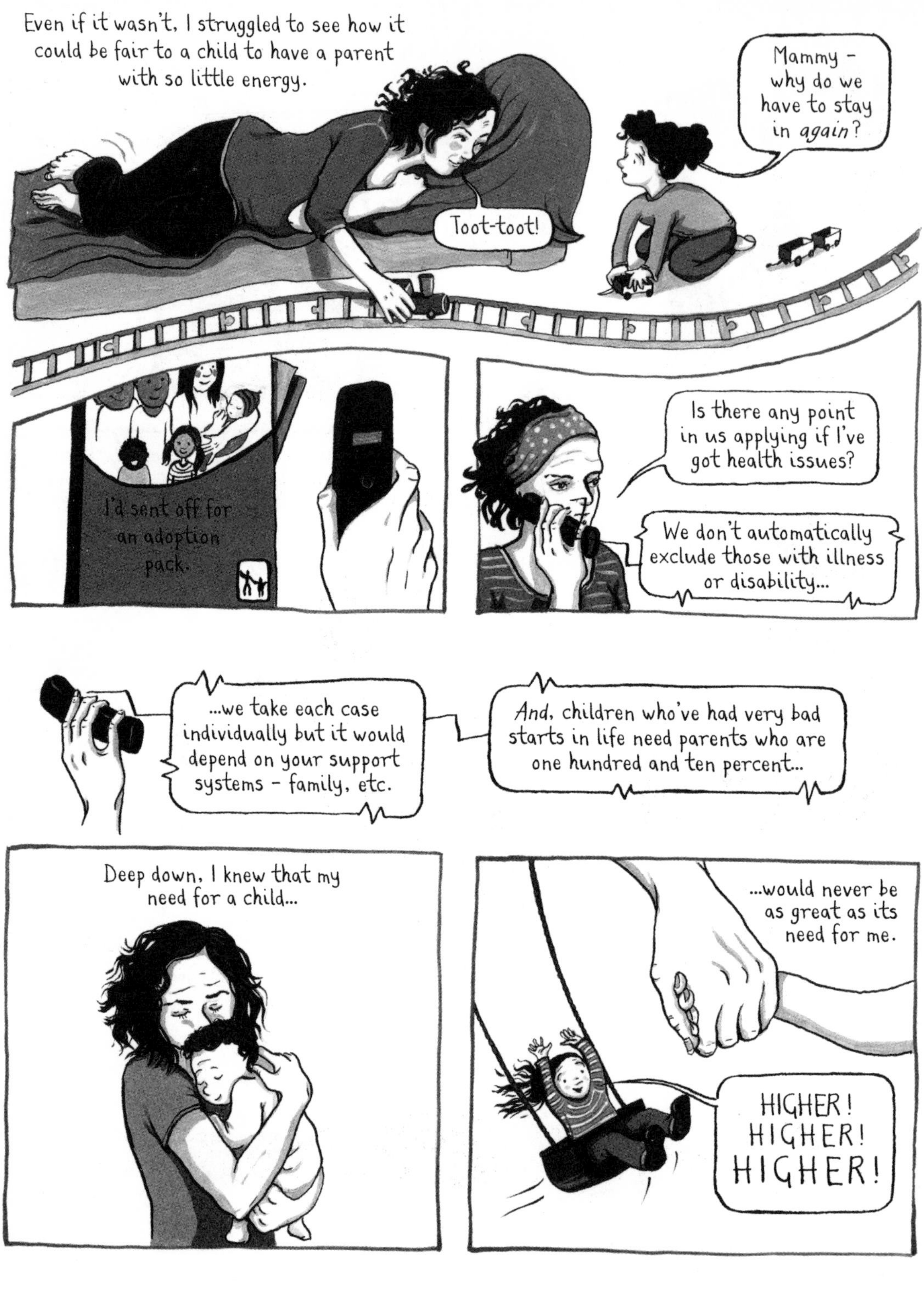
Even if it wasn't, I struggled to see how it could be fair to a child to have a parent with so little energy.
Mammy - why do we have to stay in *again*?
Toot-toot!
I'd sent off for an adoption pack.
Is there any point in us applying if I've got health issues?
We don't automatically exclude those with illness or disability...
...we take each case individually but it would depend on your support systems - family, etc.
And, children who've had very bad starts in life need parents who are one hundred and ten percent...
Deep down, I knew that my need for a child...
...would never be as great as its need for me.
HIGHER! HIGHER! HIGHER!

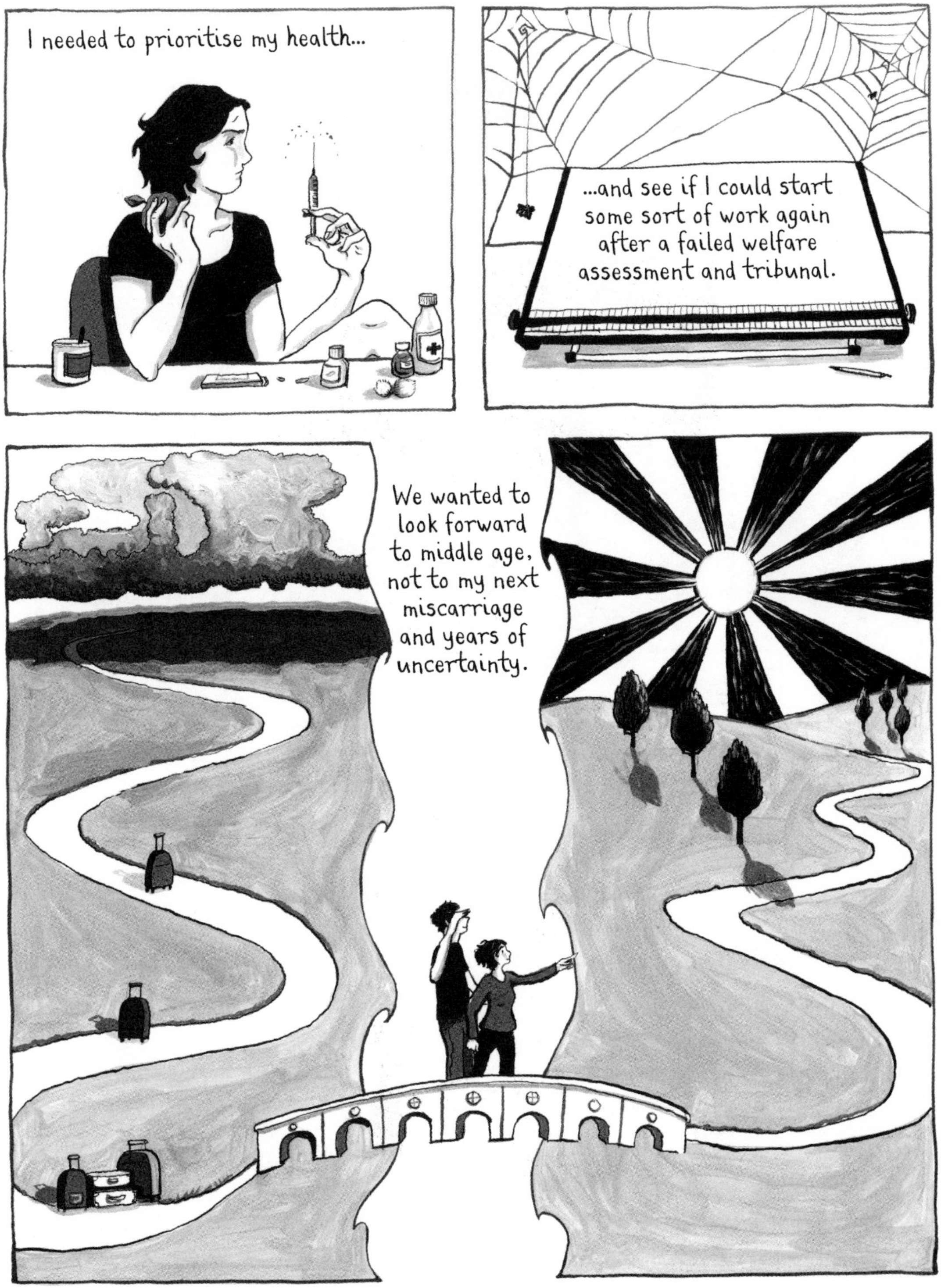
I needed to prioritise my health...
...and see if I could start some sort of work again after a failed welfare assessment and tribunal.
We wanted to look forward to middle age, not to my next miscarriage and years of uncertainty.

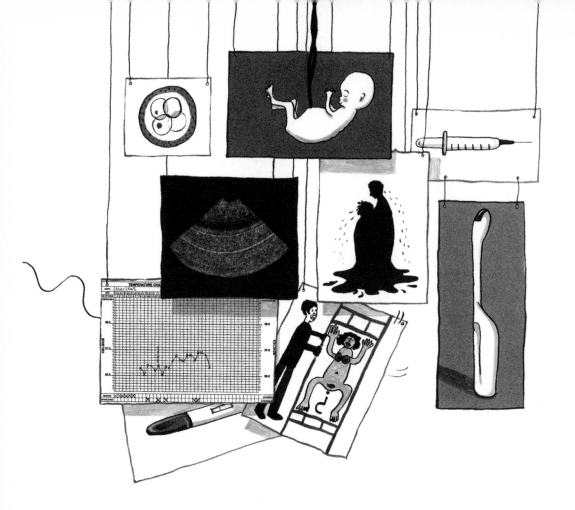

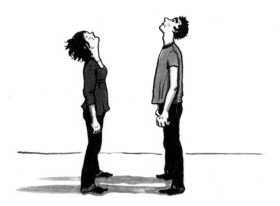

It felt like time to move on.

We can't carry on, can we?
No, I don't think so.

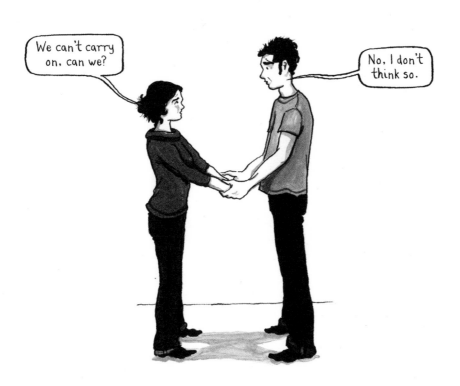

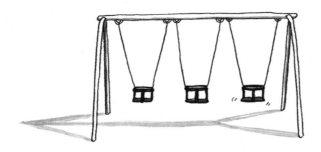

THREE

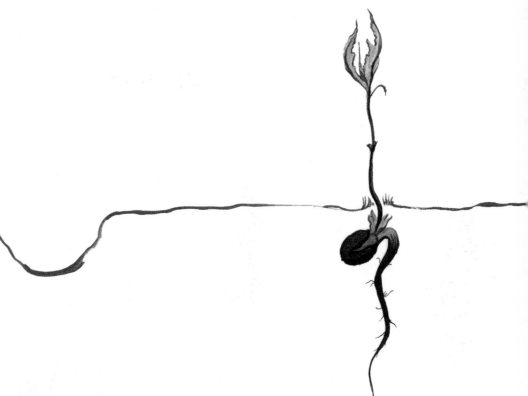

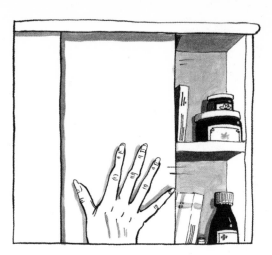

CALL FOR DONATIONS:
THE GIFTS by ALINAH AZEDEH

Do you have a small item which is pas...

emotional sell-by-date? Alinah Azedel...

...ng items, which she will use to c...

...e Gifts, an art installation of 999 v...

objects. Your item should be accomp...

by a written description of the mean...

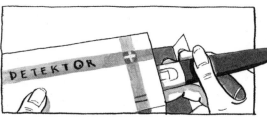

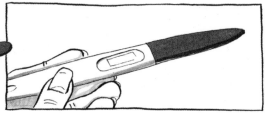

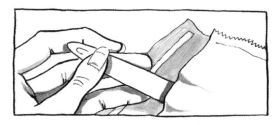

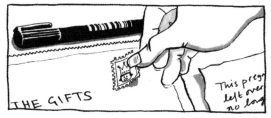

THE GIFTS

This preg...
left over
no lo...

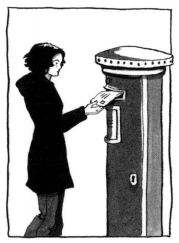

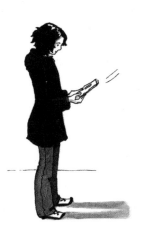

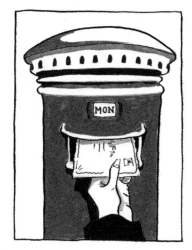

MON

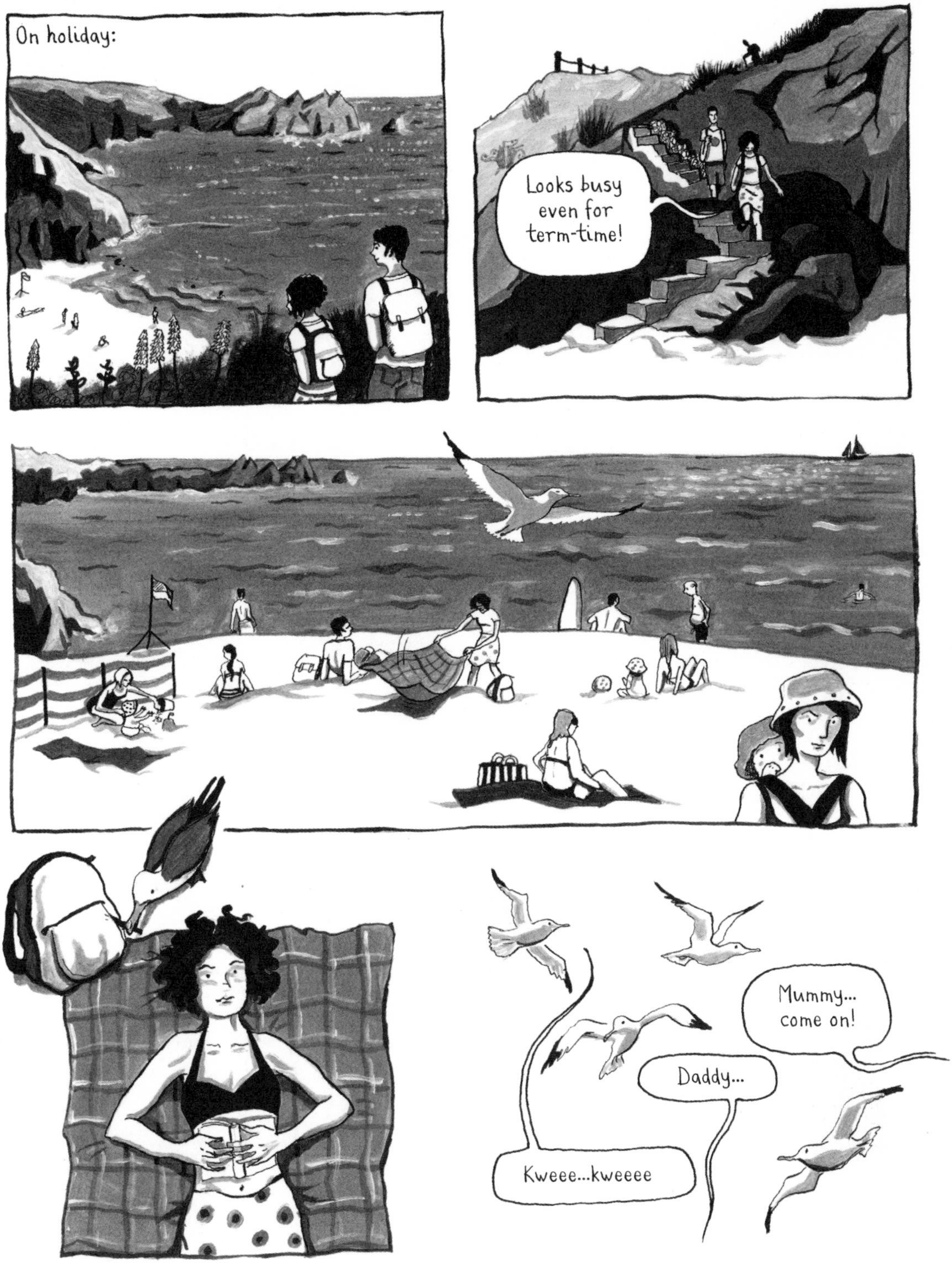
On holiday:
Looks busy even for term-time!
Mummy... come on!
Daddy...
Kweee...kweeee

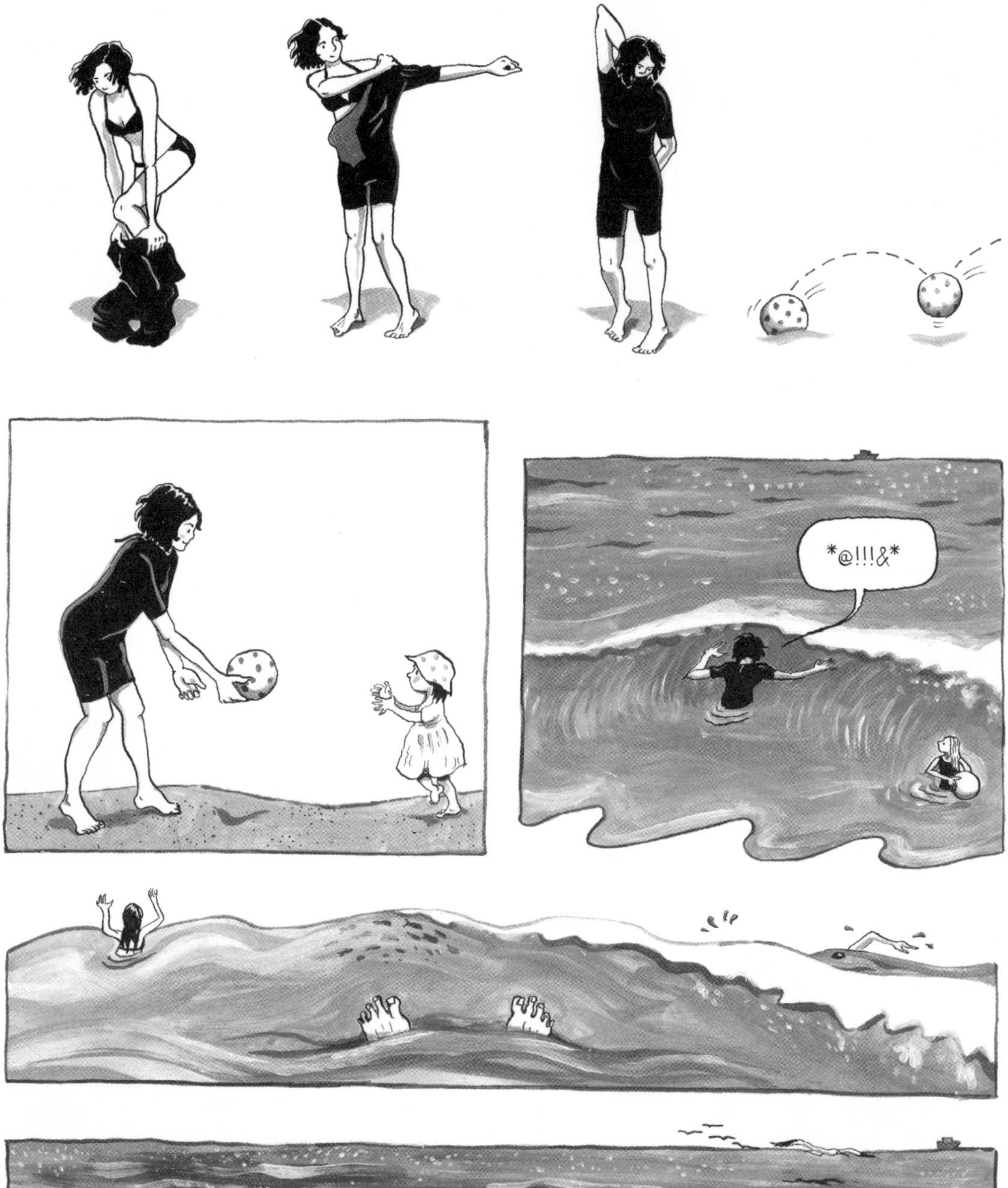
@!!!&

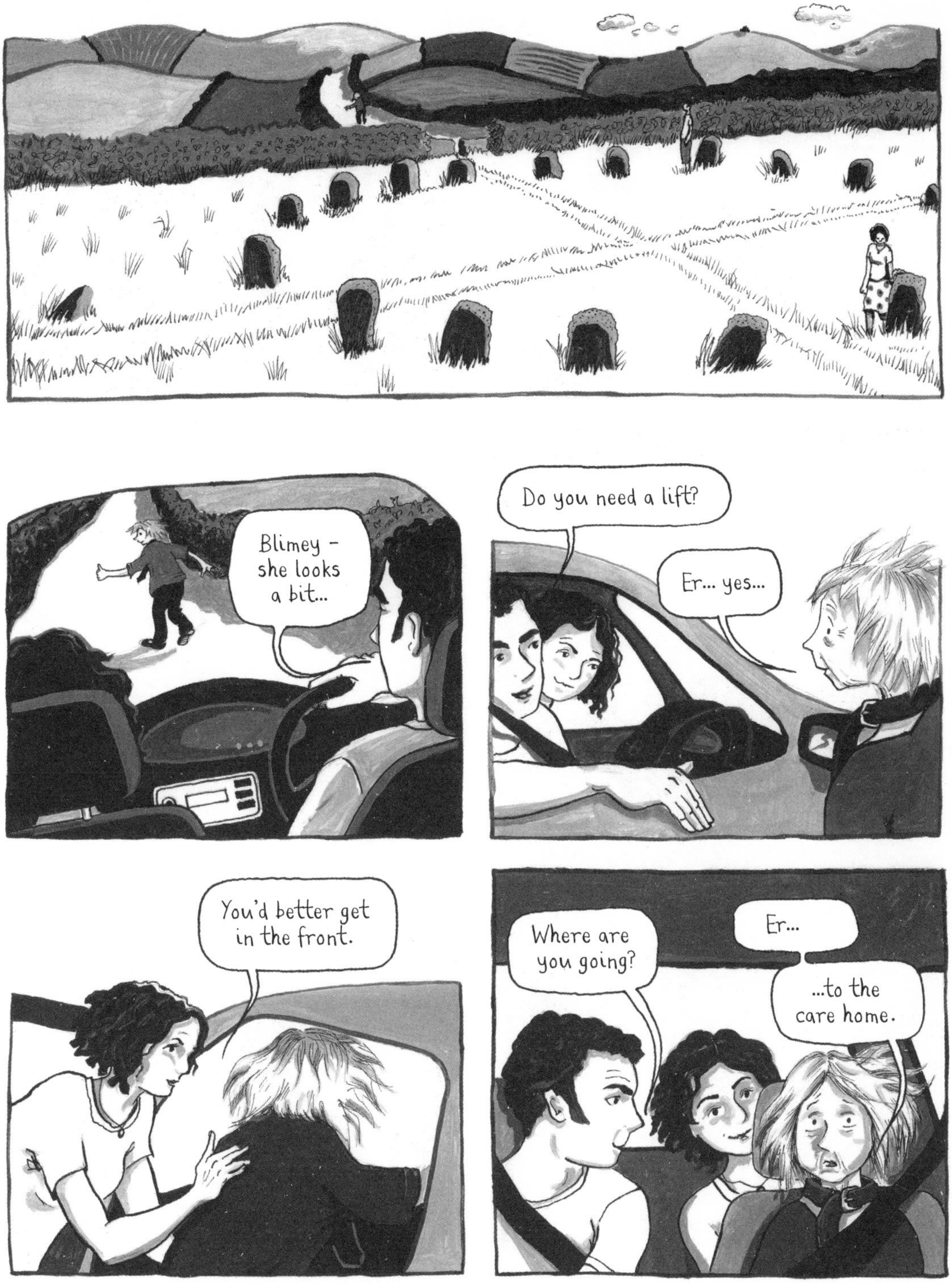
Blimey - she looks a bit...
Do you need a lift?
Er... yes...
You'd better get in the front.
Where are you going?
Er...
...to the care home.

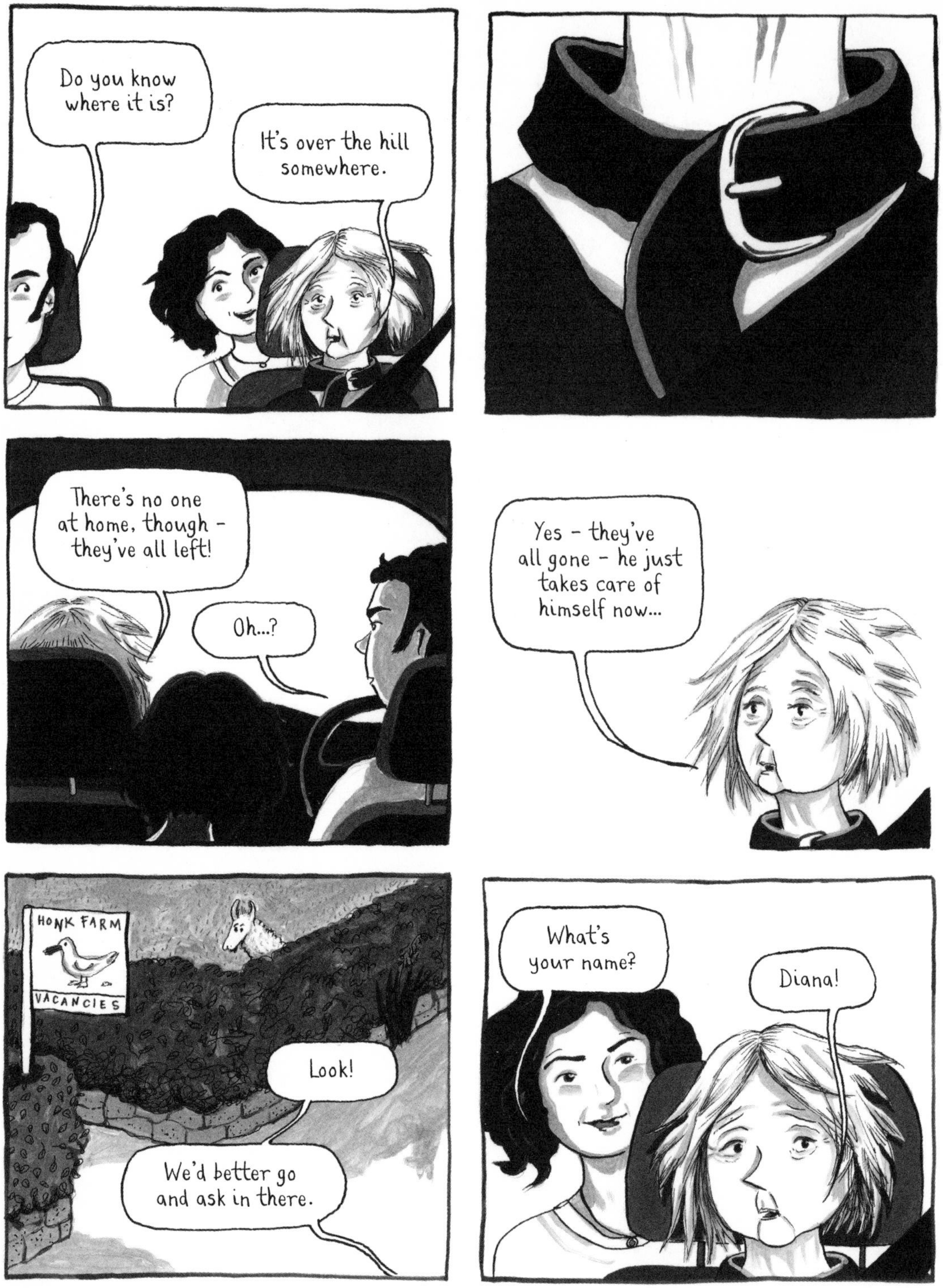
Do you know where it is?
It's over the hill somewhere.
There's no one at home, though - they've all left!
Oh...?
Yes - they've all gone - he just takes care of himself now...
HONK FARM
VACANCIES
Look!
We'd better go and ask in there.
What's your name?
Diana!

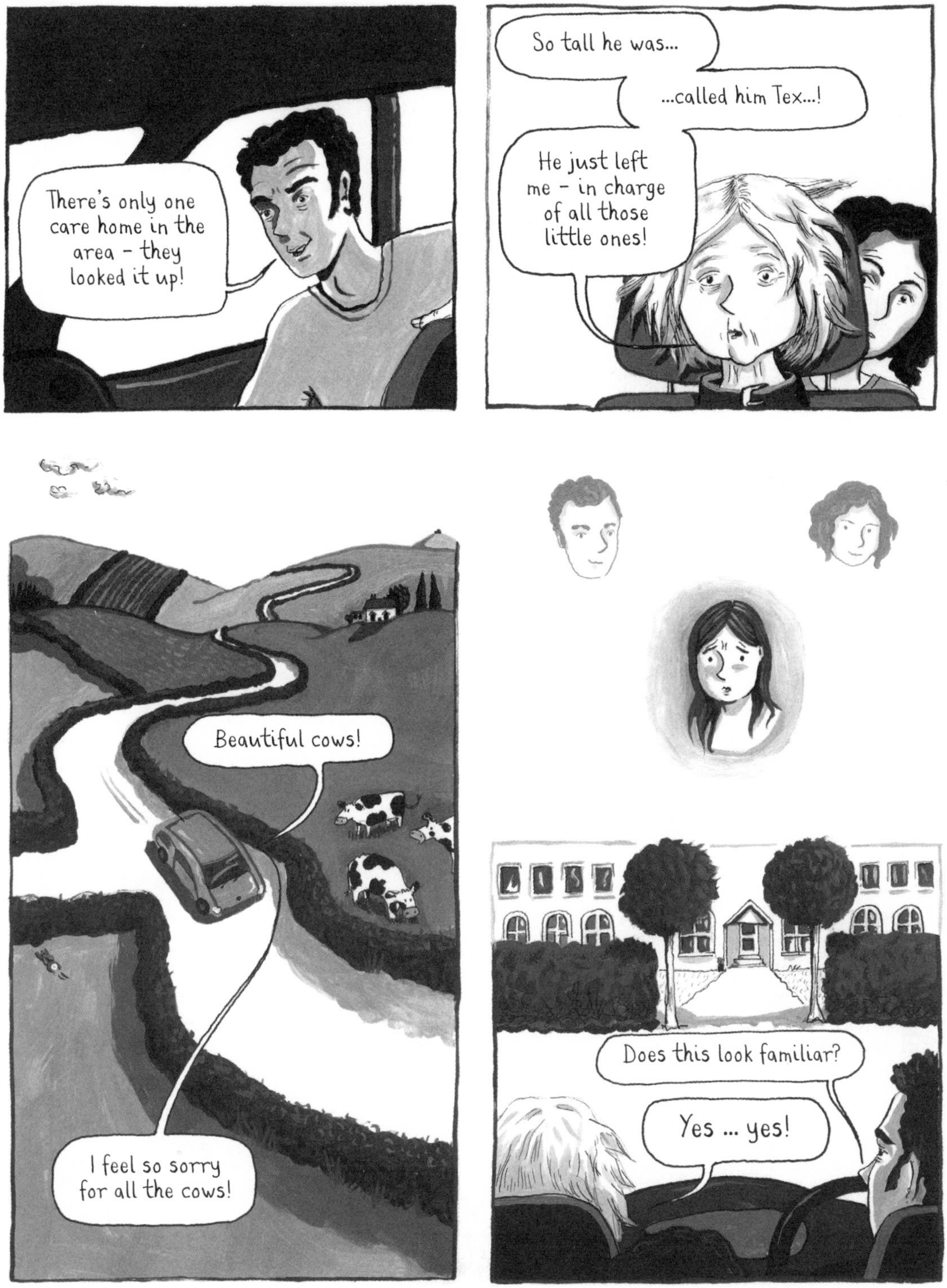
There's only one care home in the area - they looked it up!
So tall he was...
...called him Tex...!
He just left me - in charge of all those little ones!
Beautiful cows!
I feel so sorry for all the cows!
Does this look familiar?
Yes ... yes!

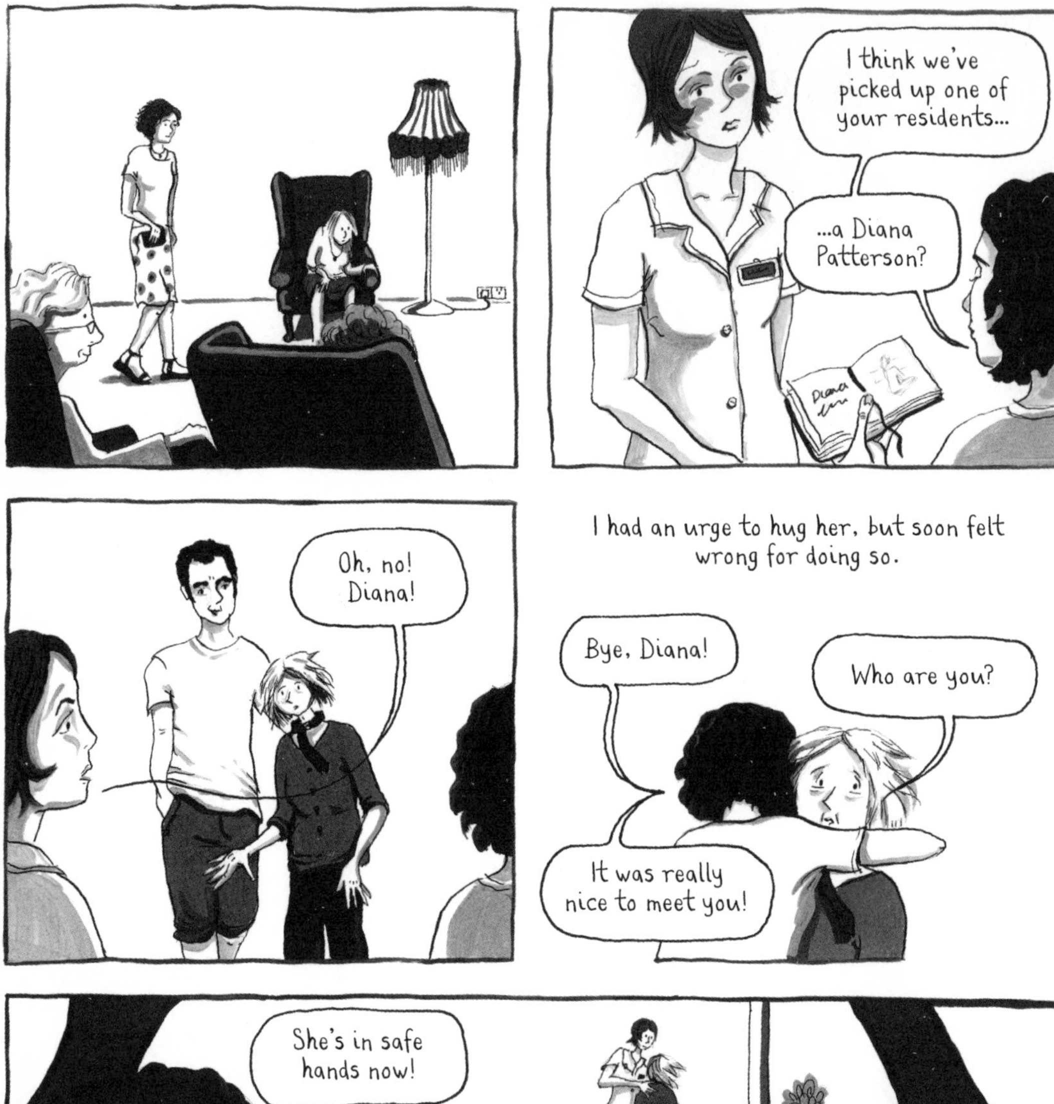
I think we've picked up one of your residents...
...a Diana Patterson?
Oh, no! Diana!
I had an urge to hug her, but soon felt wrong for doing so.
Bye, Diana!
Who are you?
It was really nice to meet you!
She's in safe hands now!
I hope so!
I wonder if she has any family?

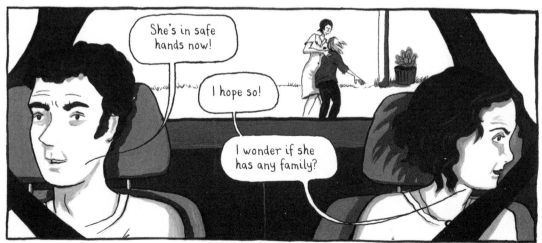

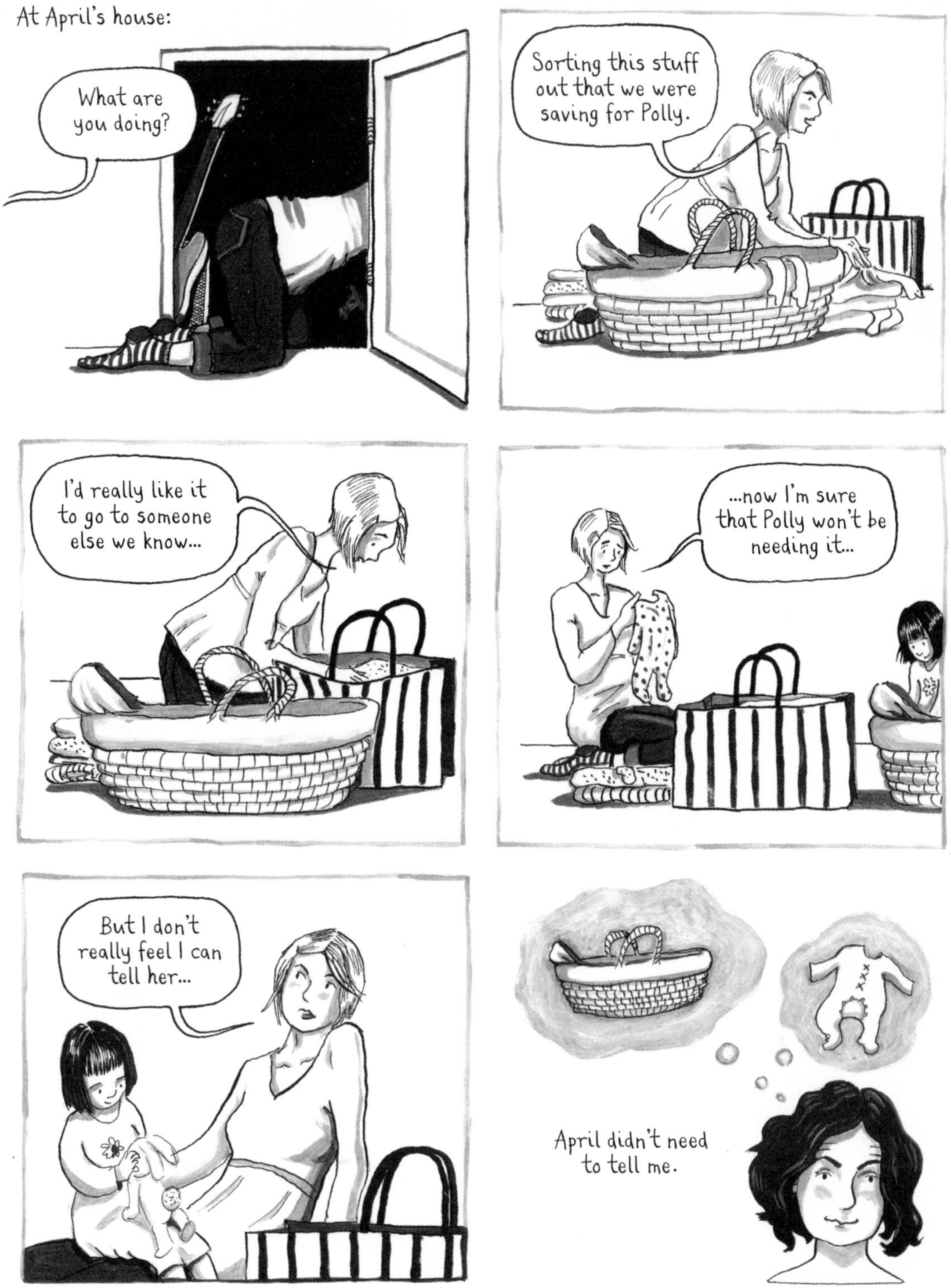
At April's house:
What are you doing?
Sorting this stuff out that we were saving for Polly.
I'd really like it to go to someone else we know...
...now I'm sure that Polly won't be needing it...
But I don't really feel I can tell her...
April didn't need to tell me.

Letting go of stuff can lighten the load, but certain things began to take on more weight, especially with no siblings or heir. What would become of precious things?

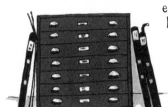

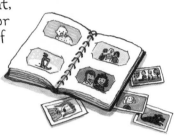

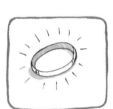

My gran's wedding ring.

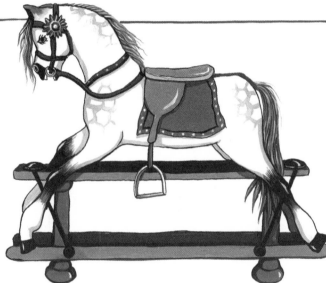

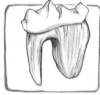

The 'lion's tooth' my dad gave me.

My mum's pressed flowers, collected in 1954.

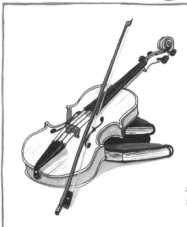

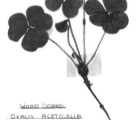

WOOD SORREL
OXALIS ACETOSELLA
FAMILY - OXALIDACEAE
FOUND:- APRIL 28TH
BARNARD CASTLE

Especially Fredbear.

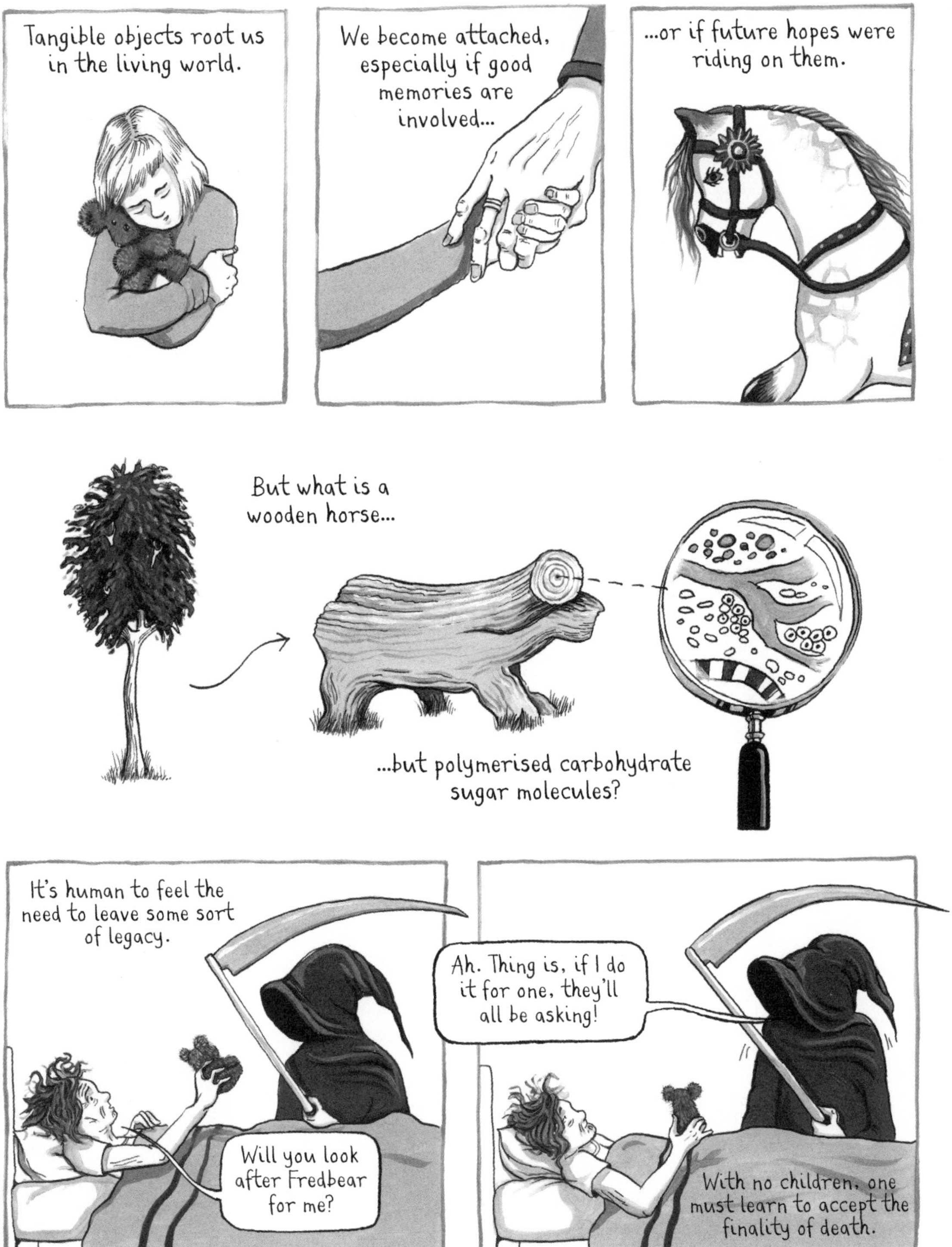
Tangible objects root us in the living world.
We become attached, especially if good memories are involved...
...or if future hopes were riding on them.
But what is a wooden horse...
...but polymerised carbohydrate sugar molecules?
It's human to feel the need to leave some sort of legacy.
Will you look after Fredbear for me?
Ah. Thing is, if I do it for one, they'll all be asking!
With no children, one must learn to accept the finality of death.

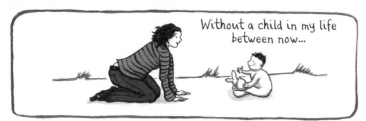

Without a child in my life between now...

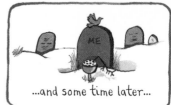

...and some time later...

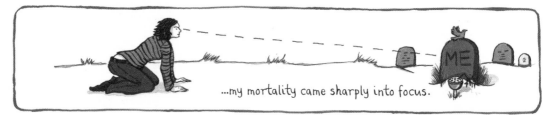

...my mortality came sharply into focus.

Part of what I thought was grief was actually a fear of the future.

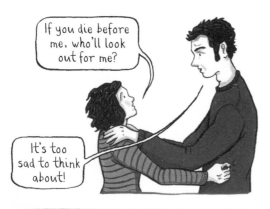

If you die before me, who'll look out for me?

It's too sad to think about!

As an only-child adult with no children, the prospect of ageing seemed bleak.

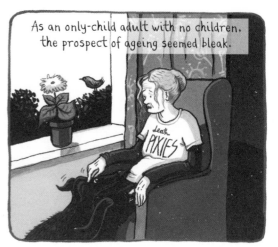

I knew that a child would have been no guarantee of company in old age.

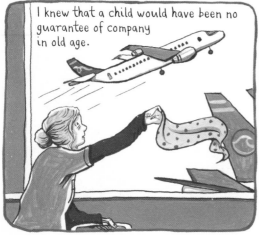

And to have one for that reason is the wrong reason.

You have to look after me now!

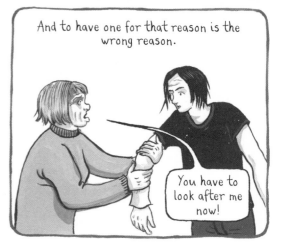

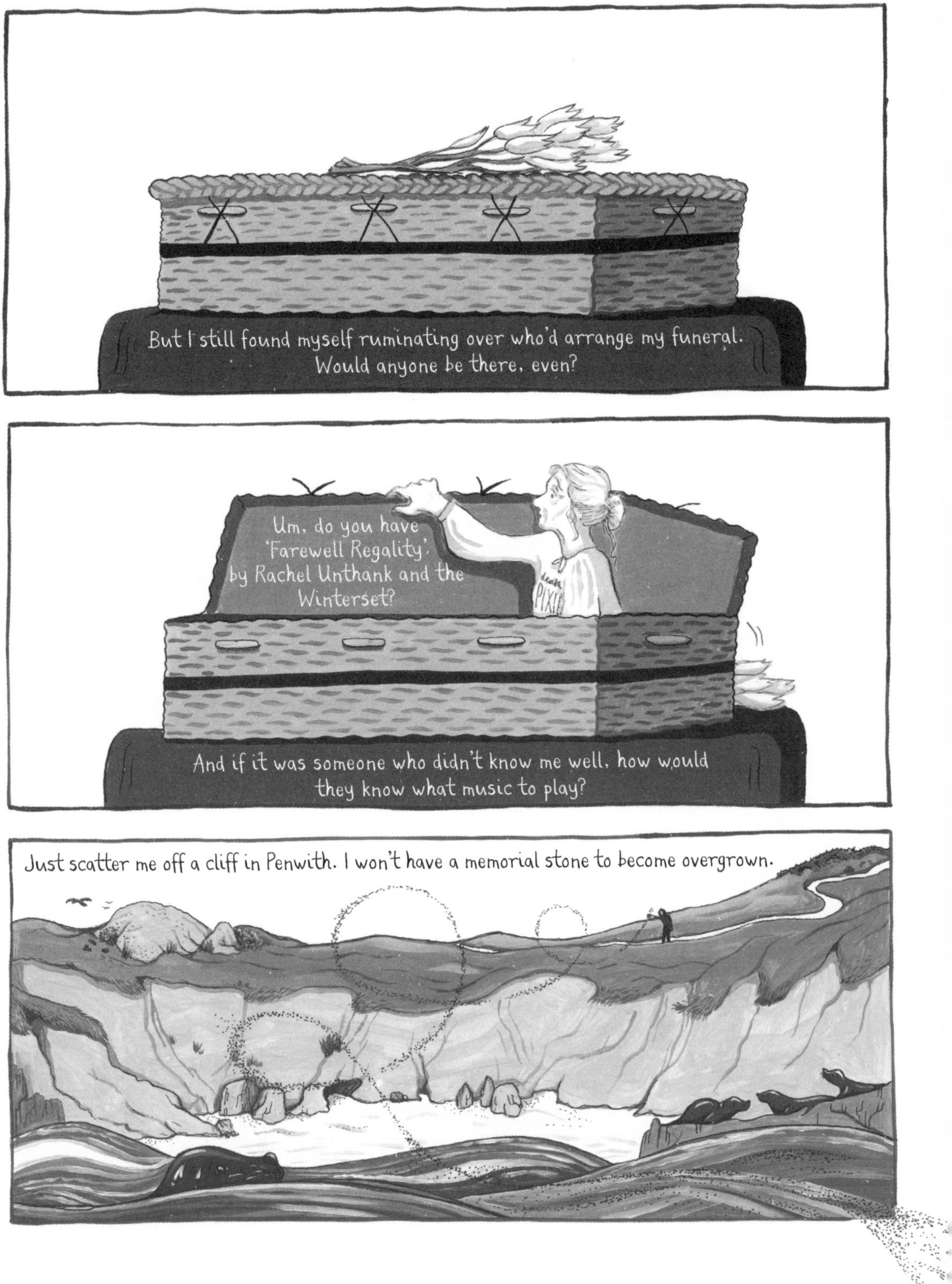
But I still found myself ruminating over who'd arrange my funeral.
Would anyone be there, even?
Um, do you have 'Farewell Regality', by Rachel Unthank and the Winterset?
And if it was someone who didn't know me well, how would they know what music to play?
Just scatter me off a cliff in Penwith. I won't have a memorial stone to become overgrown.

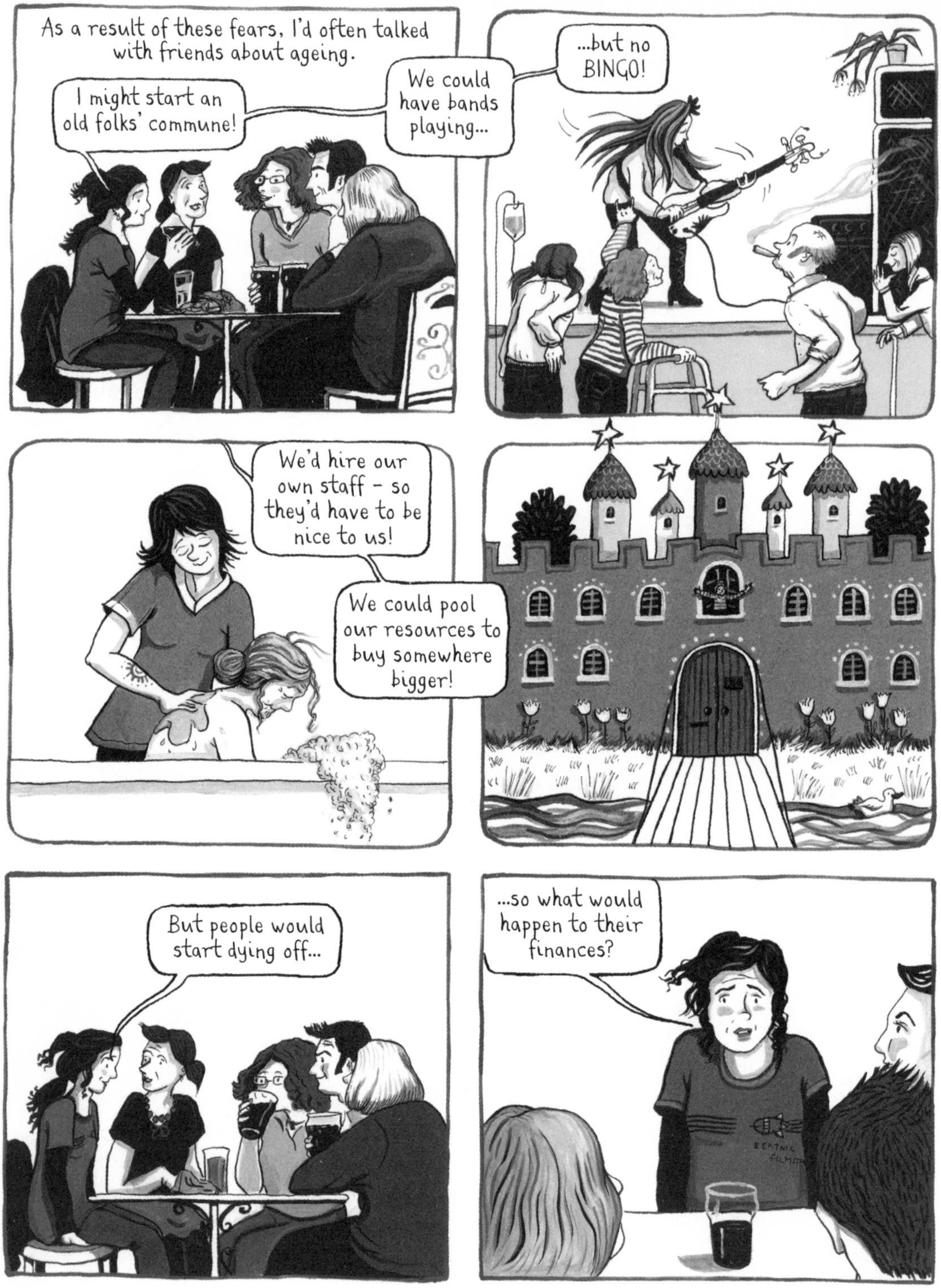
As a result of these fears, I'd often talked with friends about ageing.
I might start an old folks' commune!
We could have bands playing...
...but no BINGO!
We'd hire our own staff - so they'd have to be nice to us!
We could pool our resources to buy somewhere bigger!
But people would start dying off...
...so what would happen to their finances?

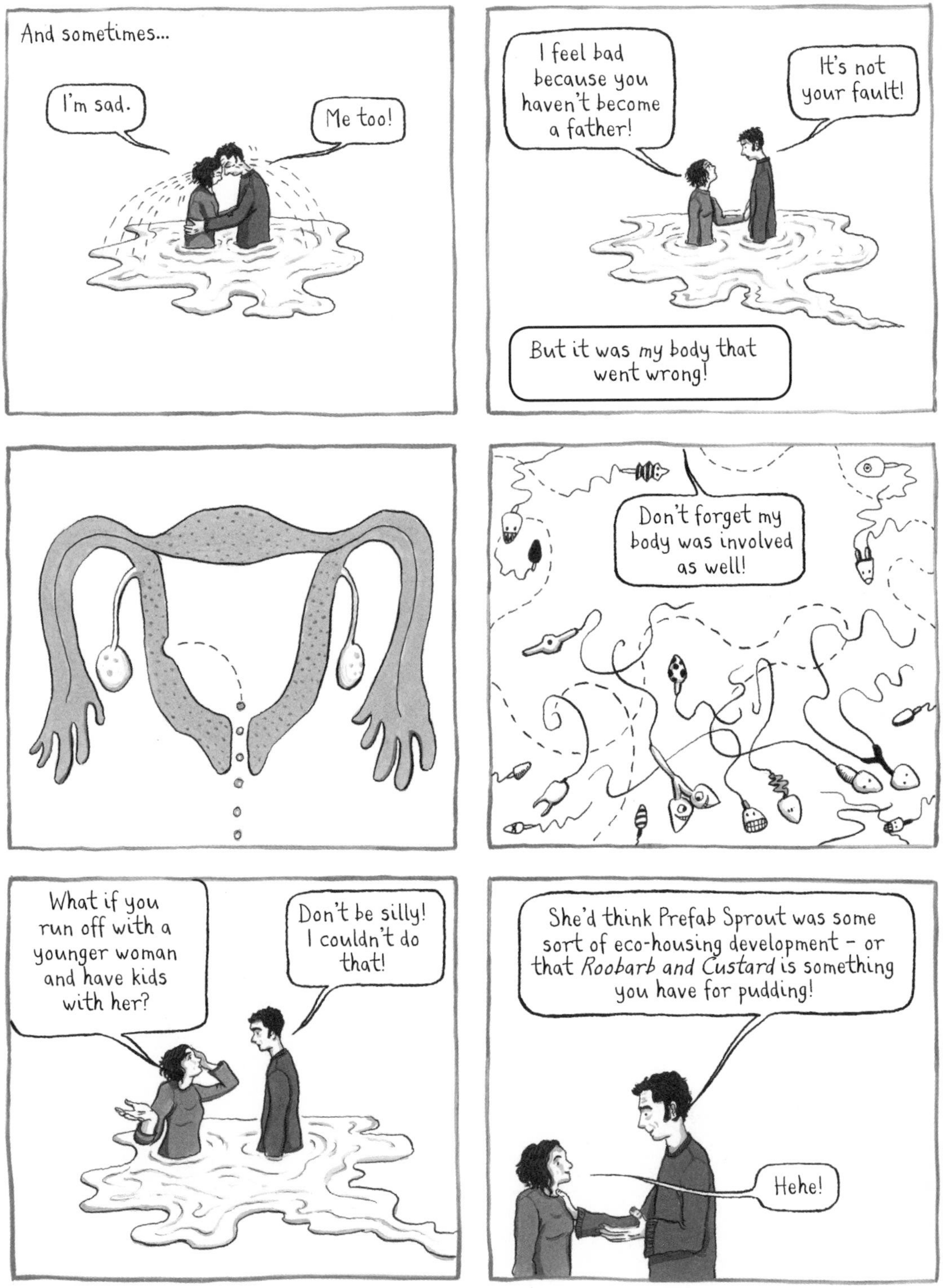
And sometimes...
I'm sad.
Me too!
I feel bad because you haven't become a father!
It's not your fault!
But it was *my* body that went wrong!
Don't forget my body was involved as well!
What if you run off with a younger woman and have kids with her?
Don't be silly! I couldn't do that!
She'd think Prefab Sprout was some sort of eco-housing development – or that *Roobarb and Custard* is something you have for pudding!
Hehe!

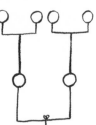

I was also sad about being the end of the line — not for my defunct genetic strain, but for lost family lore.

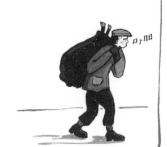

Like the one my dad told me about the black-market sheep given to my grandparents during war rationing.

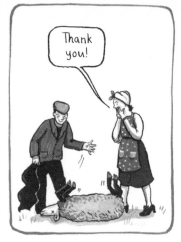

Thank you!

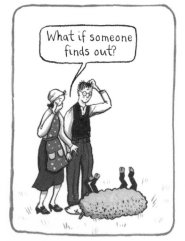

What if someone finds out?

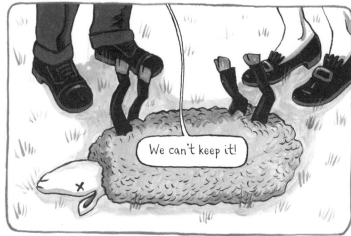

We can't keep it!

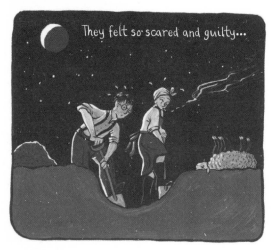

They felt so scared and guilty...

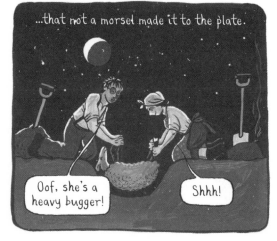

...that not a morsel made it to the plate.

Oof, she's a heavy bugger!

Shhh!

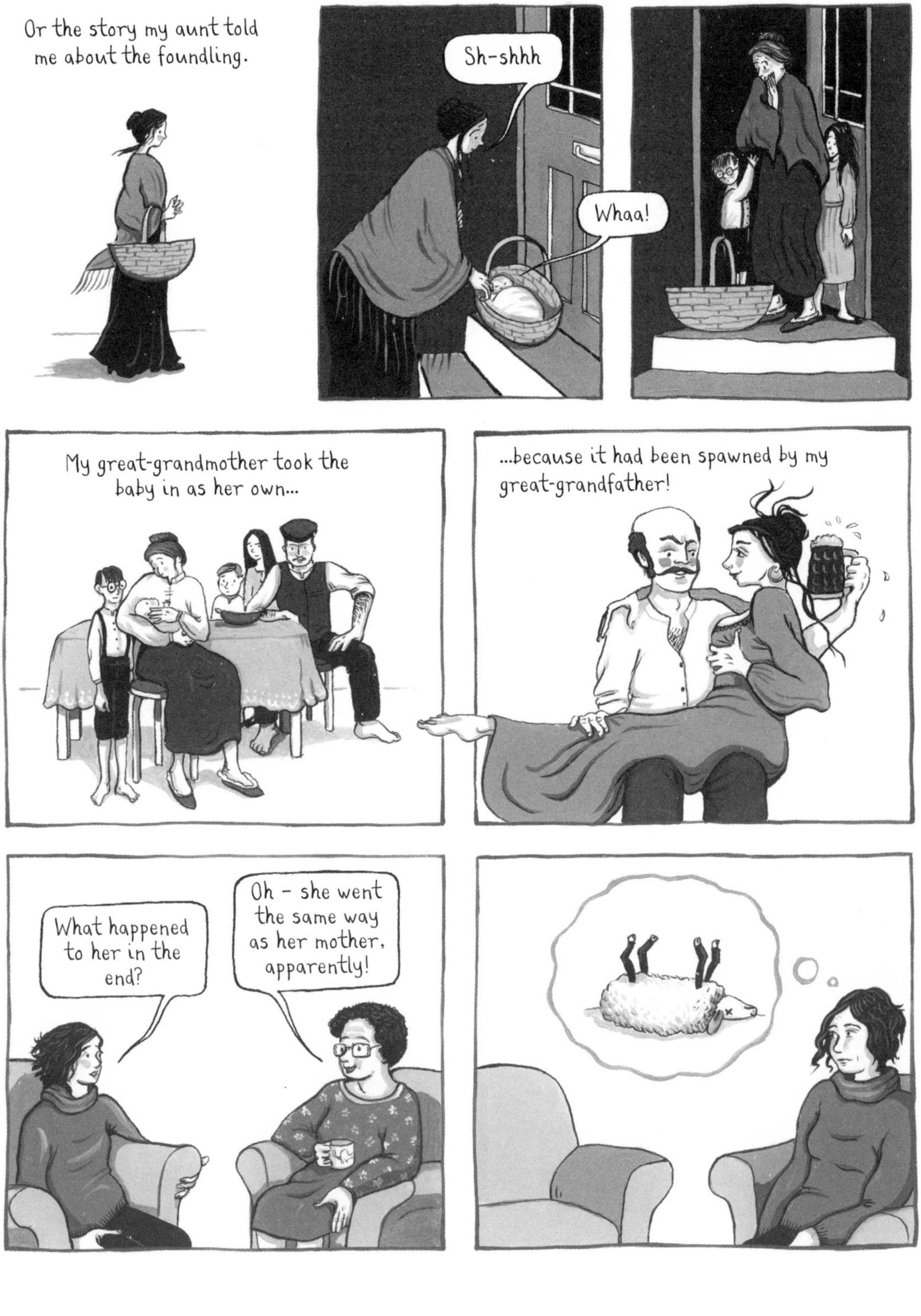
Or the story my aunt told me about the foundling.
Sh-shhh
Whaa!
My great-grandmother took the baby in as her own...
...because it had been spawned by my great-grandfather!
What happened to her in the end?
Oh - she went the same way as her mother, apparently!

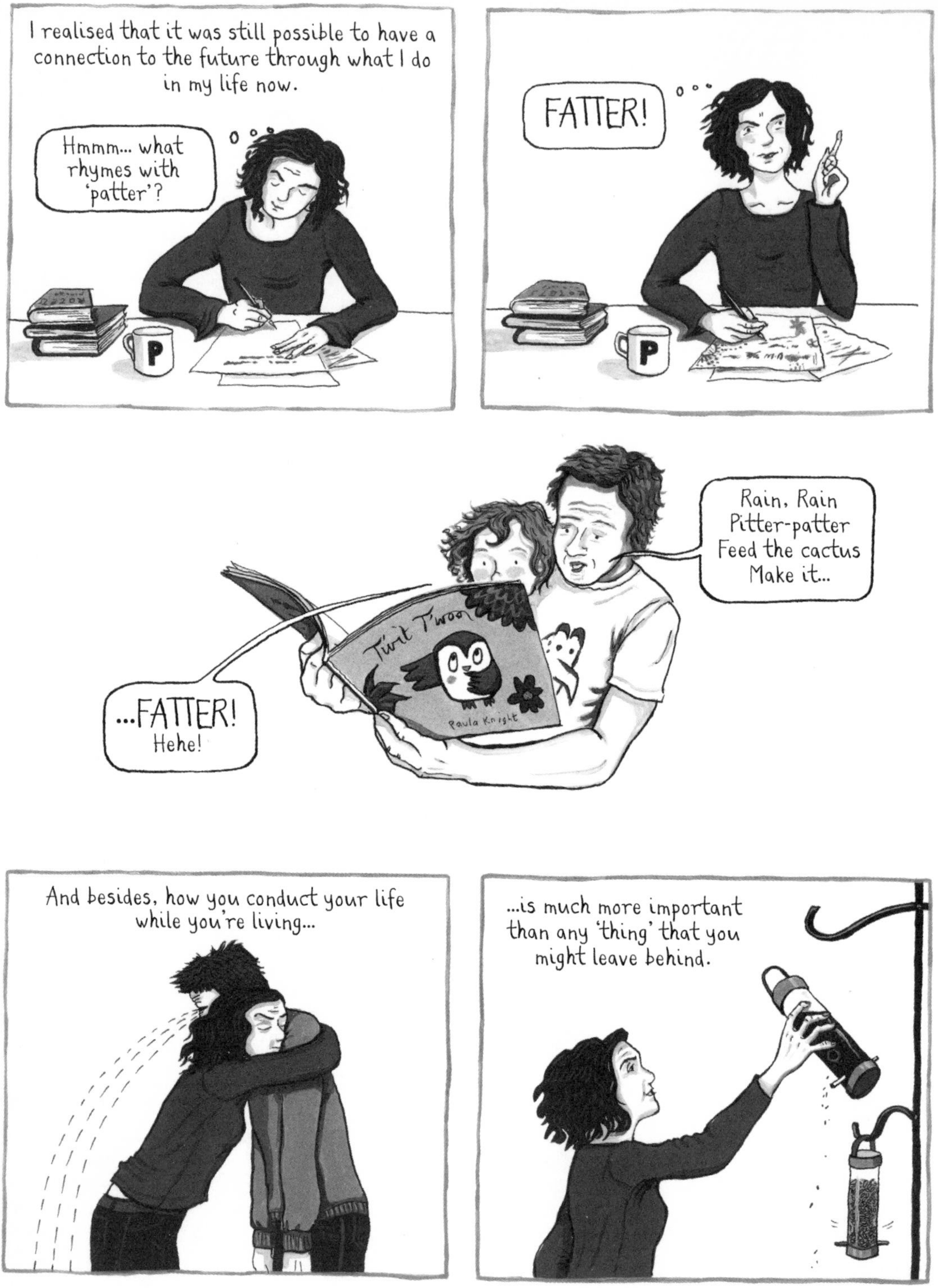
I realised that it was still possible to have a connection to the future through what I do in my life now.
Hmmm... what rhymes with 'patter'?
FATTER!
Rain, Rain
Pitter-patter
Feed the cactus
Make it...
...FATTER!
Hehe!
Twit T'woo
Paula Knight
And besides, how you conduct your life while you're living...
...is much more important than any 'thing' that you might leave behind.

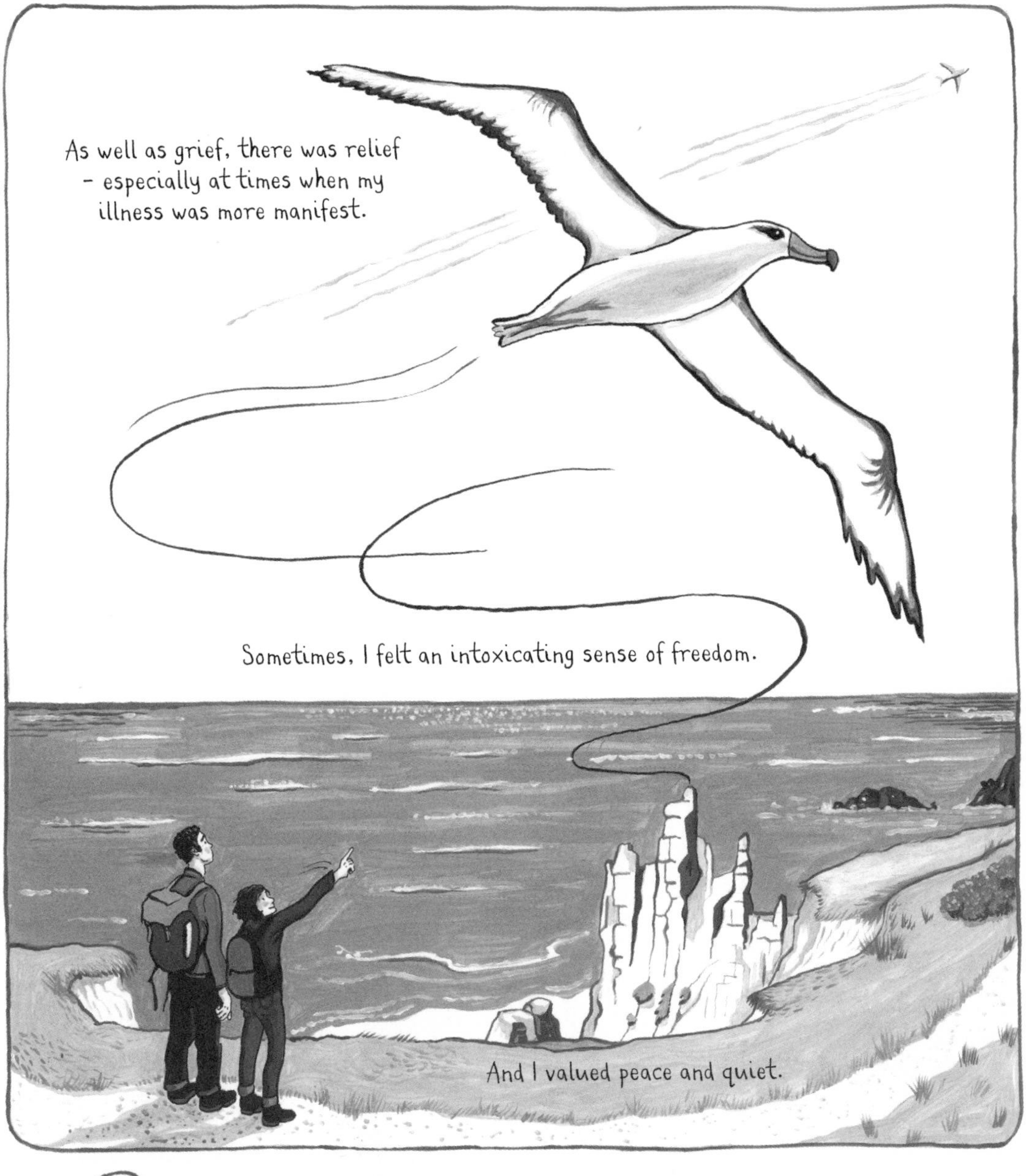
As well as grief, there was relief - especially at times when my illness was more manifest.
Sometimes, I felt an intoxicating sense of freedom.
And I valued peace and quiet.

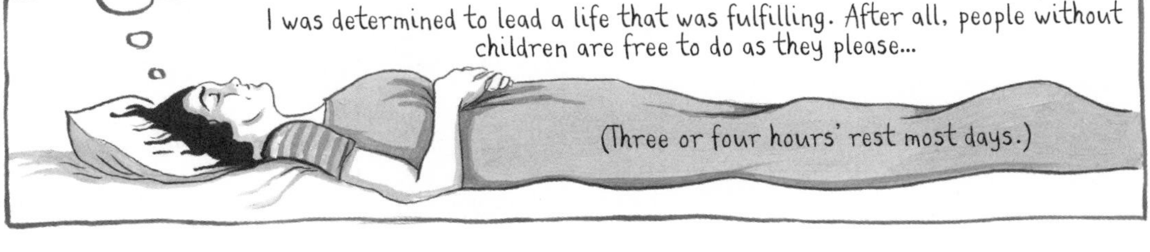
I was determined to lead a life that was fulfilling. After all, people without children are free to do as they please...
(Three or four hours' rest most days.)

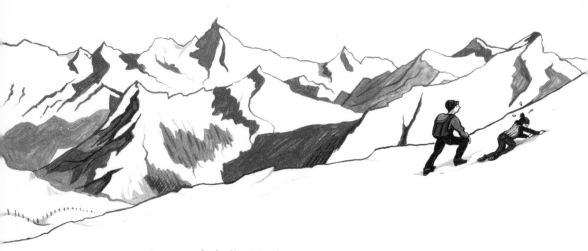

Compared to to the life I had envisaged, mine did feel empty
at times, but it wasn't the lack of a baby that made it so;
it was the lack of full health.

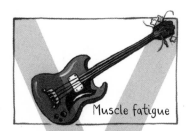

Muscle fatigue

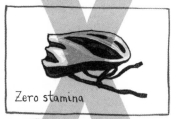

Zero stamina

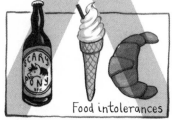

Food intolerances

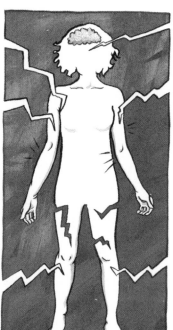

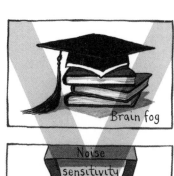

Brain fog

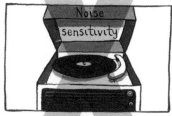

Noise sensitivity

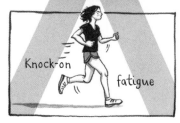

Knock-on

fatigue

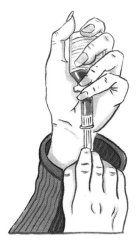

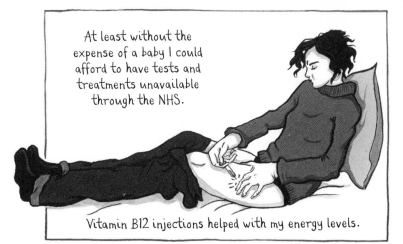

At least without the expense of a baby I could afford to have tests and treatments unavailable through the NHS.

Vitamin B12 injections helped with my energy levels.

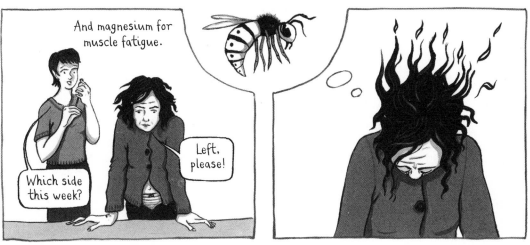

And magnesium for muscle fatigue.

Which side this week?

Left, please!

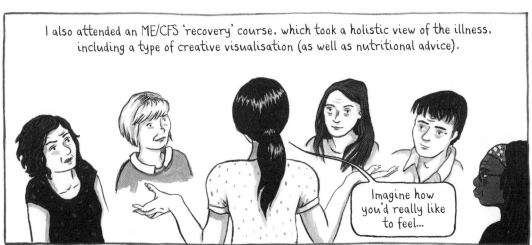

I also attended an ME/CFS 'recovery' course, which took a holistic view of the illness, including a type of creative visualisation (as well as nutritional advice).

Imagine how you'd really like to feel...

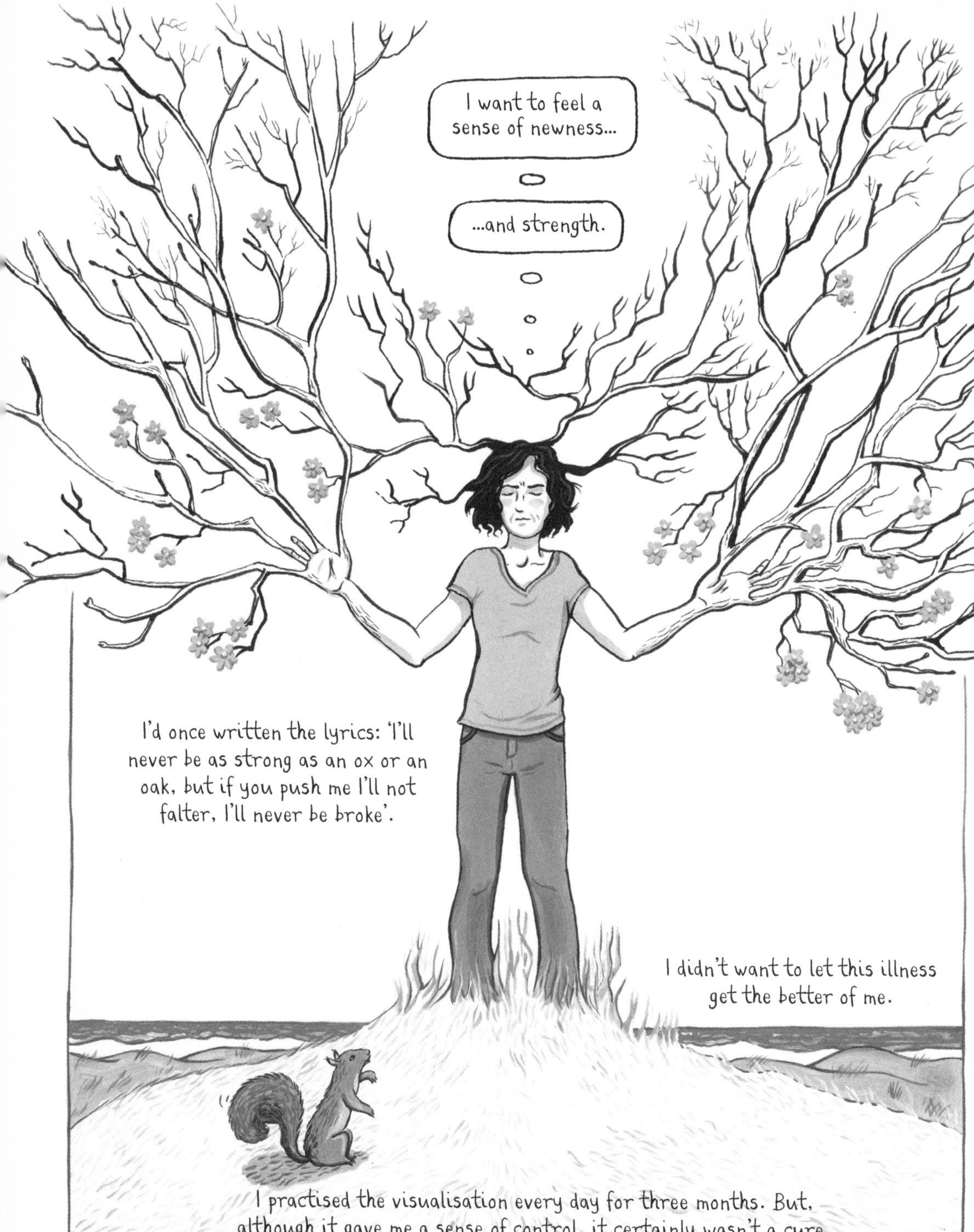
I want to feel a sense of newness...
...and strength.
I'd once written the lyrics: 'I'll never be as strong as an ox or an oak, but if you push me I'll not falter, I'll never be broke'.
I didn't want to let this illness get the better of me.
I practised the visualisation every day for three months. But, although it gave me a sense of control, it certainly wasn't a cure.

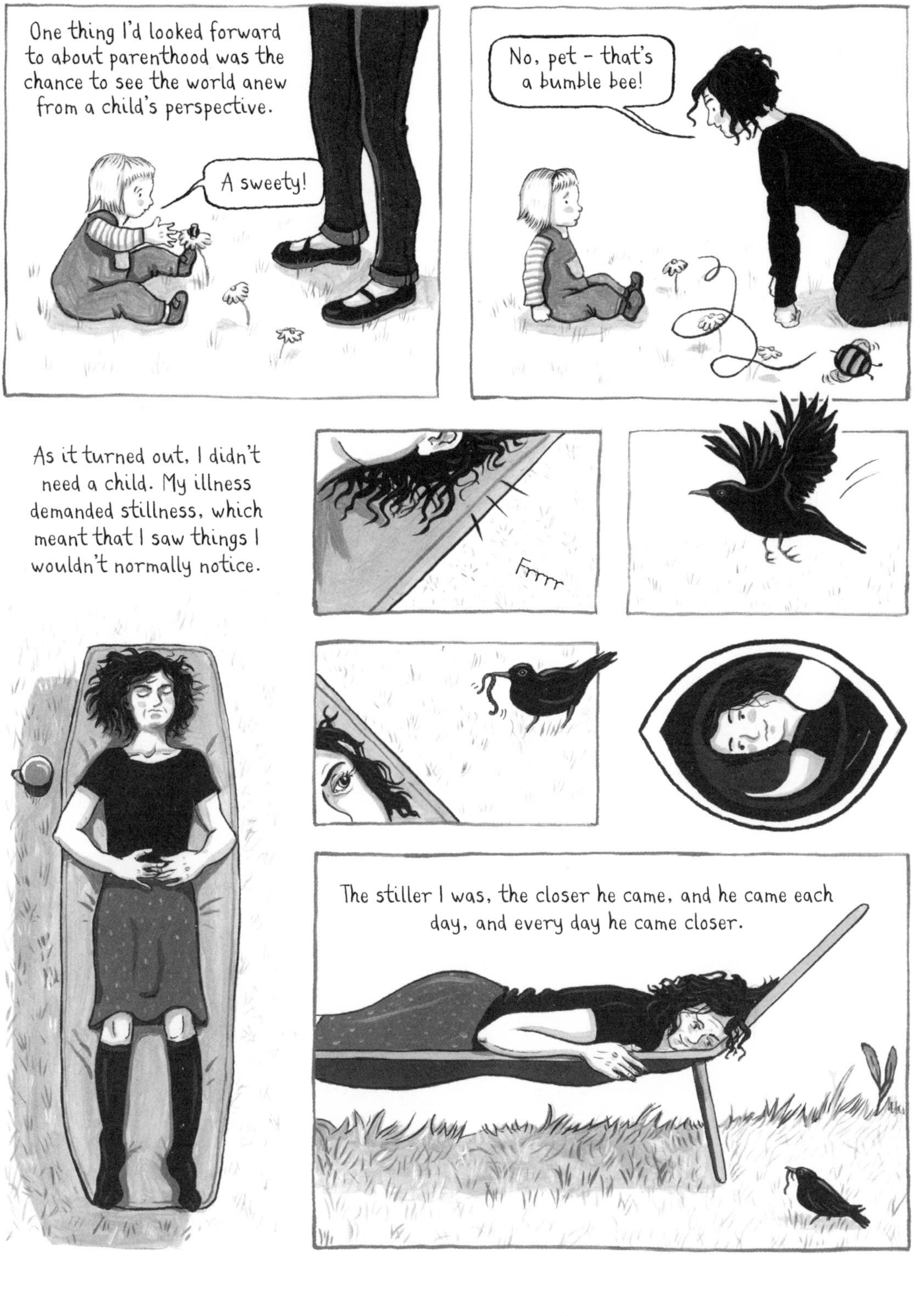
One thing I'd looked forward to about parenthood was the chance to see the world anew from a child's perspective.
A sweety!
No, pet - that's a bumble bee!
As it turned out, I didn't need a child. My illness demanded stillness, which meant that I saw things I wouldn't normally notice.
Frrrr
The stiller I was, the closer he came, and he came each day, and every day he came closer.

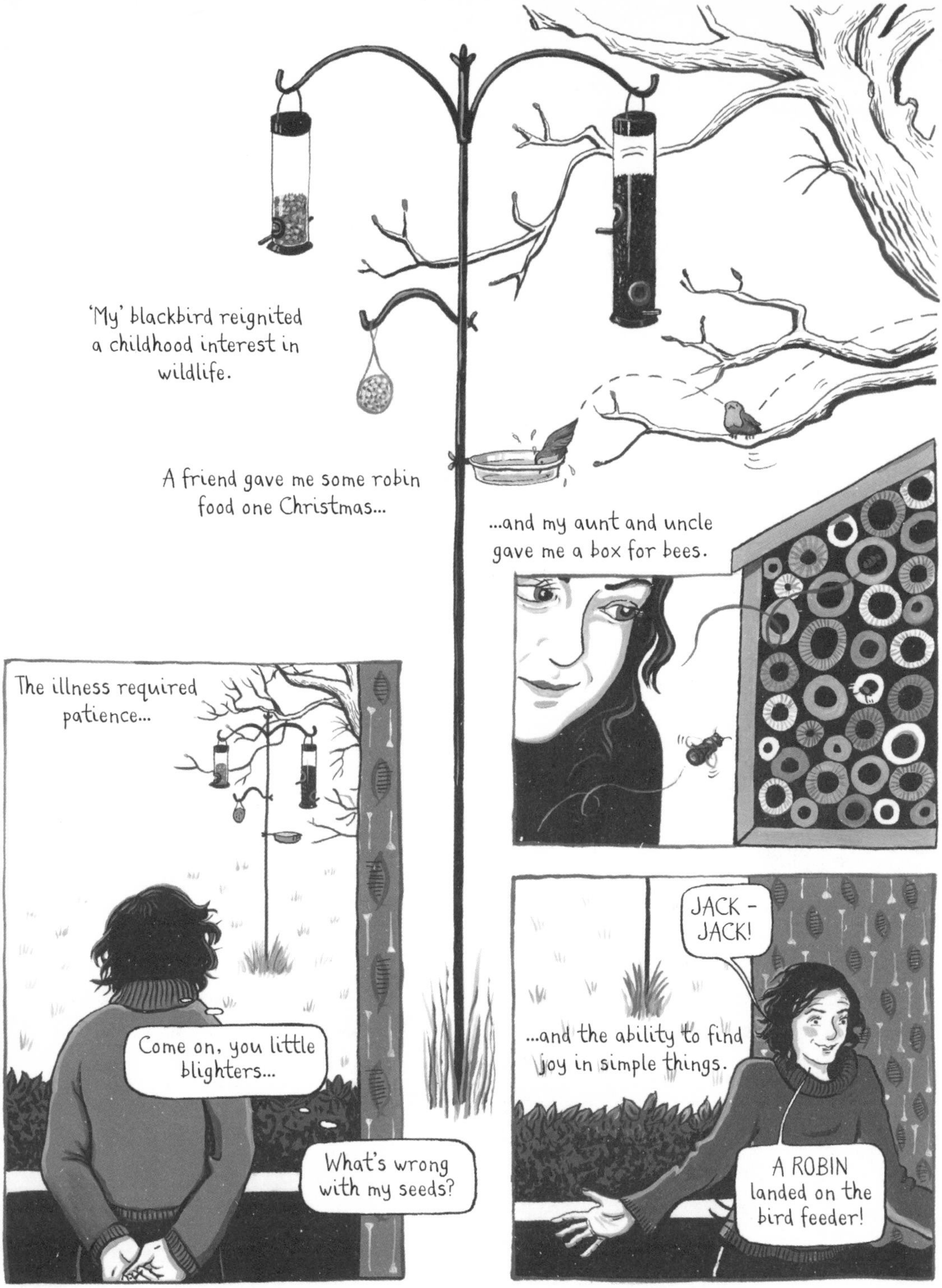
'My' blackbird reignited a childhood interest in wildlife.
A friend gave me some robin food one Christmas...
...and my aunt and uncle gave me a box for bees.
The illness required patience...
Come on, you little blighters...
What's wrong with my seeds?
JACK - JACK!
...and the ability to find joy in simple things.
A ROBIN landed on the bird feeder!

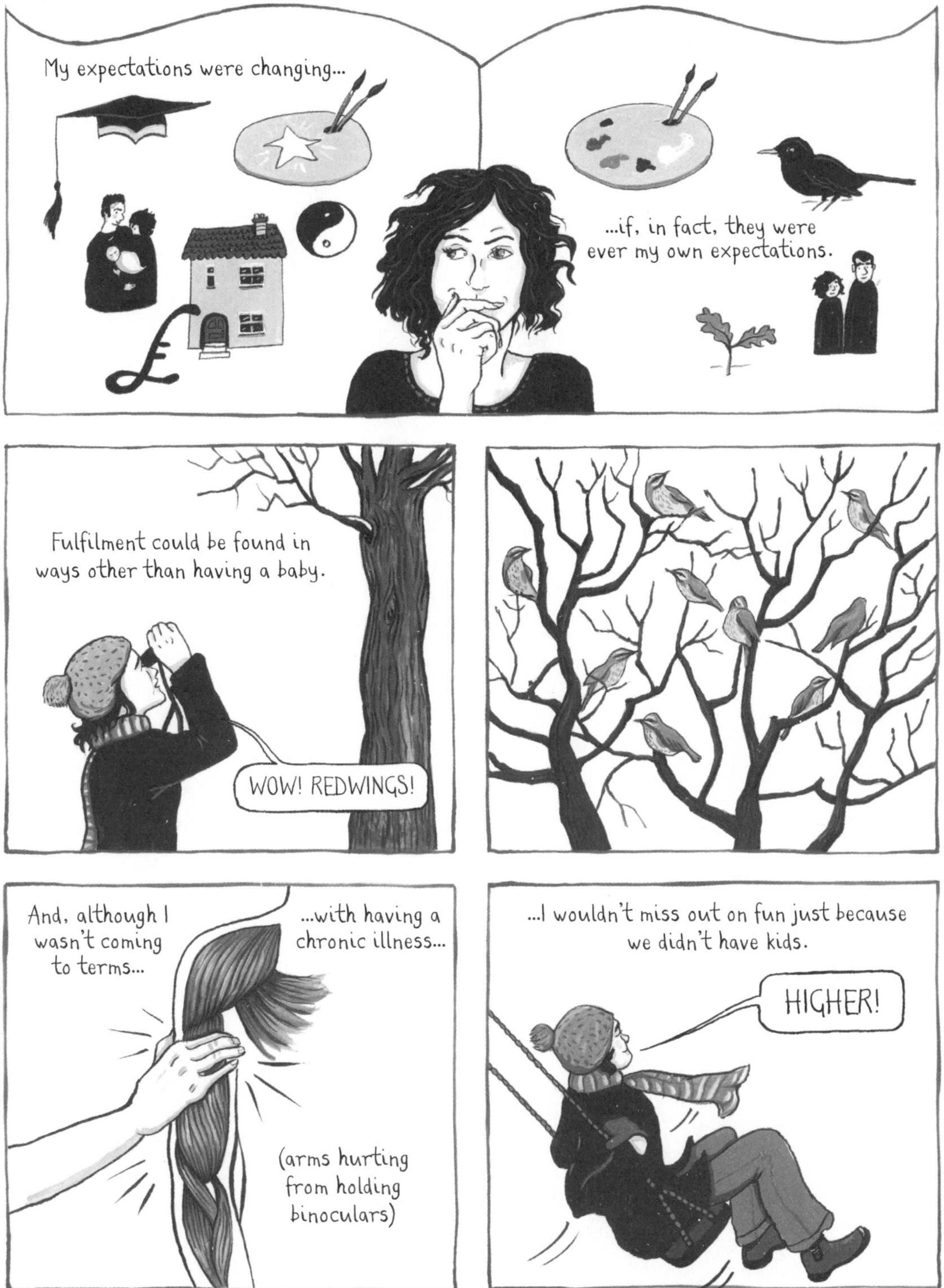
My expectations were changing...
...if, in fact, they were ever my own expectations.
Fulfilment could be found in ways other than having a baby.
WOW! REDWINGS!
And, although I wasn't coming to terms...
...with having a chronic illness...
(arms hurting from holding binoculars)
...I wouldn't miss out on fun just because we didn't have kids.
HIGHER!

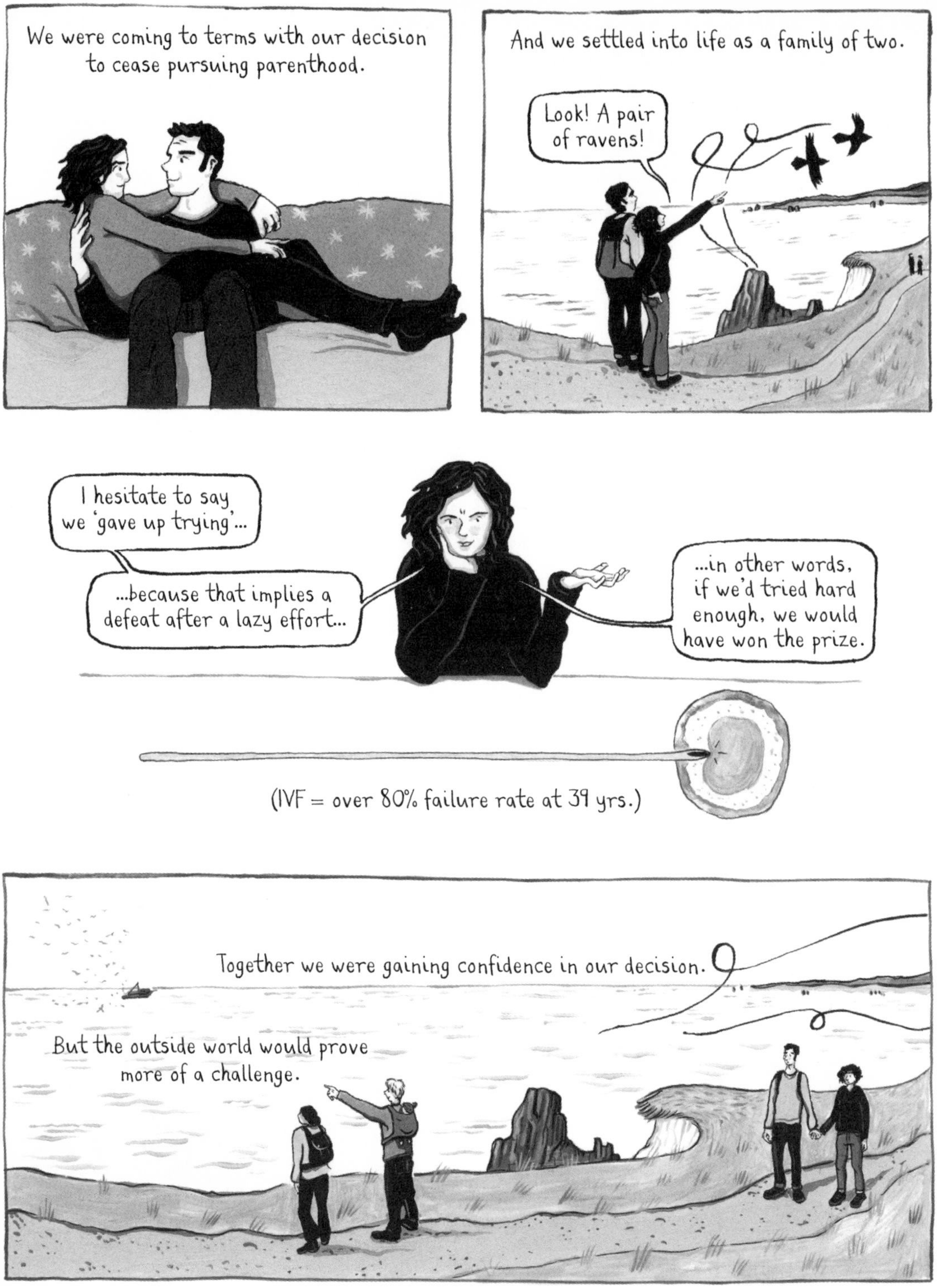
We were coming to terms with our decision to cease pursuing parenthood.
And we settled into life as a family of two.
Look! A pair of ravens!
I hesitate to say we 'gave up trying'...
...because that implies a defeat after a lazy effort...
...in other words, if we'd tried hard enough, we would have won the prize.
(IVF = over 80% failure rate at 39 yrs.)
Together we were gaining confidence in our decision.
But the outside world would prove more of a challenge.

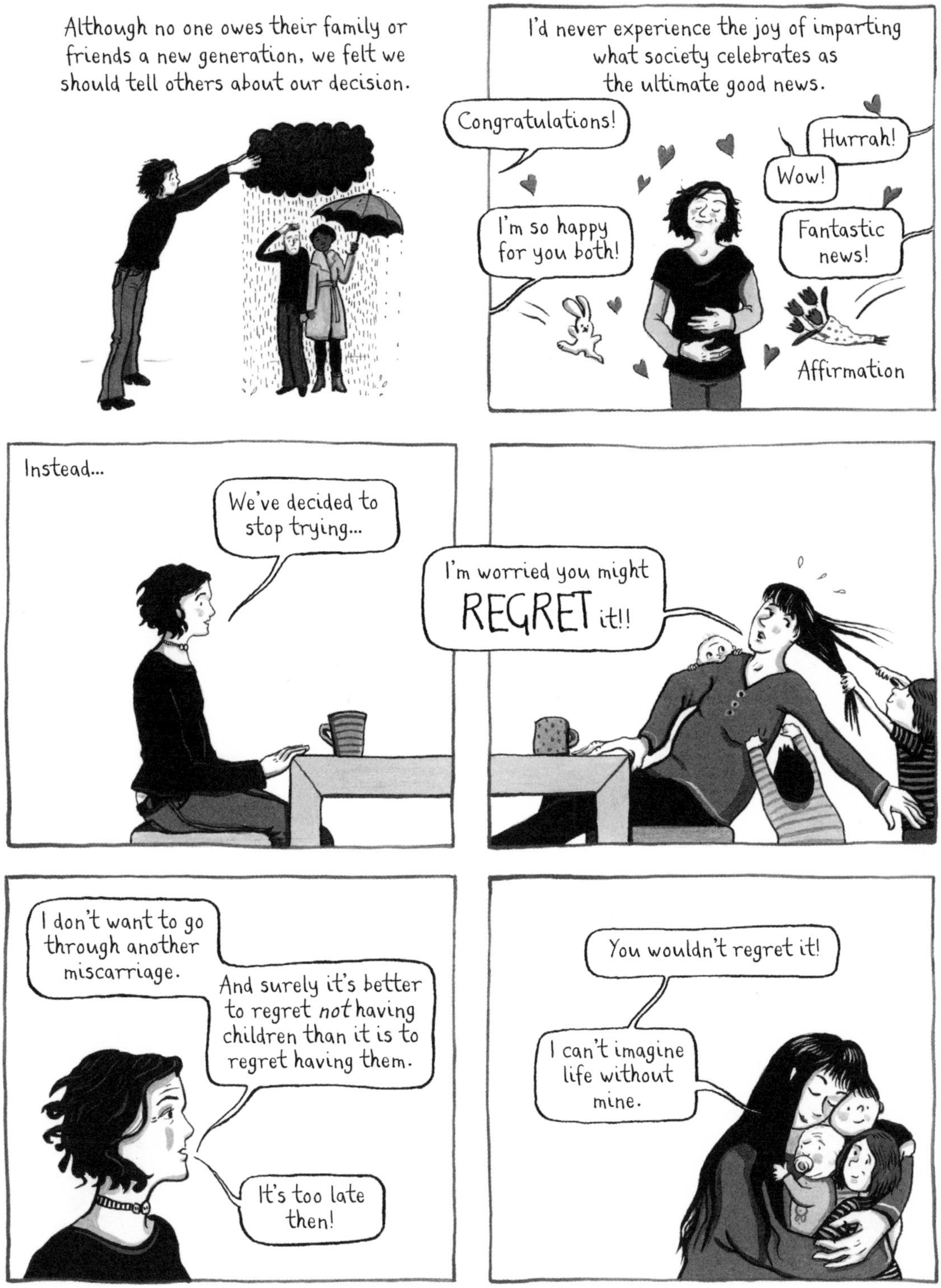
Although no one owes their family or friends a new generation, we felt we should tell others about our decision.
I'd never experience the joy of imparting what society celebrates as the ultimate good news.
Congratulations!
I'm so happy for you both!
Hurrah!
Wow!
Fantastic news!
Affirmation
Instead...
We've decided to stop trying...
I'm worried you might REGRET it!!
I don't want to go through another miscarriage.
And surely it's better to regret *not* having children than it is to regret having them.
It's too late then!
You wouldn't regret it!
I can't imagine life without mine.

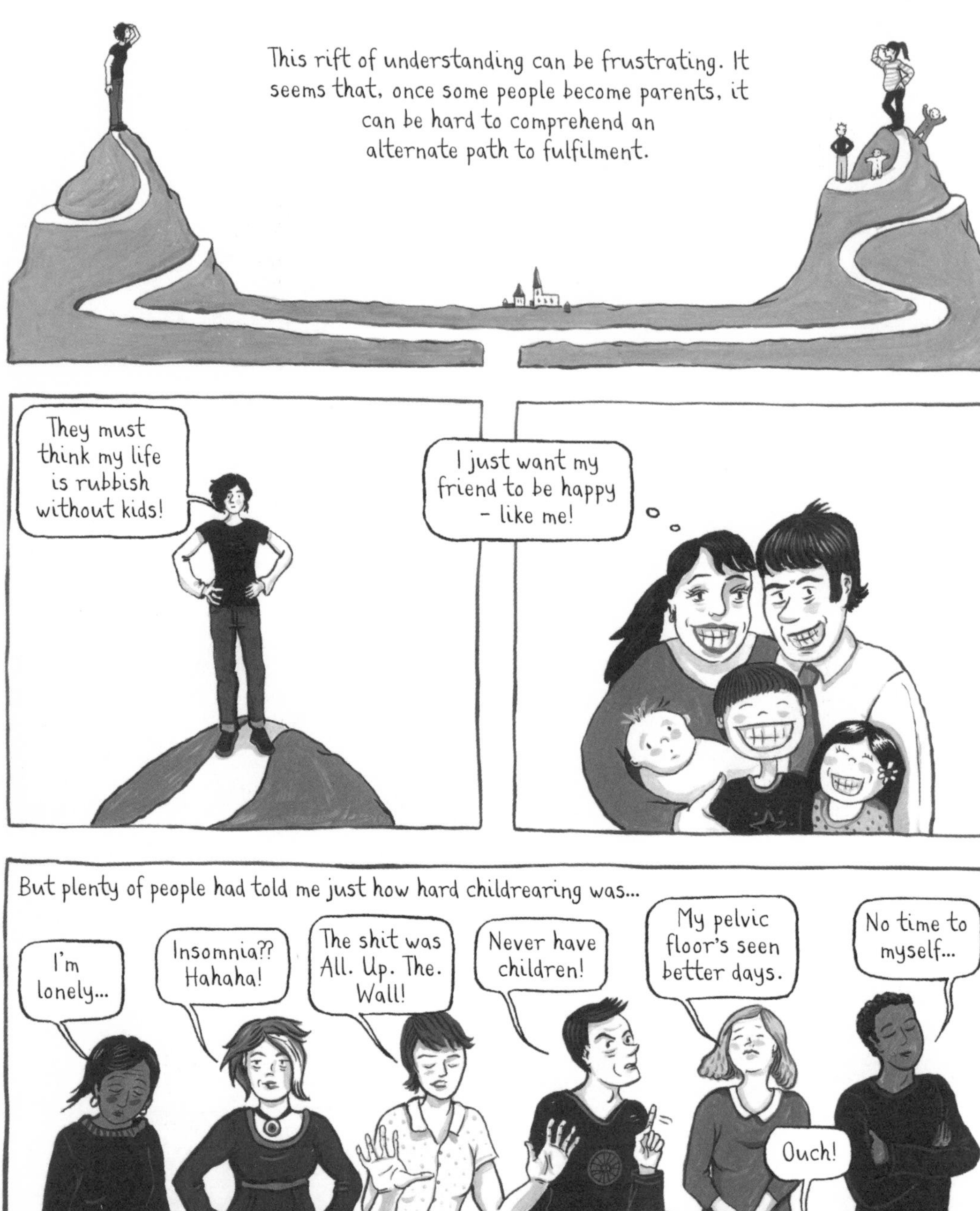
This rift of understanding can be frustrating. It seems that, once some people become parents, it can be hard to comprehend an alternate path to fulfilment.
They must think my life is rubbish without kids!
I just want my friend to be happy – like me!
But plenty of people had told me just how hard childrearing was...
I'm lonely...
Insomnia?? Hahaha!
The shit was All. Up. The. Wall!
Oh no!
Never have children!
OK...
My pelvic floor's seen better days.
Ouch!
No time to myself...

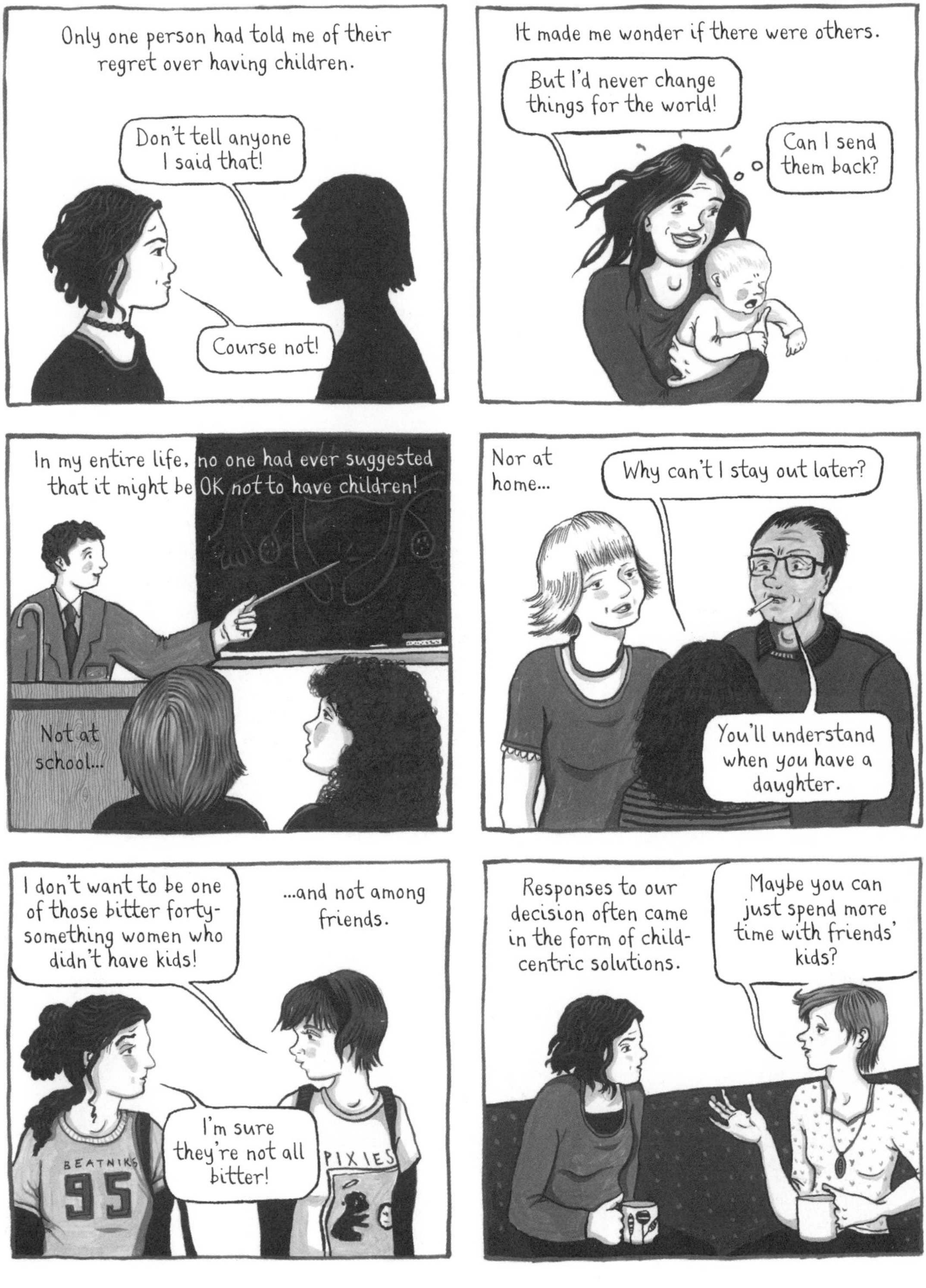
Only one person had told me of their regret over having children.
Don't tell anyone I said that!
Course not!
It made me wonder if there were others.
But I'd never change things for the world!
Can I send them back?
In my entire life, no one had ever suggested that it might be OK not to have children!
Not at school...
Nor at home...
Why can't I stay out later?
You'll understand when you have a daughter.
I don't want to be one of those bitter forty-something women who didn't have kids!
...and not among friends.
I'm sure they're not all bitter!
BEATNIKS
95
PIXIES
Responses to our decision often came in the form of child-centric solutions.
Maybe you can just spend more time with friends' kids?

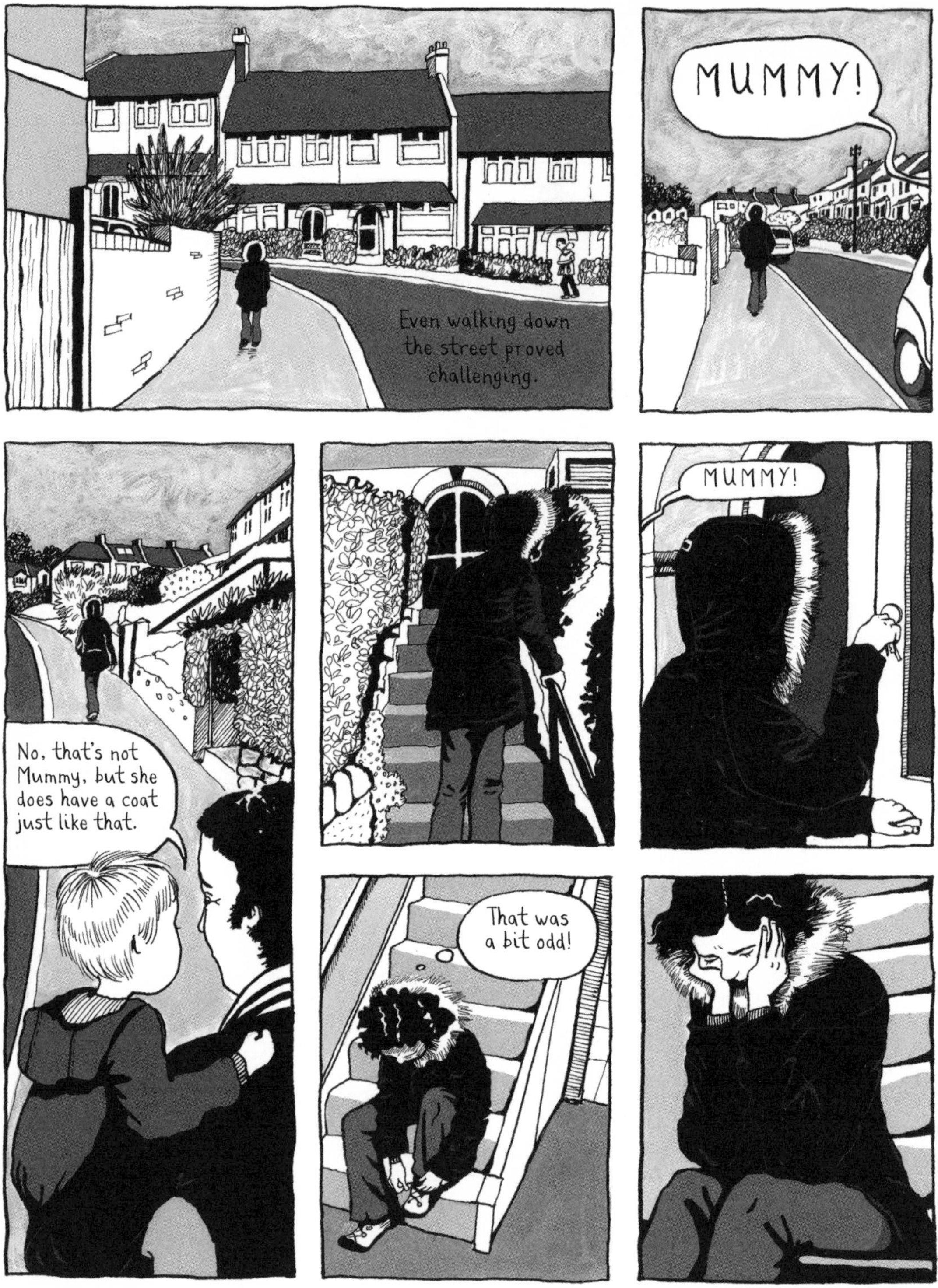

Even walking down the street proved challenging.
MUMMY!
MUMMY!
No, that's not Mummy, but she does have a coat just like that.
That was a bit odd!

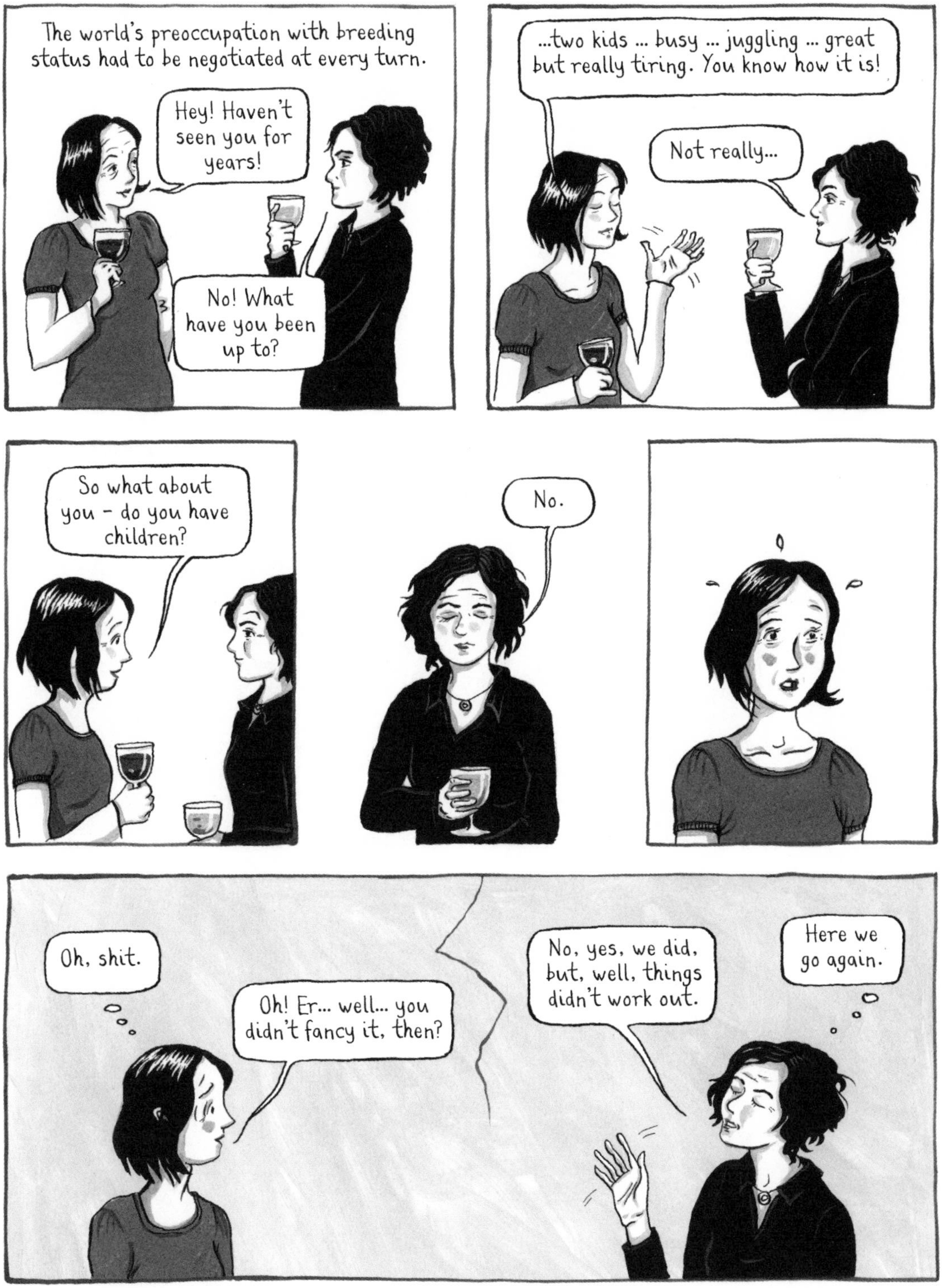

The world's preoccupation with breeding status had to be negotiated at every turn.
Hey! Haven't seen you for years!
No! What have you been up to?
...two kids ... busy ... juggling ... great but really tiring. You know how it is!
Not really...
So what about you - do you have children?
No.
Oh, shit.
Oh! Er... well... you didn't fancy it, then?
No, yes, we did, but, well, things didn't work out.
Here we go again.

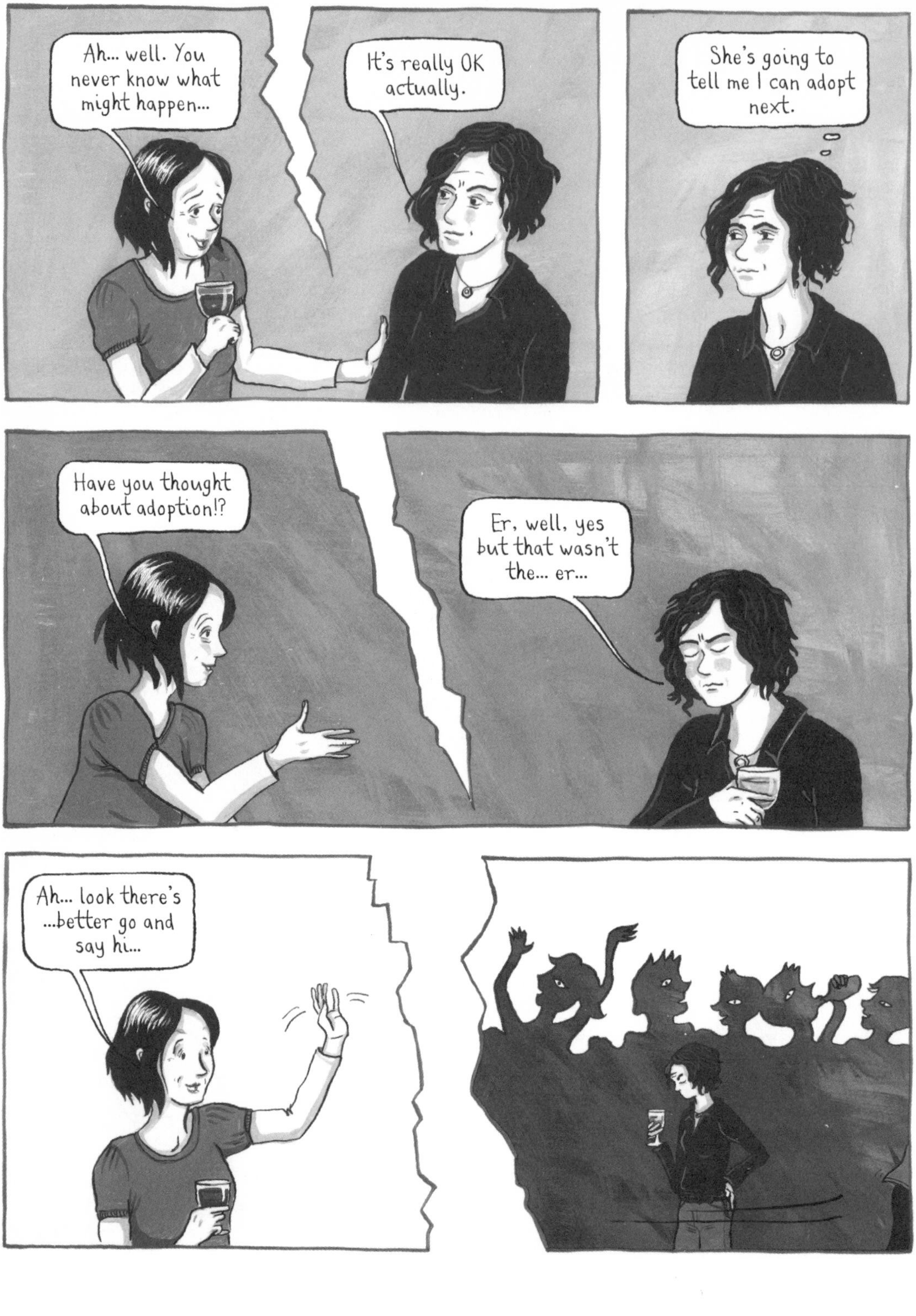
Ah... well. You never know what might happen...
It's really OK actually.
She's going to tell me I can adopt next.
Have you thought about adoption!?
Er, well, yes but that wasn't the... er...
Ah... look there's ...better go and say hi...

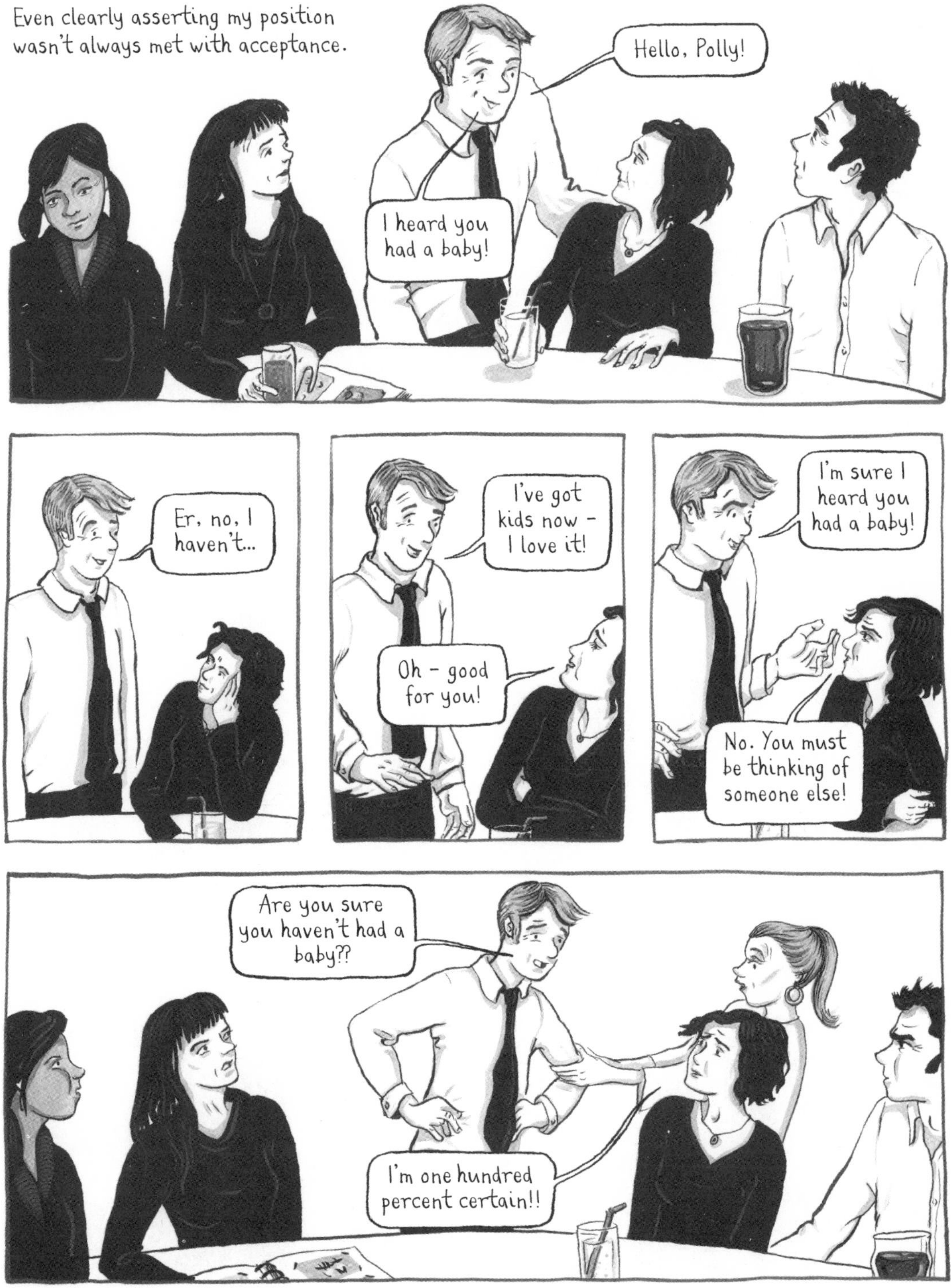
Even clearly asserting my position wasn't always met with acceptance.
Hello, Polly!
I heard you had a baby!
Er, no, I haven't...
I've got kids now - I love it!
Oh - good for you!
I'm sure I heard you had a baby!
No. You must be thinking of someone else!
Are you sure you haven't had a baby??
I'm one hundred percent certain!!

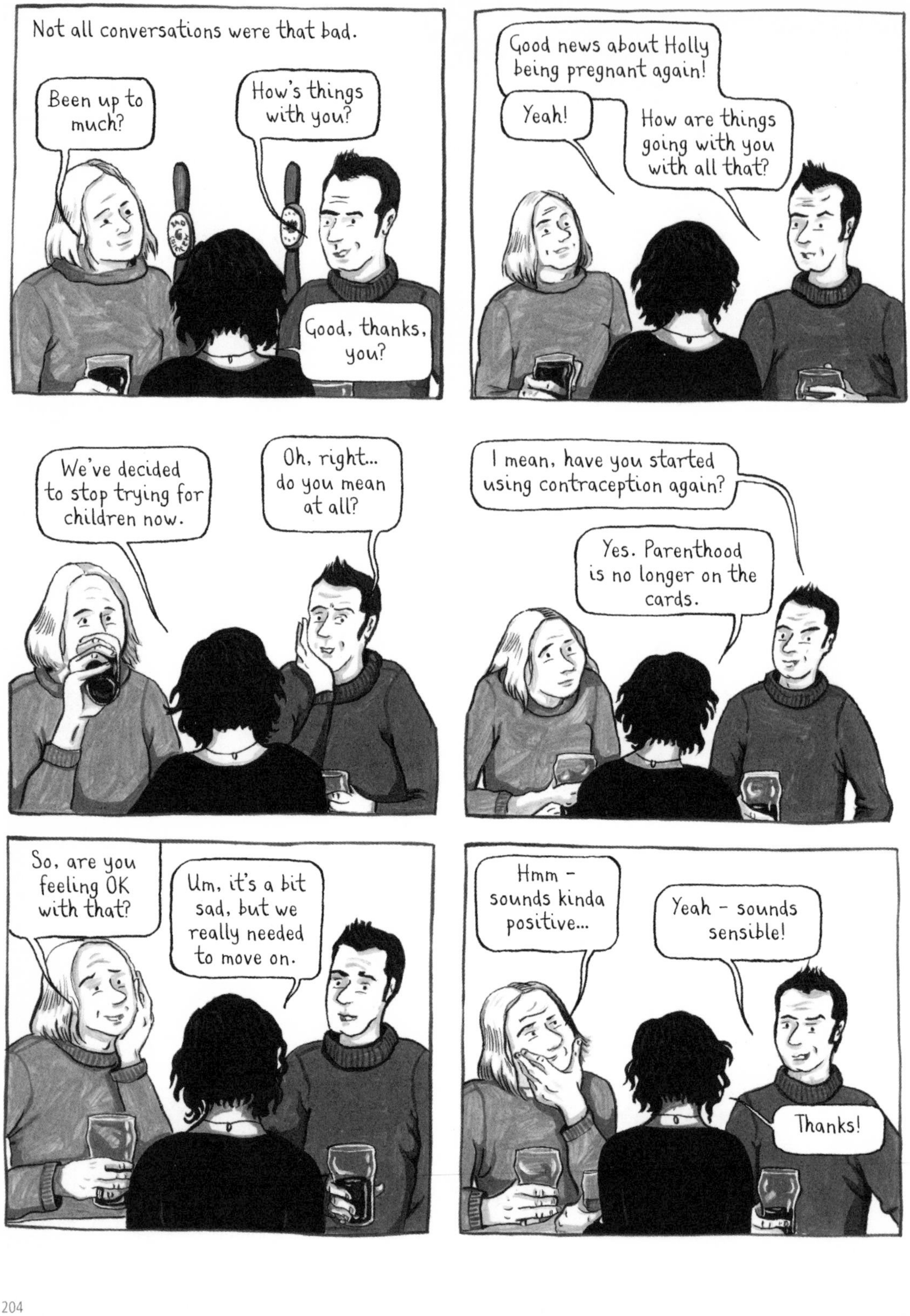
Not all conversations were that bad.
Been up to much?
How's things with you?
Good, thanks, you?
Good news about Holly being pregnant again!
Yeah!
How are things going with you with all that?
We've decided to stop trying for children now.
Oh, right... do you mean at all?
I mean, have you started using contraception again?
Yes. Parenthood is no longer on the cards.
So, are you feeling OK with that?
Um, it's a bit sad, but we really needed to move on.
Hmm - sounds kinda positive...
Yeah - sounds sensible!
Thanks!

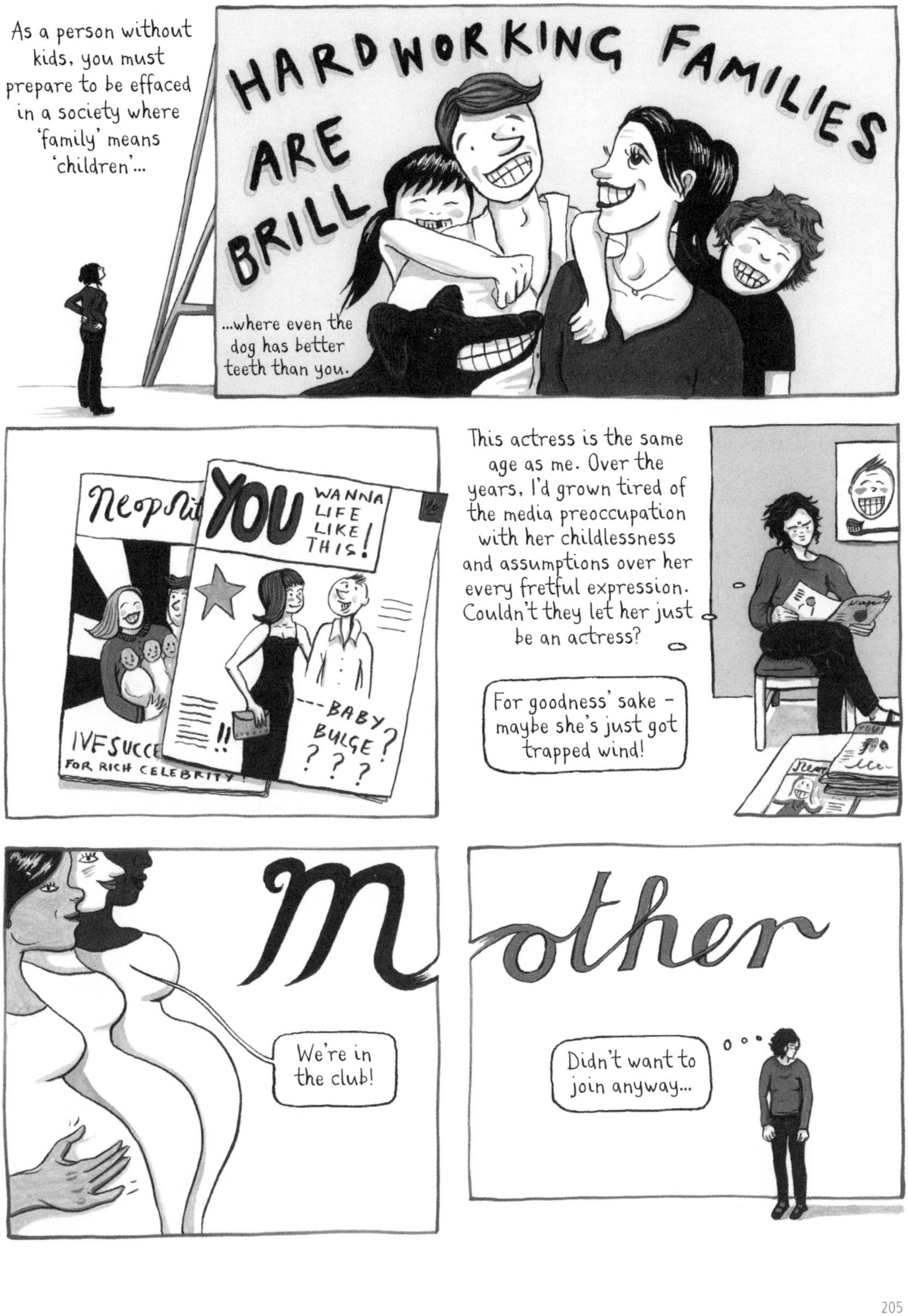

As a person without kids, you must prepare to be effaced in a society where 'family' means 'children'...
HARDWORKING FAMILIES ARE BRILL
...where even the dog has better teeth than you.
Neop
YOU WANNA LIFE LIKE THIS!
IVF SUCC
FOR RICH CELEBRITY!
BABY BULGE? ???
This actress is the same age as me. Over the years, I'd grown tired of the media preoccupation with her childlessness and assumptions over her every fretful expression. Couldn't they let her just be an actress?
For goodness' sake - maybe she's just got trapped wind!
Mother
We're in the club!
Didn't want to join anyway...

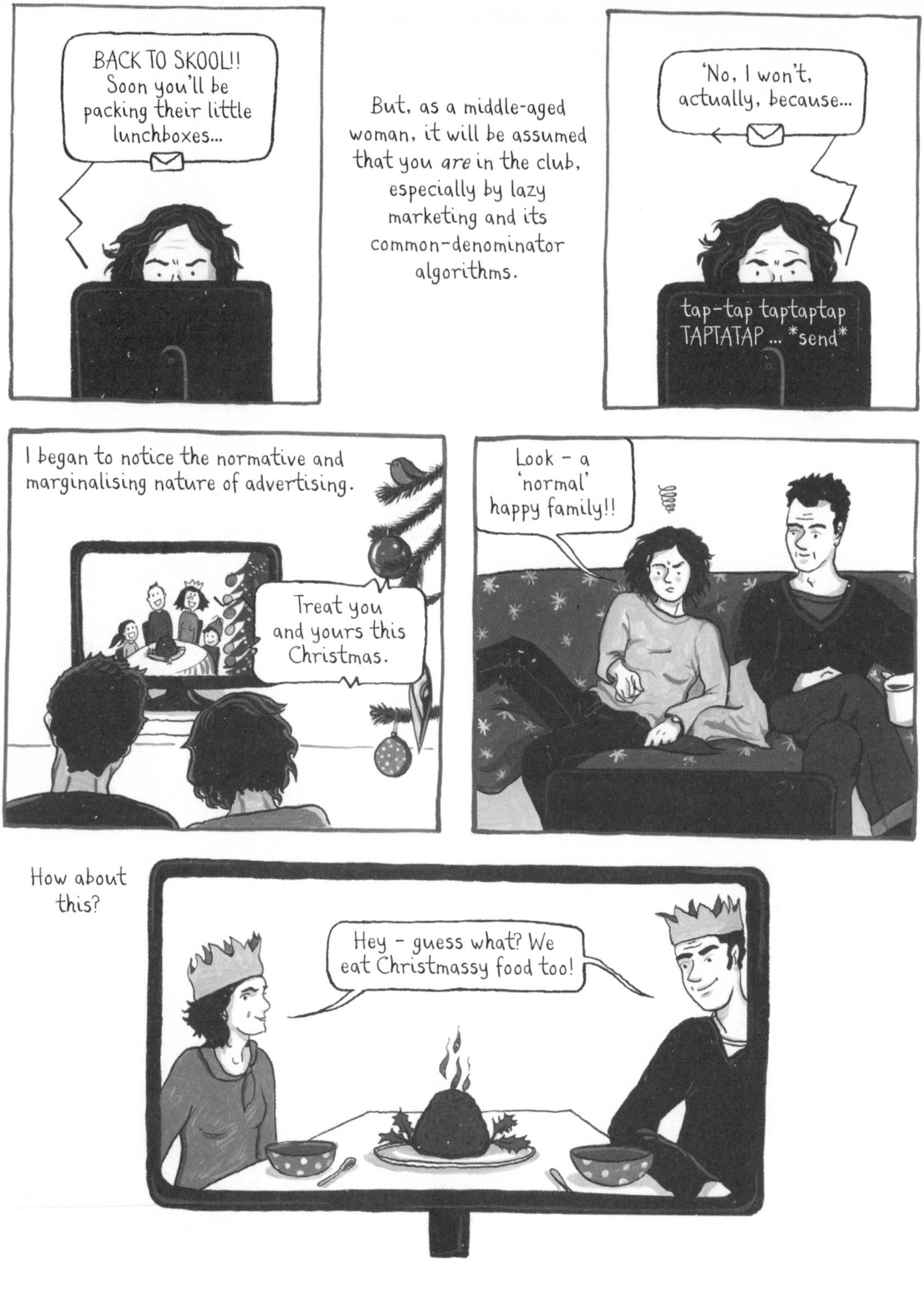
BACK TO SKOOL!! Soon you'll be packing their little lunchboxes...
But, as a middle-aged woman, it will be assumed that you *are* in the club, especially by lazy marketing and its common-denominator algorithms.
'No, I won't, actually, because...
tap-tap taptaptap TAPTATAP ... *send*
I began to notice the normative and marginalising nature of advertising.
Treat you and yours this Christmas.
Look – a 'normal' happy family!!
How about this?
Hey – guess what? We eat Christmassy food too!

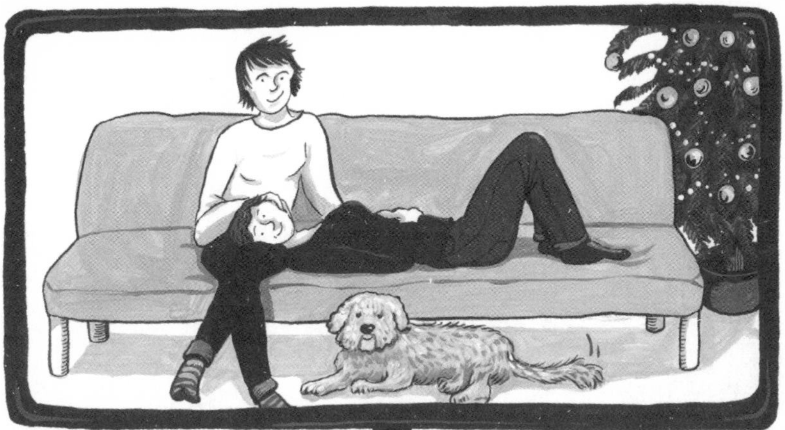

Or this?

(Oops, silly me – Christmas is all about the children...)

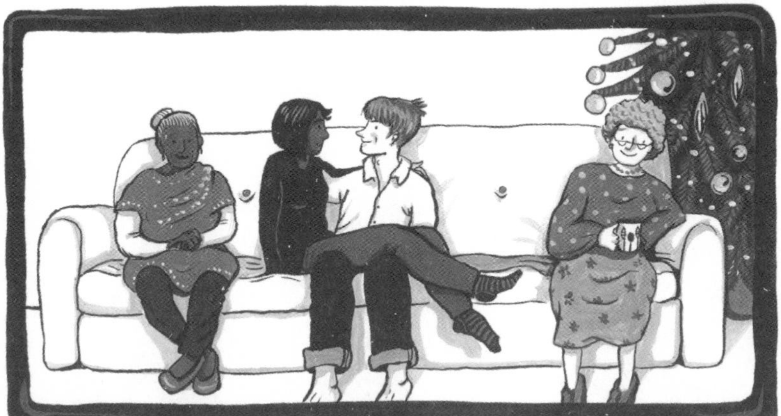

Or this?

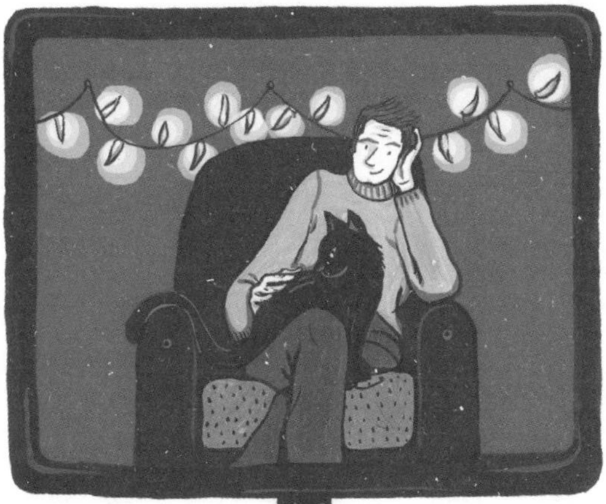

Or this?

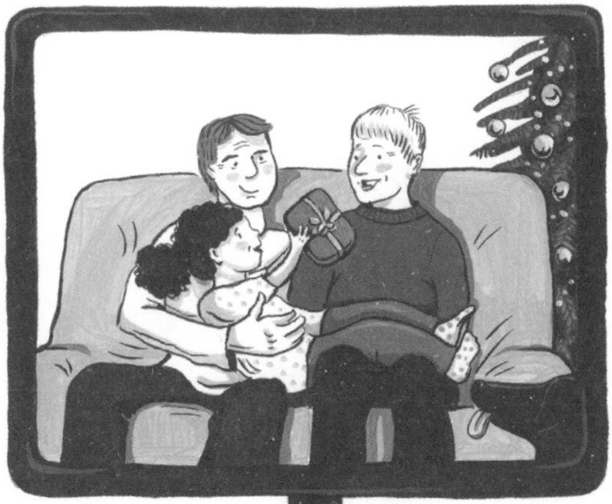

Or this?

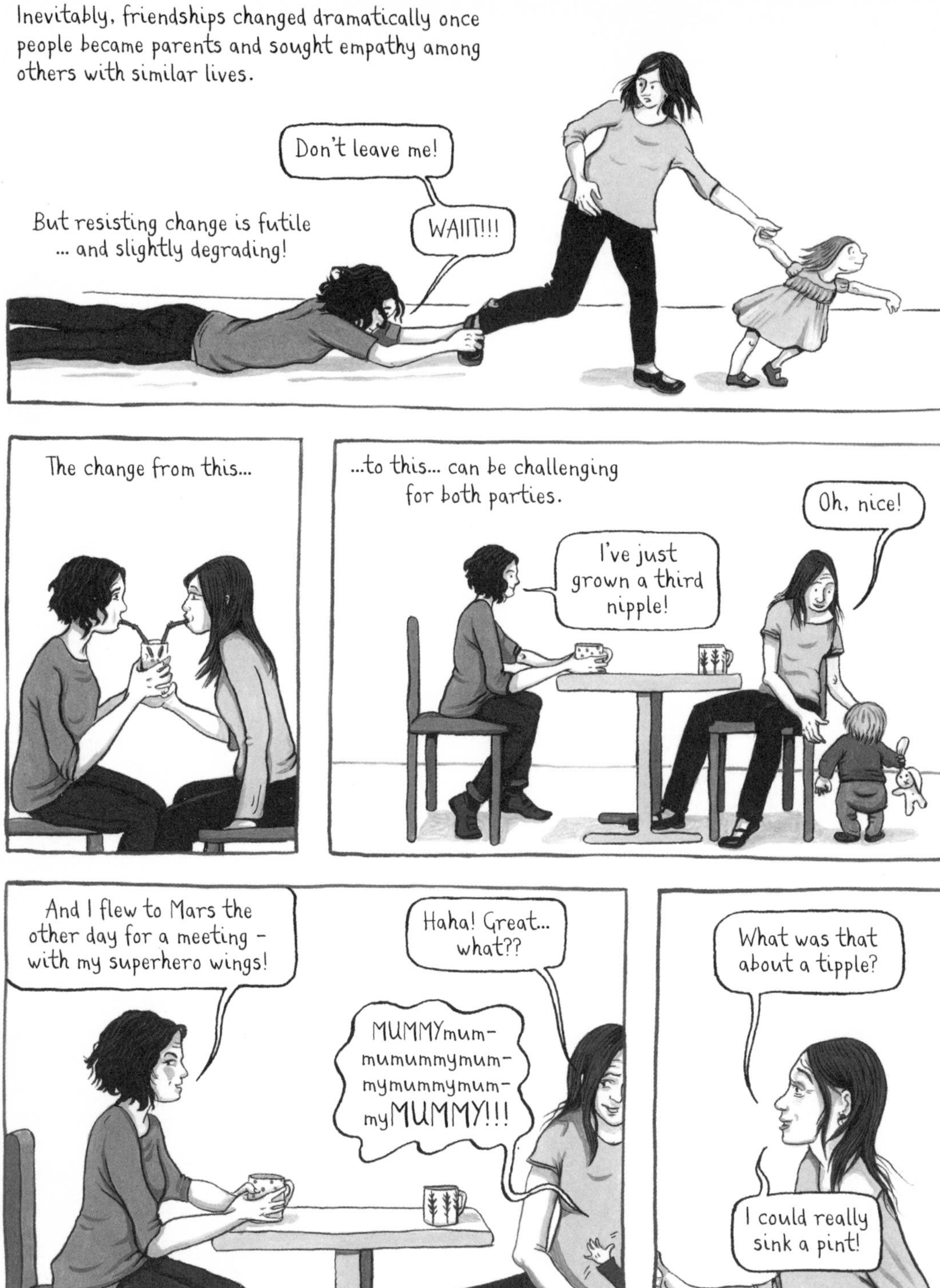
Inevitably, friendships changed dramatically once people became parents and sought empathy among others with similar lives.
But resisting change is futile ... and slightly degrading!
Don't leave me!
WAIIT!!!
The change from this...
...to this... can be challenging for both parties.
I've just grown a third nipple!
Oh, nice!
And I flew to Mars the other day for a meeting - with my superhero wings!
Haha! Great... what??
MUMMYmum-mumummymum-mymummymum-myMUMMY!!!
What was that about a tipple?
I could really sink a pint!

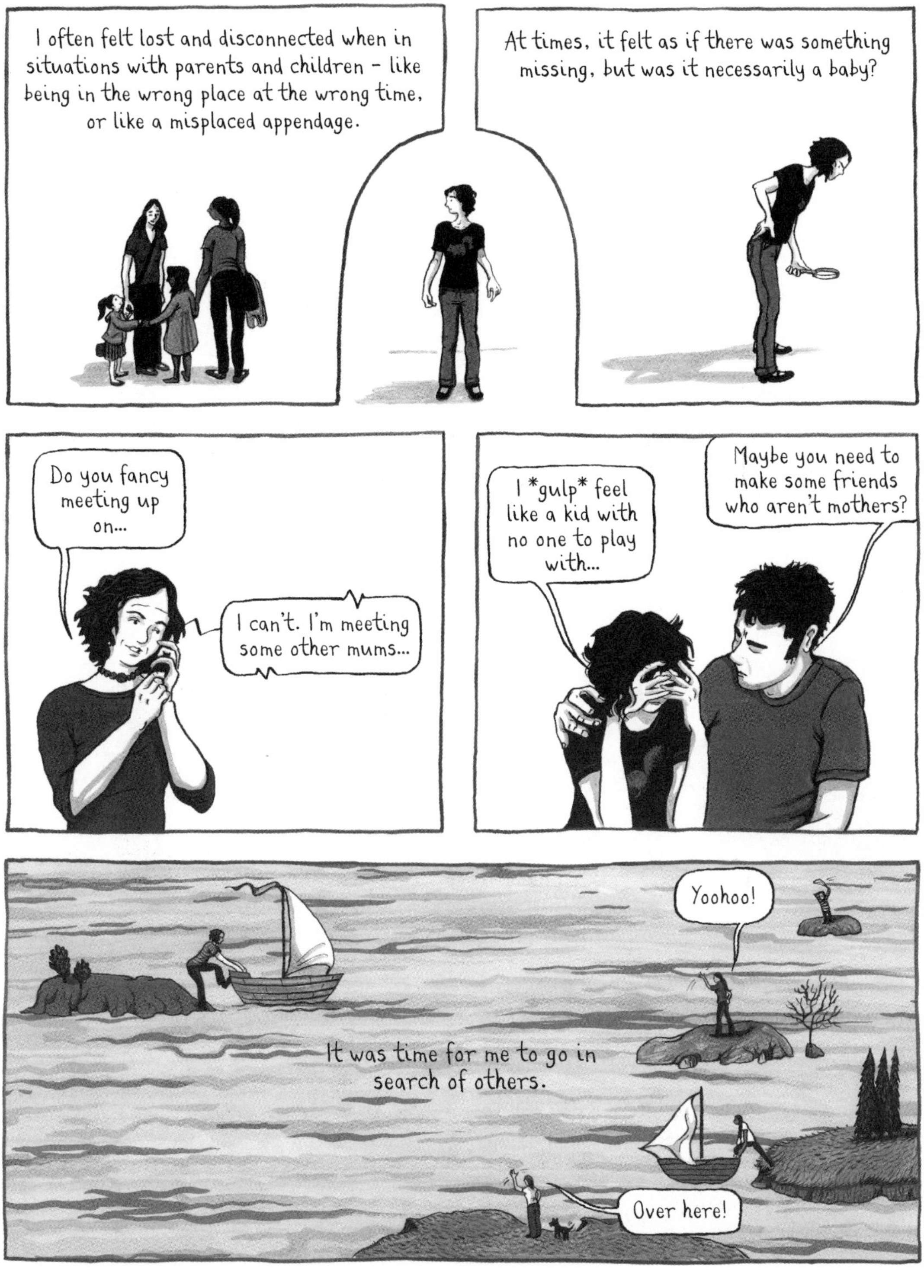
I often felt lost and disconnected when in situations with parents and children – like being in the wrong place at the wrong time, or like a misplaced appendage.
At times, it felt as if there was something missing, but was it necessarily a baby?
Do you fancy meeting up on...
I can't. I'm meeting some other mums...
I *gulp* feel like a kid with no one to play with...
Maybe you need to make some friends who aren't mothers?
It was time for me to go in search of others.
Yoohoo!
Over here!

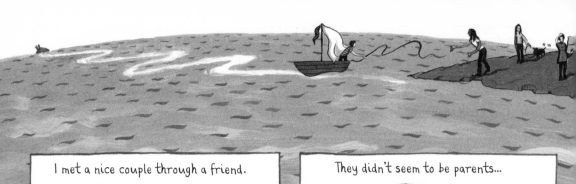

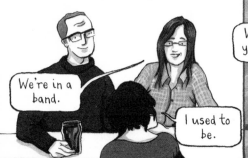
I met a nice couple through a friend.

We're in a band.

I used to be.

What do you play?

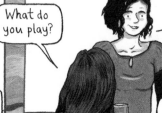

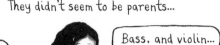
They didn't seem to be parents...

Bass, and violin...

but I'm out of practice.

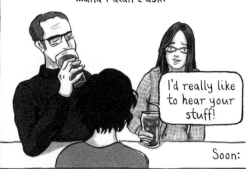
...and I didn't ask.

I'd really like to hear your stuff!

Soon:

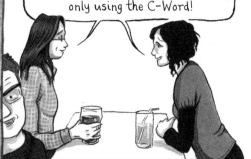
HahaHA! We could write a whole song only using the C-Word!

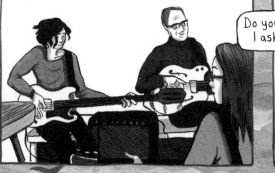
A few weeks later.

Do you mind if I ask you...?

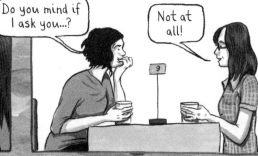
Hazel and I bonded over non-parenthood.

Not at all!

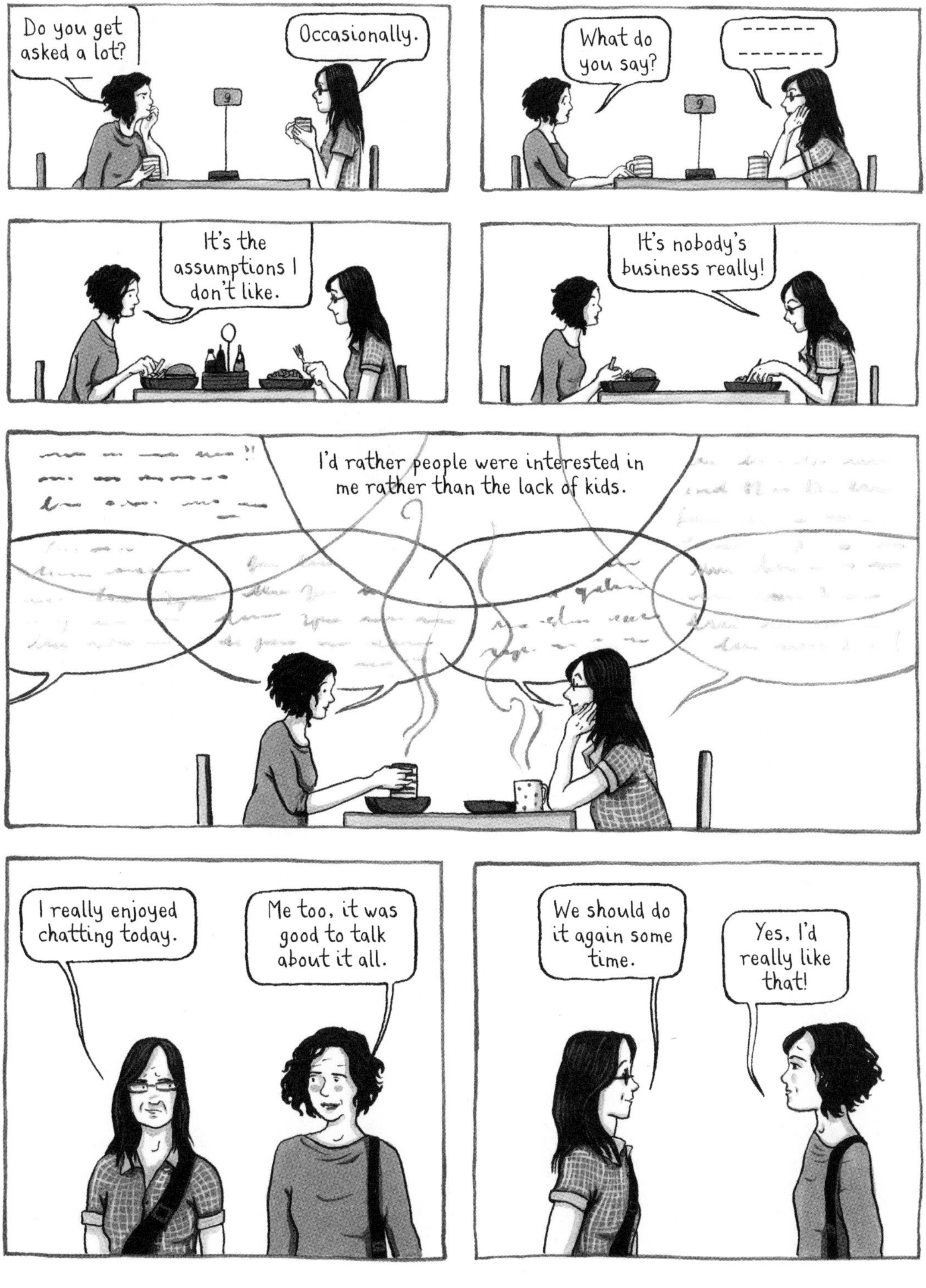
Do you get asked a lot?
Occasionally.
What do you say?
It's the assumptions I don't like.
It's nobody's business really!
I'd rather people were interested in me rather than the lack of kids.
I really enjoyed chatting today.
Me too, it was good to talk about it all.
We should do it again some time.
Yes, I'd really like that!

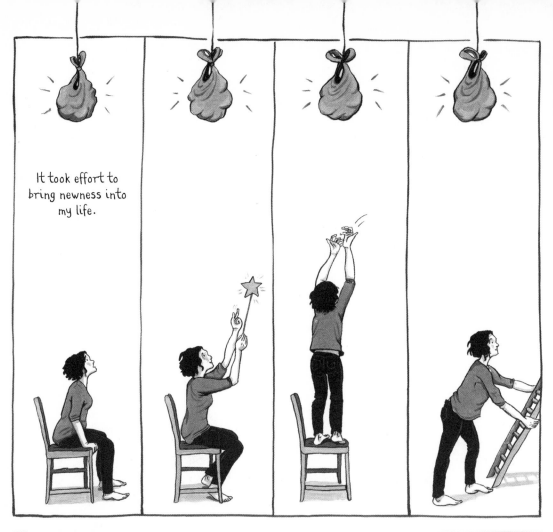

It took effort to
bring newness into
my life.

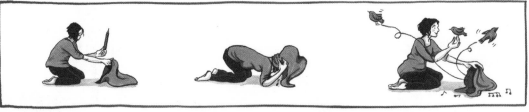

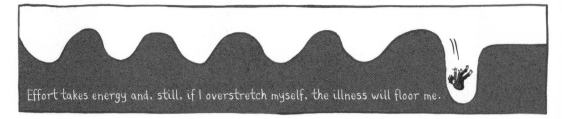

Effort takes energy and, still, if I overstretch myself, the illness will floor me.

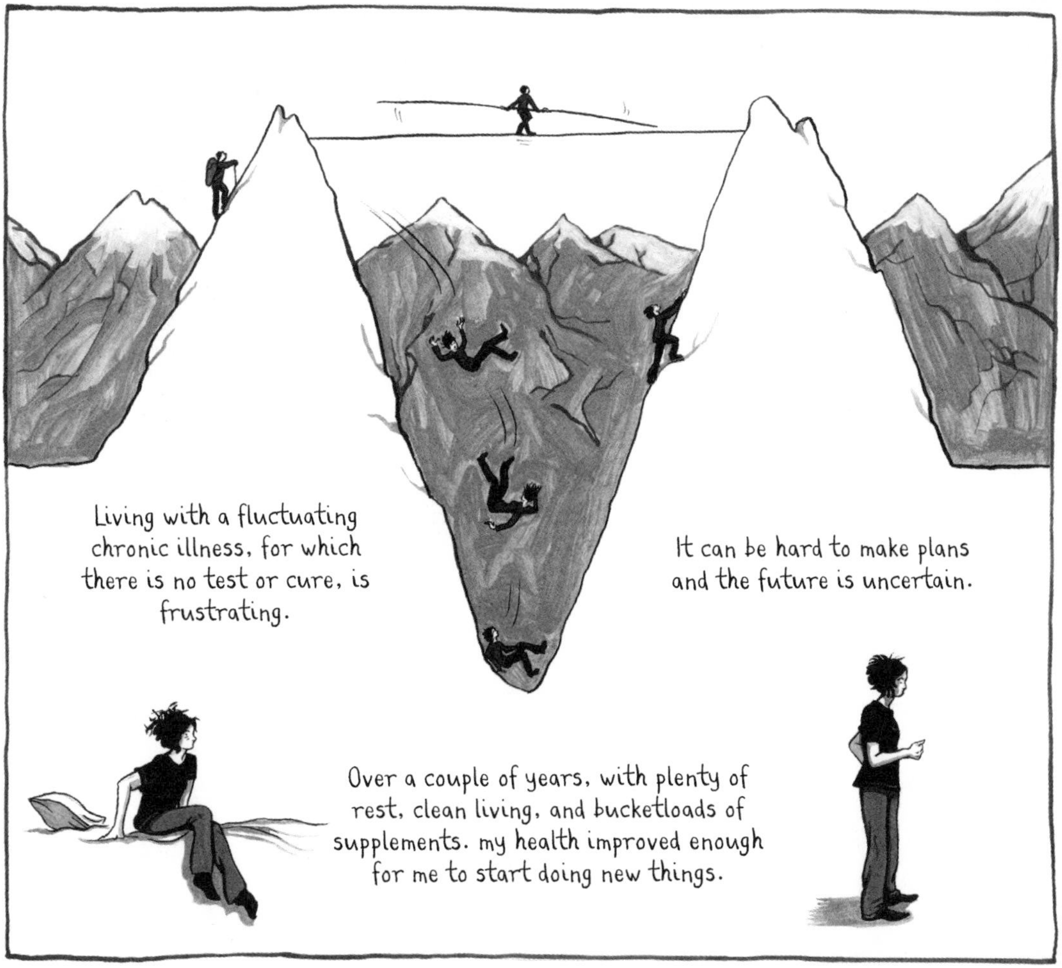
Living with a fluctuating chronic illness, for which there is no test or cure, is frustrating.
It can be hard to make plans and the future is uncertain.
Over a couple of years, with plenty of rest, clean living, and bucketloads of supplements. my health improved enough for me to start doing new things.

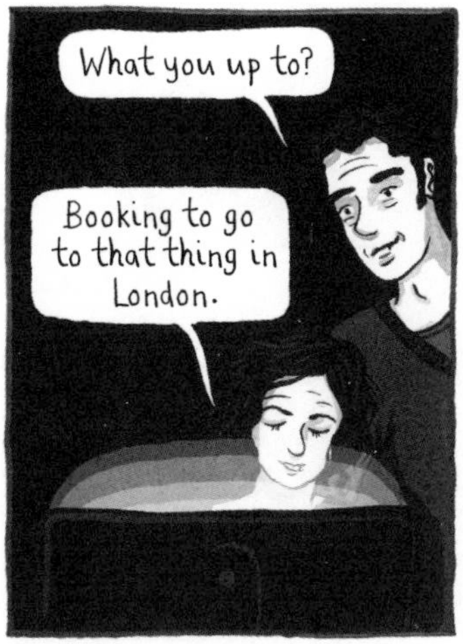
What you up to?
Booking to go to that thing in London.

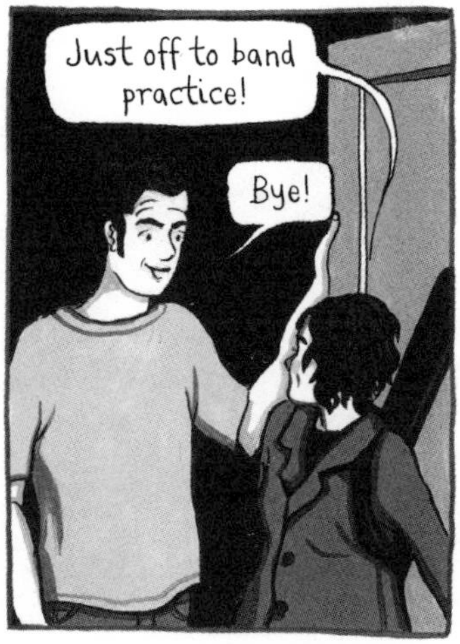
Just off to band practice!
Bye!

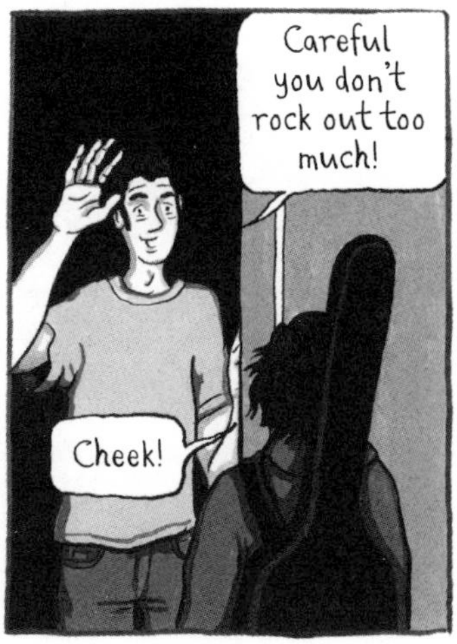
Careful you don't rock out too much!
Cheek!

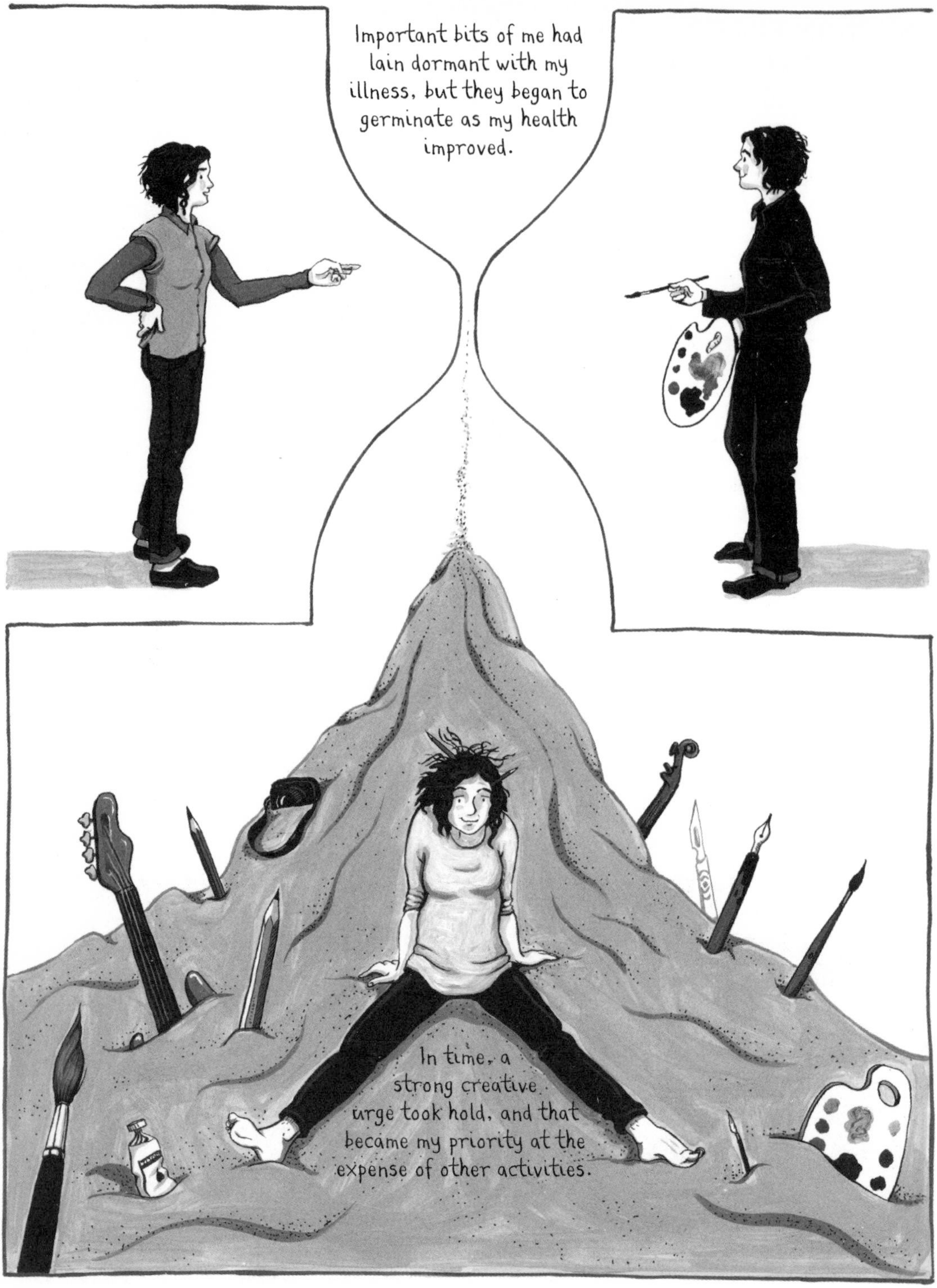
Important bits of me had lain dormant with my illness, but they began to germinate as my health improved.
In time, a strong creative urge took hold, and that became my priority at the expense of other activities.

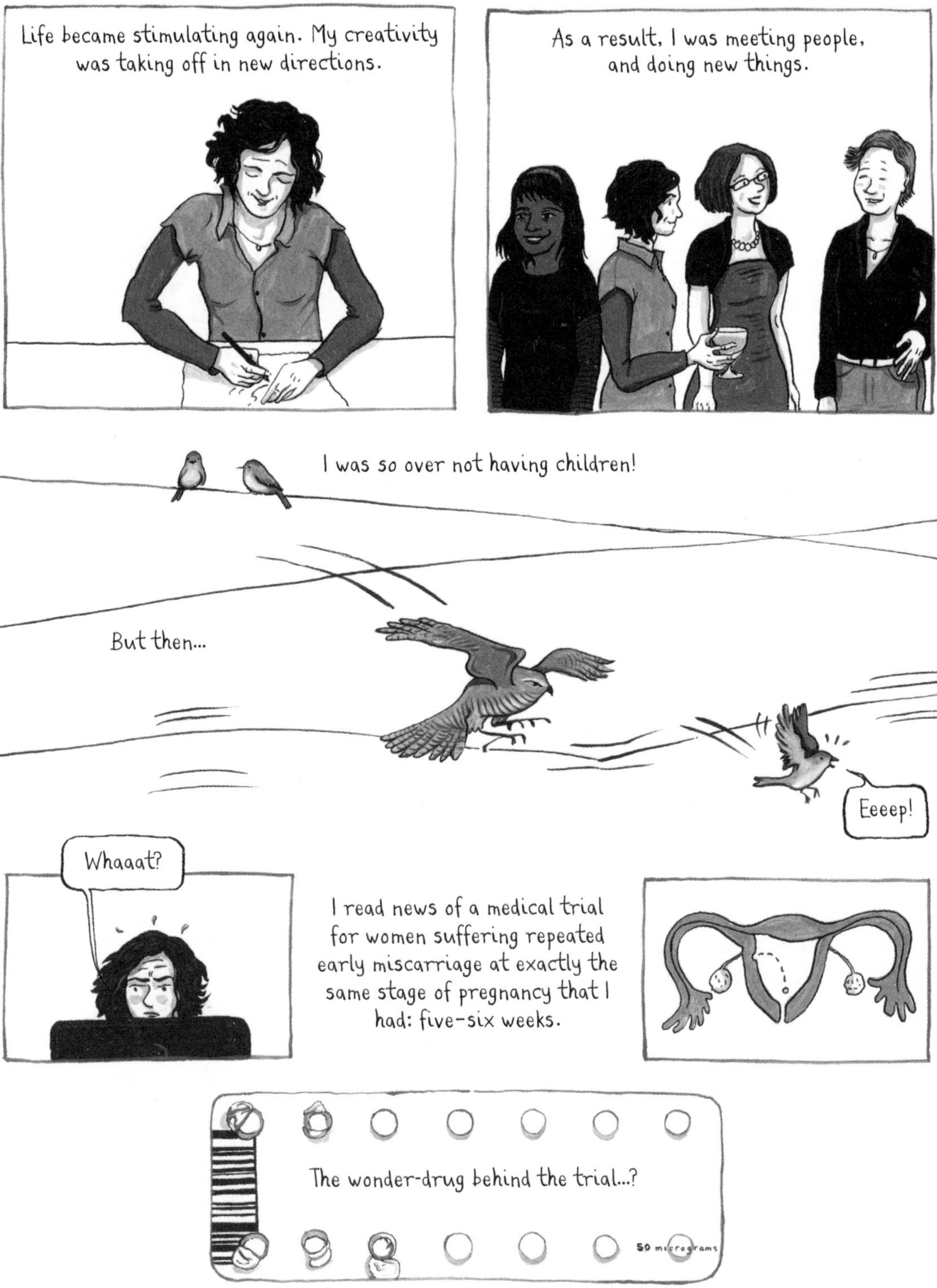
Life became stimulating again. My creativity was taking off in new directions.
As a result, I was meeting people, and doing new things.
I was so over not having children!
But then...
Eeeep!
Whaaat?
I read news of a medical trial for women suffering repeated early miscarriage at exactly the same stage of pregnancy that I had: five-six weeks.
The wonder-drug behind the trial...?
50 micrograms

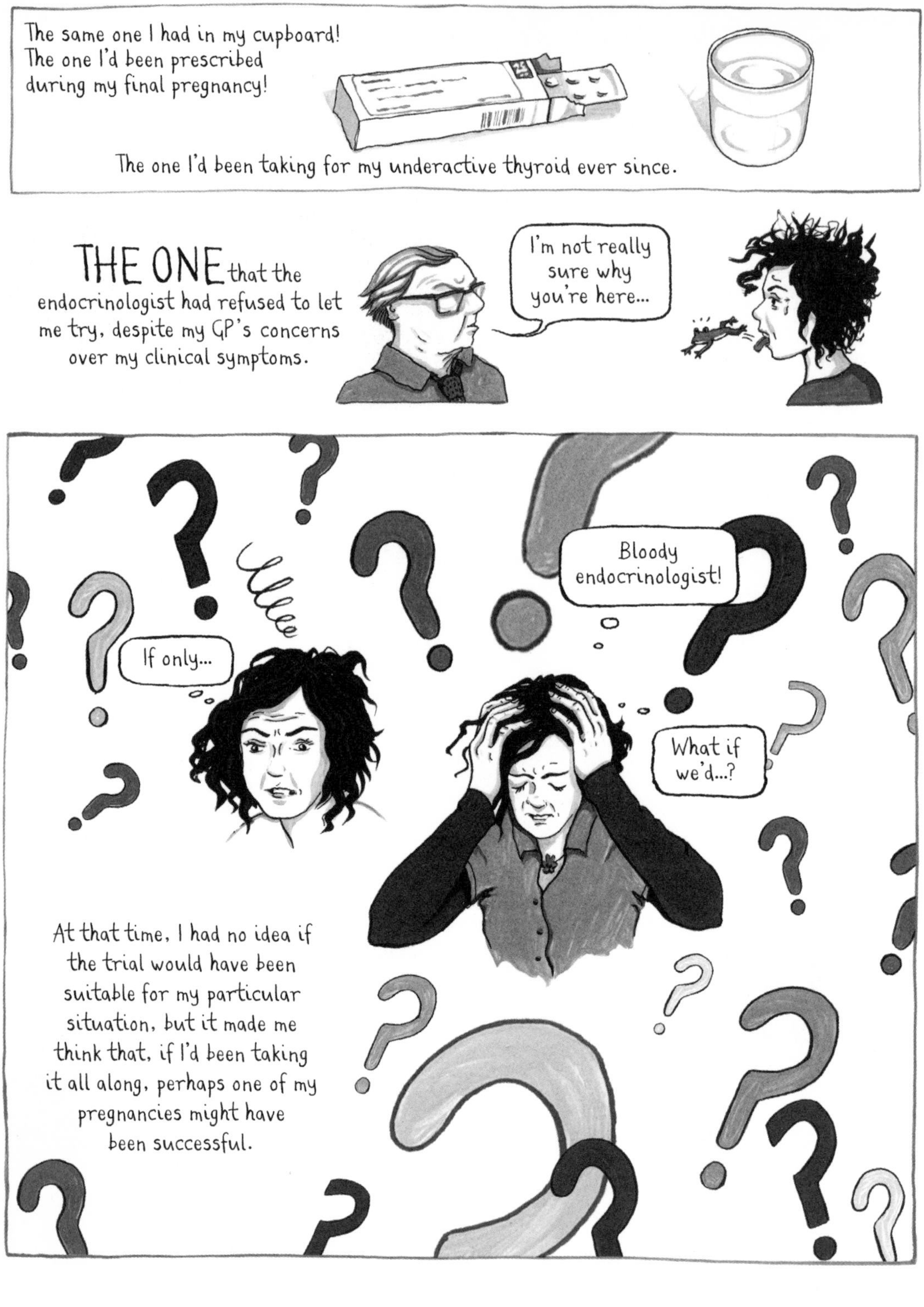
The same one I had in my cupboard! The one I'd been prescribed during my final pregnancy!
The one I'd been taking for my underactive thyroid ever since.
THE ONE that the endocrinologist had refused to let me try, despite my GP's concerns over my clinical symptoms.
I'm not really sure why you're here...
If only...
Bloody endocrinologist!
What if we'd...?
At that time, I had no idea if the trial would have been suitable for my particular situation, but it made me think that, if I'd been taking it all along, perhaps one of my pregnancies might have been successful.

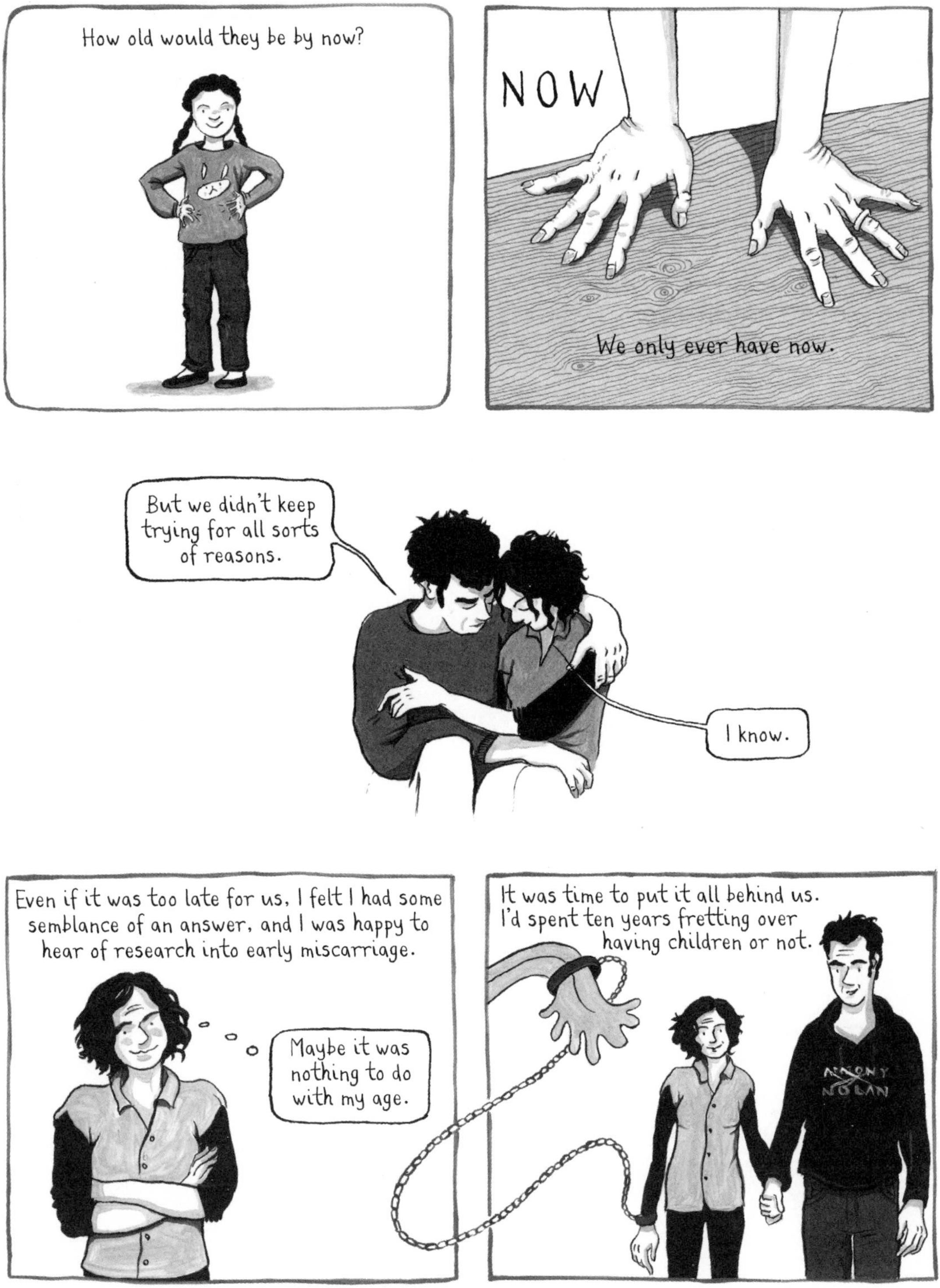
How old would they be by now?
NOW
We only ever have now.
But we didn't keep trying for all sorts of reasons.
I know.
Even if it was too late for us, I felt I had some semblance of an answer, and I was happy to hear of research into early miscarriage.
Maybe it was nothing to do with my age.
It was time to put it all behind us. I'd spent ten years fretting over having children or not.

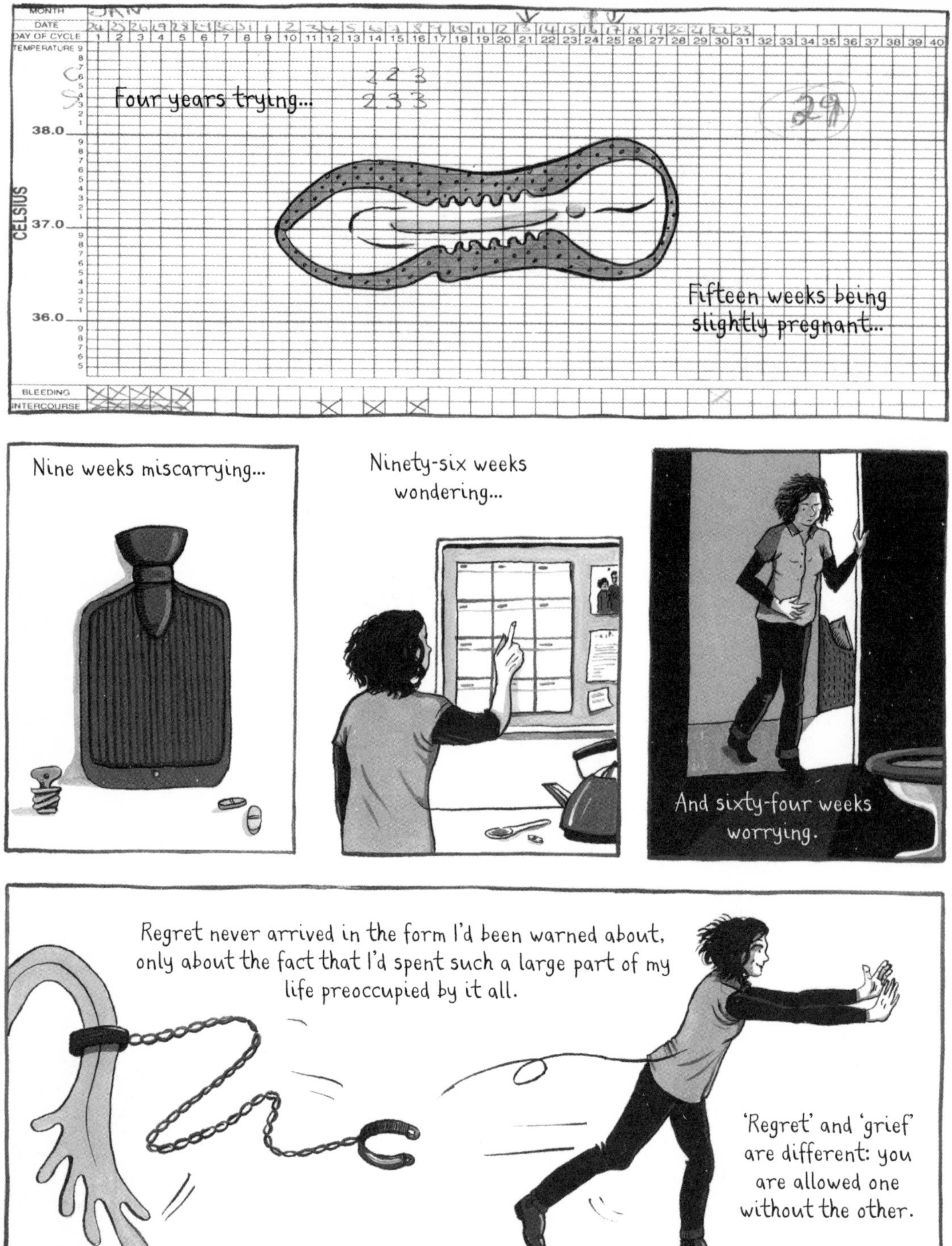
MONTH
DATE
DAY OF CYCLE
TEMPERATURE
Four years trying...
38.0
CELSIUS
37.0
36.0
Fifteen weeks being slightly pregnant...
BLEEDING
INTERCOURSE
Nine weeks miscarrying...
Ninety-six weeks wondering...
And sixty-four weeks worrying.
Regret never arrived in the form I'd been warned about, only about the fact that I'd spent such a large part of my life preoccupied by it all.
'Regret' and 'grief' are different: you are allowed one without the other.

Although I'd accepted not having children, I was finding a society where 'mum's the word' hard to swallow – a society where even the simple task of serving a drink evokes motherhood.

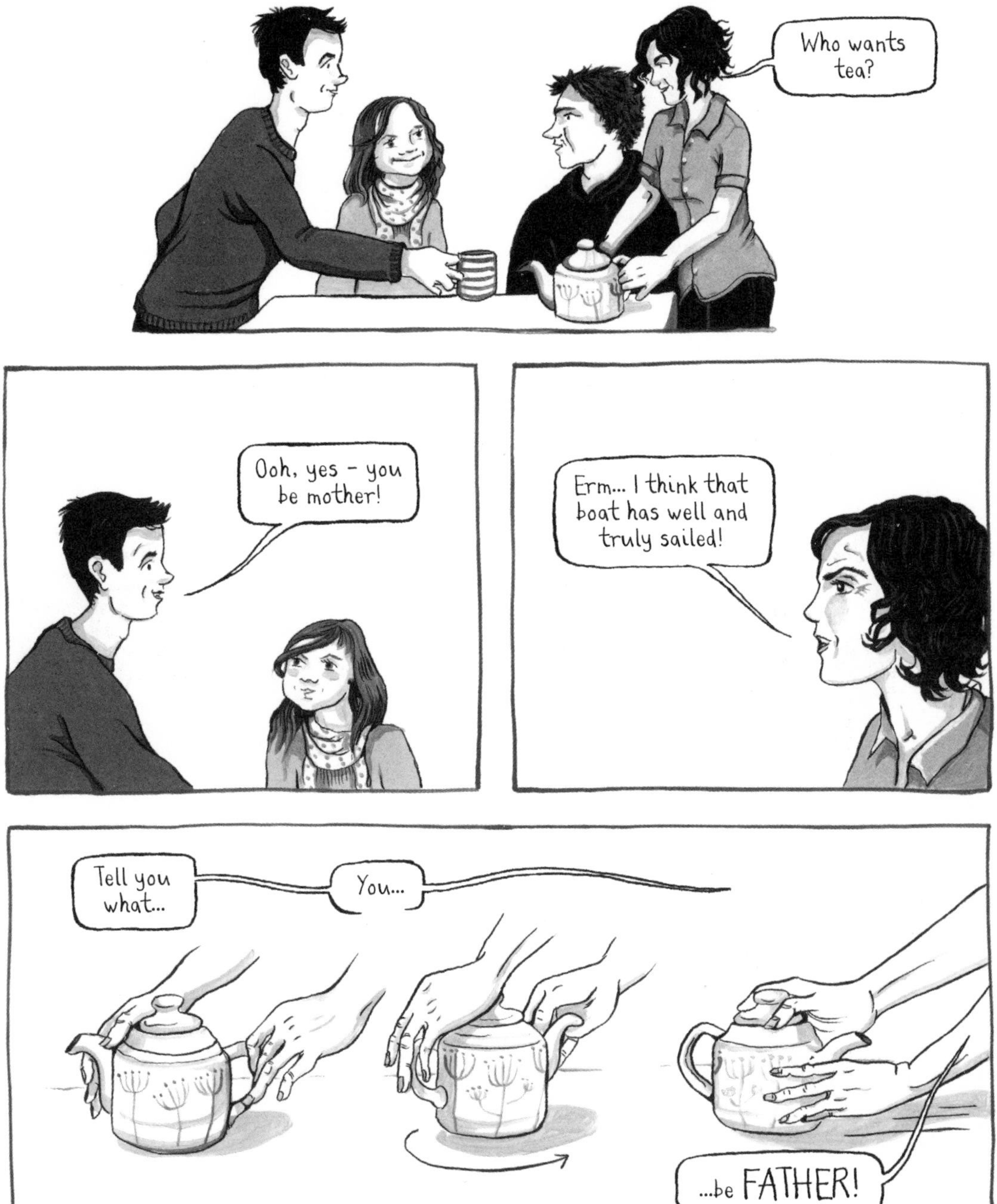
Who wants tea?
Ooh, yes – you be mother!
Erm... I think that boat has well and truly sailed!
Tell you what...
You...
...be FATHER!

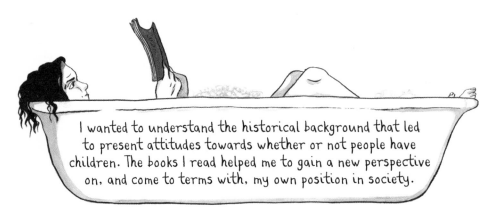

I wanted to understand the historical background that led to present attitudes towards whether or not people have children. The books I read helped me to gain a new perspective on, and come to terms with, my own position in society.

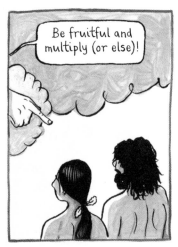

Be fruitful and multiply (or else)!

I learnt about pronatalism, a religious, political and cultural ideology that encourages people to reproduce. This was useful in times when there weren't many humans...

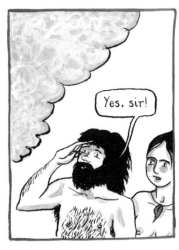

Yes, sir!

...or when population levels dropped, such as during the early 1900s after the worldwide flu pandemic.

In a bid to encourage women to feel that motherhood was their destiny, the status of motherhood was elevated.

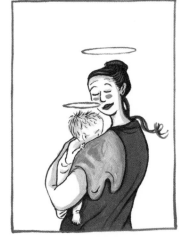

Pregnancy and motherhood became sentimentalised. (You never hear much about Mary dealing with Baby Jesus's stinky nappies, do you?)

I wonder if this also informed a conspiracy of silence over the dangers and problems regarding pregnancy, childbirth and the troubles associated with childrearing, the volume only now beginning to increase with social media.

Keep it quiet...
...or they won't breed!

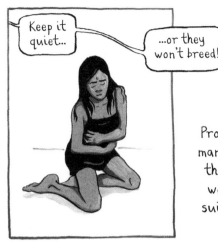

Pronatalism has also manifested in policies that have corralled women's lives, but suited governments.

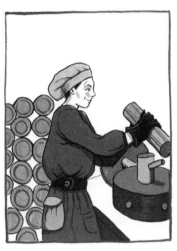

For example, in WWII, childcare was state-funded when women's labour was required, but removed after the war, making it hard for women to continue to combine work and childrearing.

Moooo!

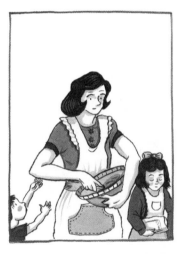

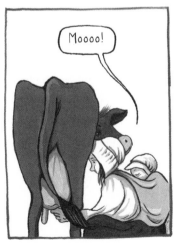

This division of work and home was a result of the Industrial Revolution. In rural societies, work, domestic and social lives existed in the same space. This was no longer possible in industrial societies, factories being no place for babies.

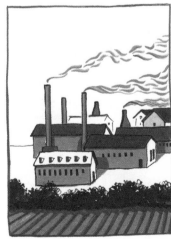

It doesn't make sense to me that, despite the world's population heading towards 9bn by 2040...

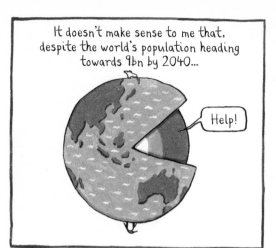

Help!

...pronatal ideology is still rife.

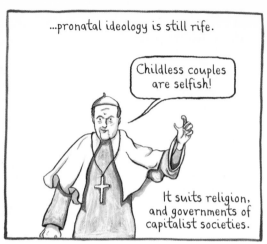

Childless couples are selfish!

It suits religion, and governments of capitalist societies.

Future flock...

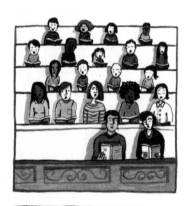

Future voters and taxpayers...

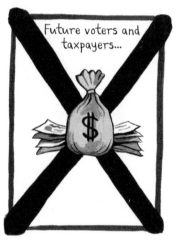

Future consumers of stuff and resources.

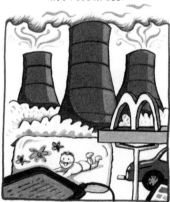

Although it would have been nice to have had one child, these facts nudged me towards a childfree mentality at times.

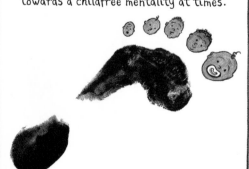

At least I still have a moderately sparkling carbon footprint.

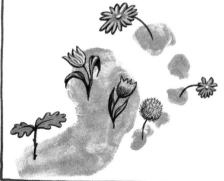

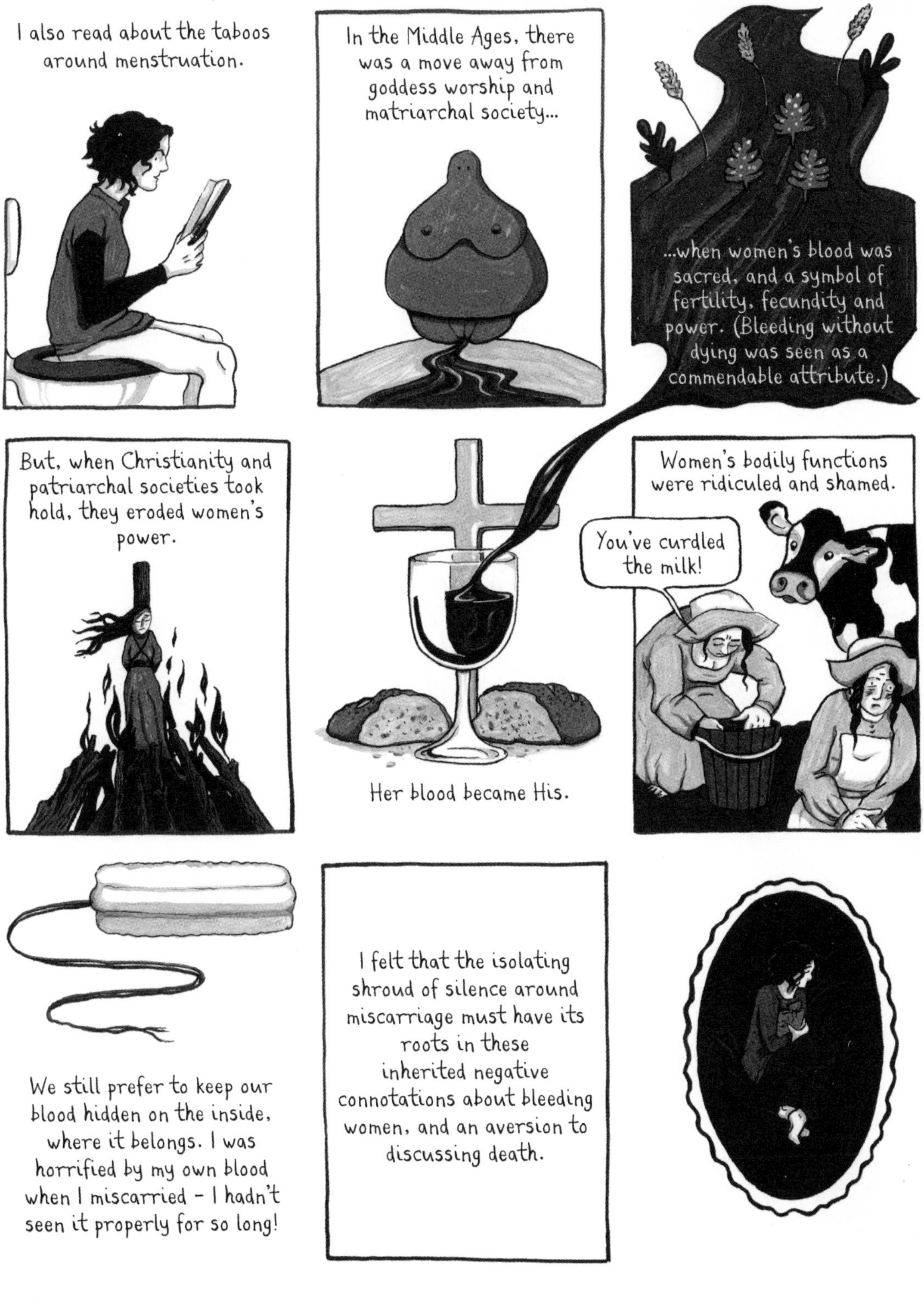
I also read about the taboos around menstruation.
In the Middle Ages, there was a move away from goddess worship and matriarchal society...
...when women's blood was sacred, and a symbol of fertility, fecundity and power. (Bleeding without dying was seen as a commendable attribute.)
But, when Christianity and patriarchal societies took hold, they eroded women's power.
Her blood became His.
Women's bodily functions were ridiculed and shamed.
You've curdled the milk!
We still prefer to keep our blood hidden on the inside, where it belongs. I was horrified by my own blood when I miscarried – I hadn't seen it properly for so long!
I felt that the isolating shroud of silence around miscarriage must have its roots in these inherited negative connotations about bleeding women, and an aversion to discussing death.

I also read about Second Wave Feminism, which was gathering momentum at the time I was born. This movement voiced a growing dissatisfaction among some housewives – a longing to escape the boredom of the domestic servitude apportioned to them since the two World Wars.

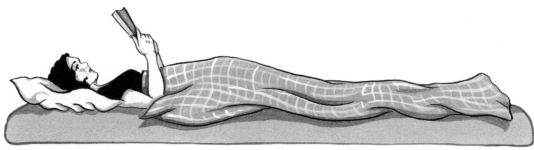

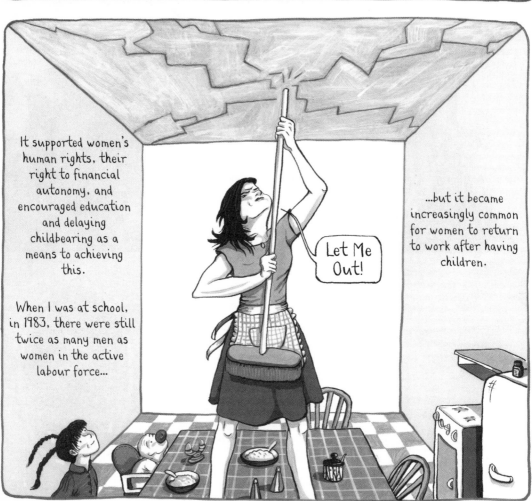

It supported women's human rights, their right to financial autonomy, and encouraged education and delaying childbearing as a means to achieving this.

When I was at school, in 1983, there were still twice as many men as women in the active labour force...

Let Me Out!

...but it became increasingly common for women to return to work after having children.

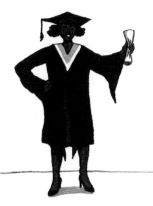

As a result of better access to contraception, the birth rate had been falling in the 1970s, especially in women under the age of nineteen.

It was this group who were responsible for the rise in women enrolling for higher education in the 1970s and '80s, including myself.

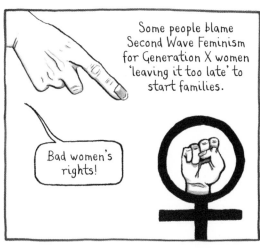

Some people blame Second Wave Feminism for Generation X women 'leaving it too late' to start families.

Bad women's rights!

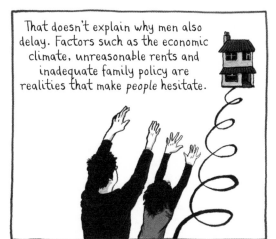

That doesn't explain why men also delay. Factors such as the economic climate, unreasonable rents and inadequate family policy are realities that make *people* hesitate.

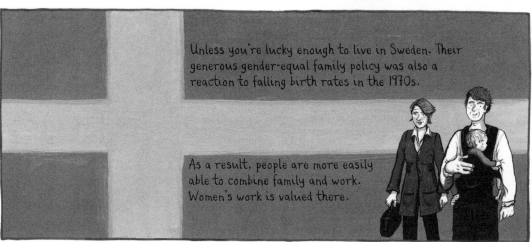

Unless you're lucky enough to live in Sweden. Their generous gender-equal family policy was also a reaction to falling birth rates in the 1970s.

As a result, people are more easily able to combine family and work. Women's work is valued there.

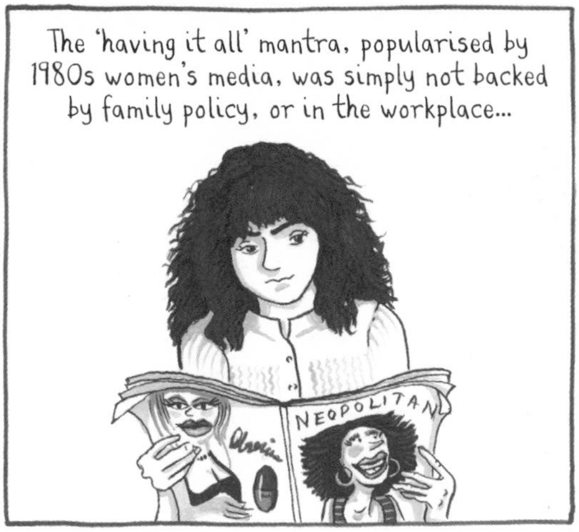
The 'having it all' mantra, popularised by 1980s women's media, was simply not backed by family policy, or in the workplace...
NEOPOLITAN

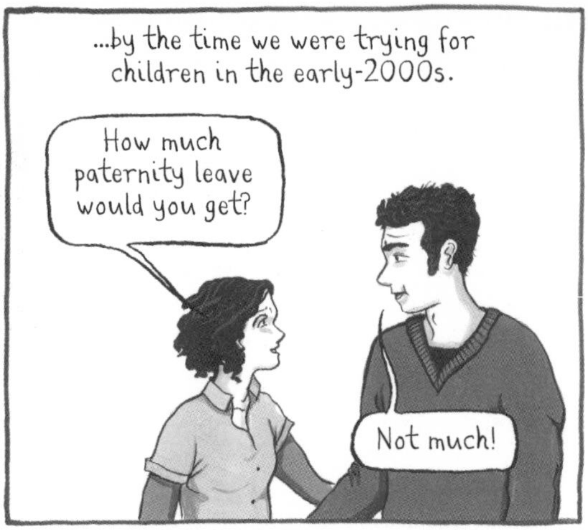
...by the time we were trying for children in the early-2000s.
How much paternity leave would you get?
Not much!

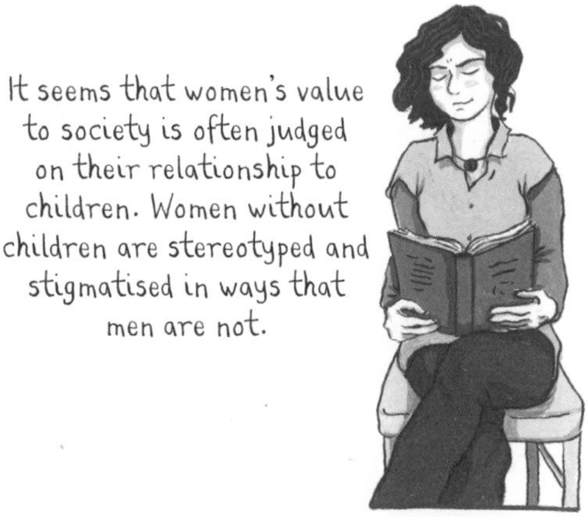
It seems that women's value to society is often judged on their relationship to children. Women without children are stereotyped and stigmatised in ways that men are not.

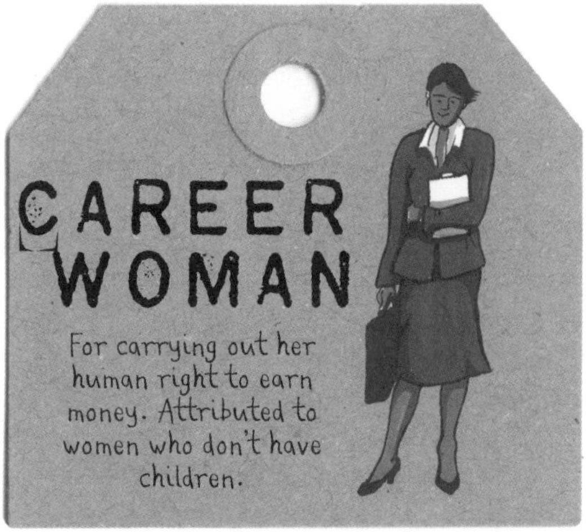
CAREER WOMAN
For carrying out her human right to earn money. Attributed to women who don't have children.

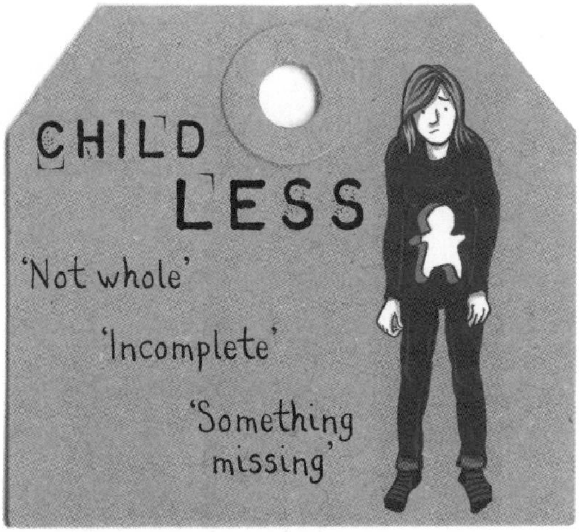
CHILD LESS
'Not whole'
'Incomplete'
'Something missing'

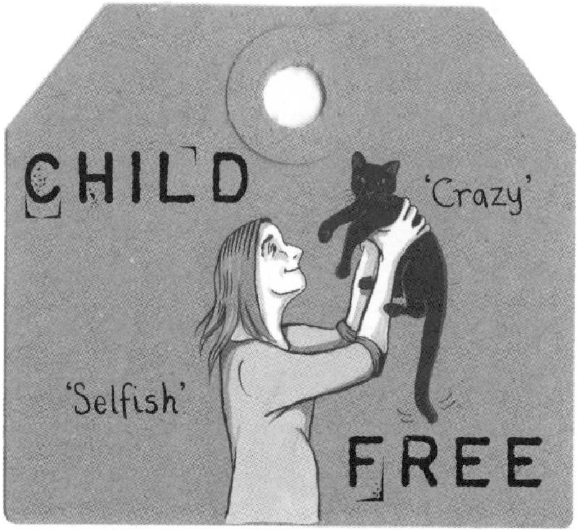
CHILD
'Crazy'
'Selfish'
FREE

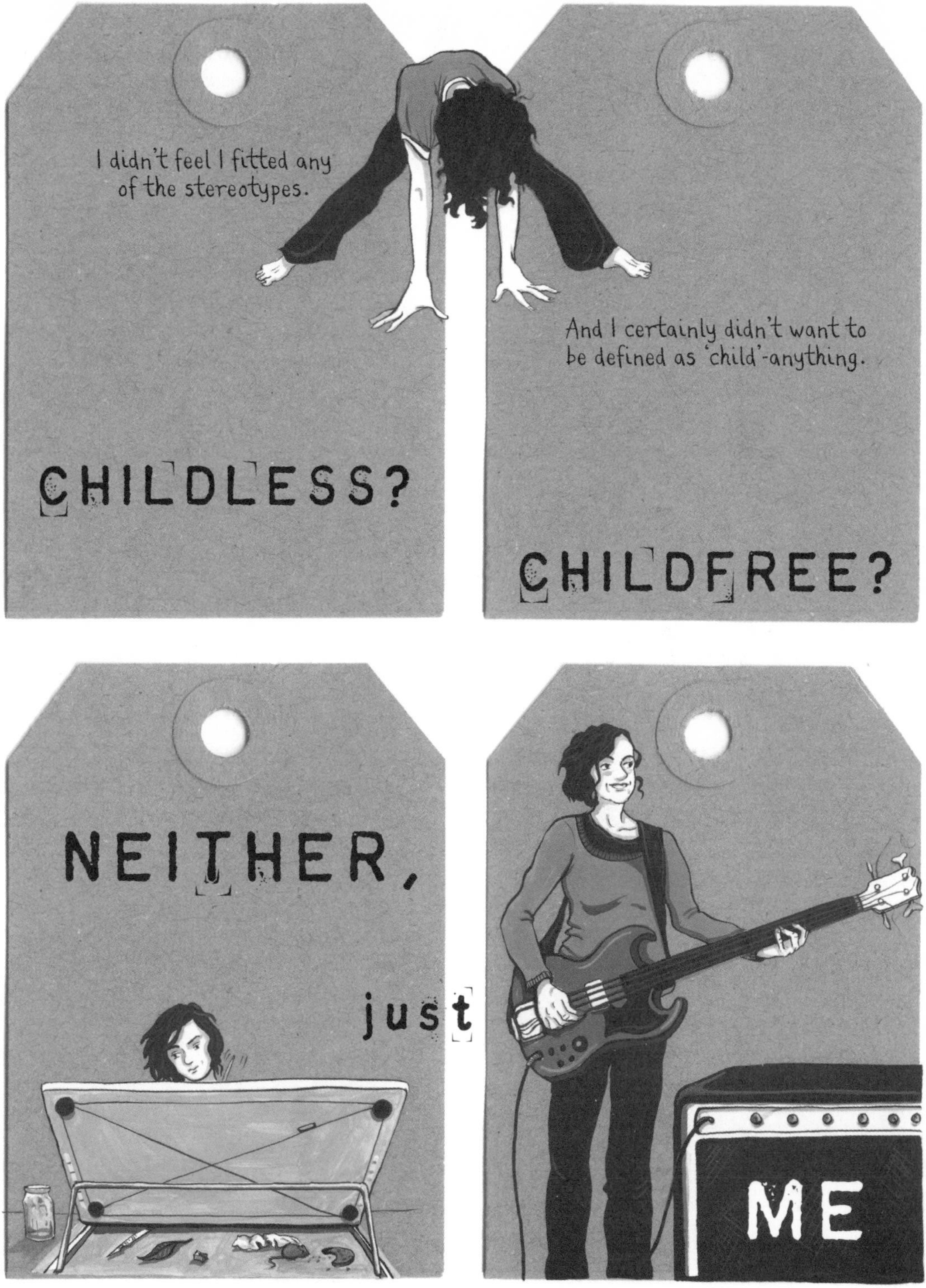

I didn't feel I fitted any of the stereotypes.
CHILDLESS?
And I certainly didn't want to be defined as 'child'-anything.
CHILDFREE?
NEITHER,
just
ME

Does an innate biological urge to procreate actually exist? According to scientists, we do have hormonal urges, especially in oestrus.

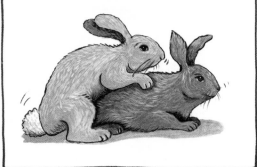

If you stir that in with cultural conditioning...

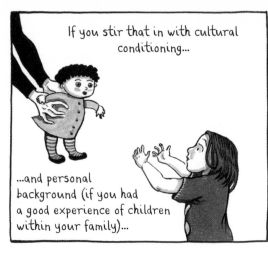

...and personal background (if you had a good experience of children within your family)...

...our attraction to cuteness...

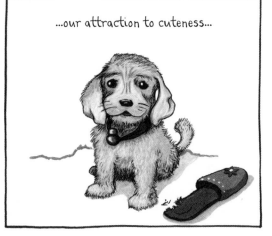

...a sense of time running out...

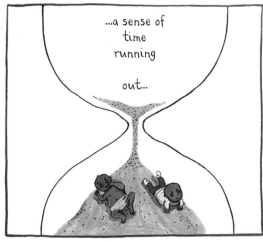

...of feeling left out, and peer pressure, it can all amount to powerful feelings that we may interpret as a 'biological urge'.

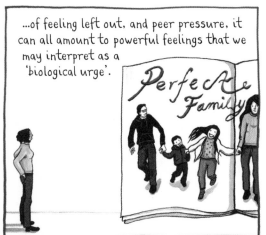

But if it were truly a biological imperative, we wouldn't be making choices.

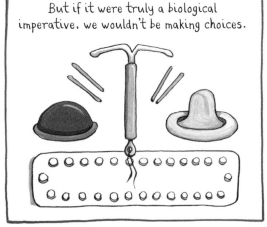

We are the only species that can choose not to perpetuate our DNA – our consciousness allows it.

If this choice is part of human nature, it must, therefore, be natural.

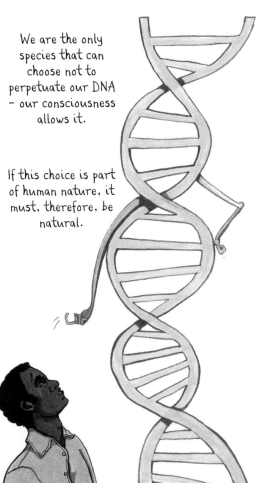

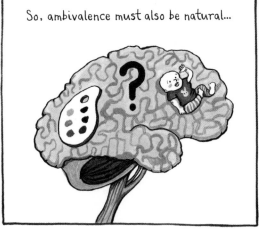

So, ambivalence must also be natural...

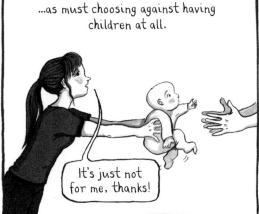

...as must choosing against having children at all.

It's just not for me, thanks!

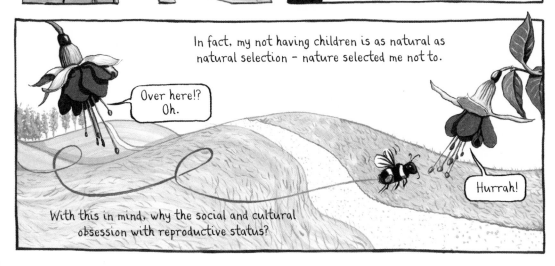

In fact, my not having children is as natural as natural selection – nature selected me not to.

Over here!? Oh.

Hurrah!

With this in mind, why the social and cultural obsession with reproductive status?

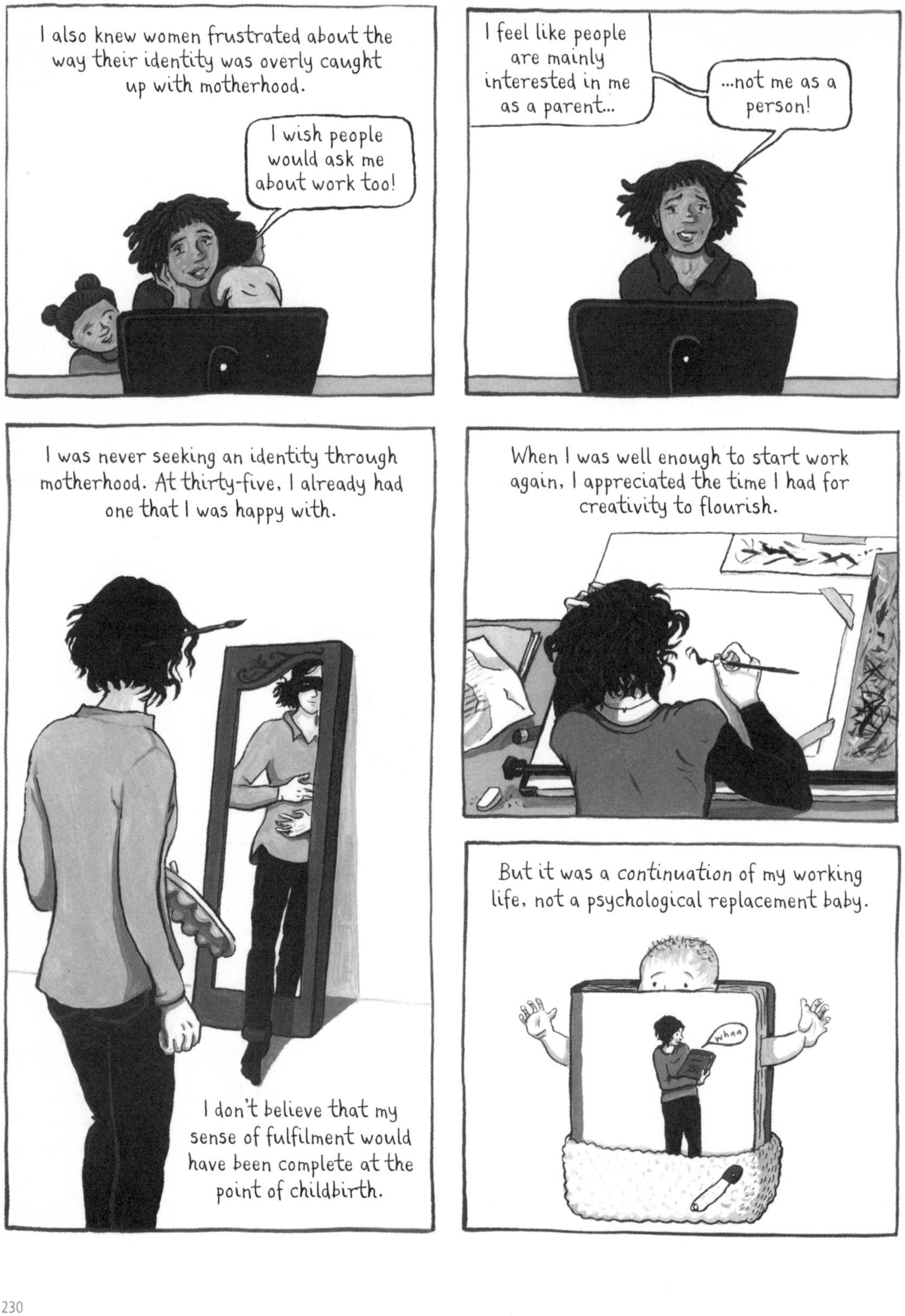
I also knew women frustrated about the way their identity was overly caught up with motherhood.
I wish people would ask me about work too!
I feel like people are mainly interested in me as a parent...
...not me as a person!
I was never seeking an identity through motherhood. At thirty-five, I already had one that I was happy with.
I don't believe that my sense of fulfilment would have been complete at the point of childbirth.
When I was well enough to start work again, I appreciated the time I had for creativity to flourish.
But it was a continuation of my working life, not a psychological replacement baby.
whaa

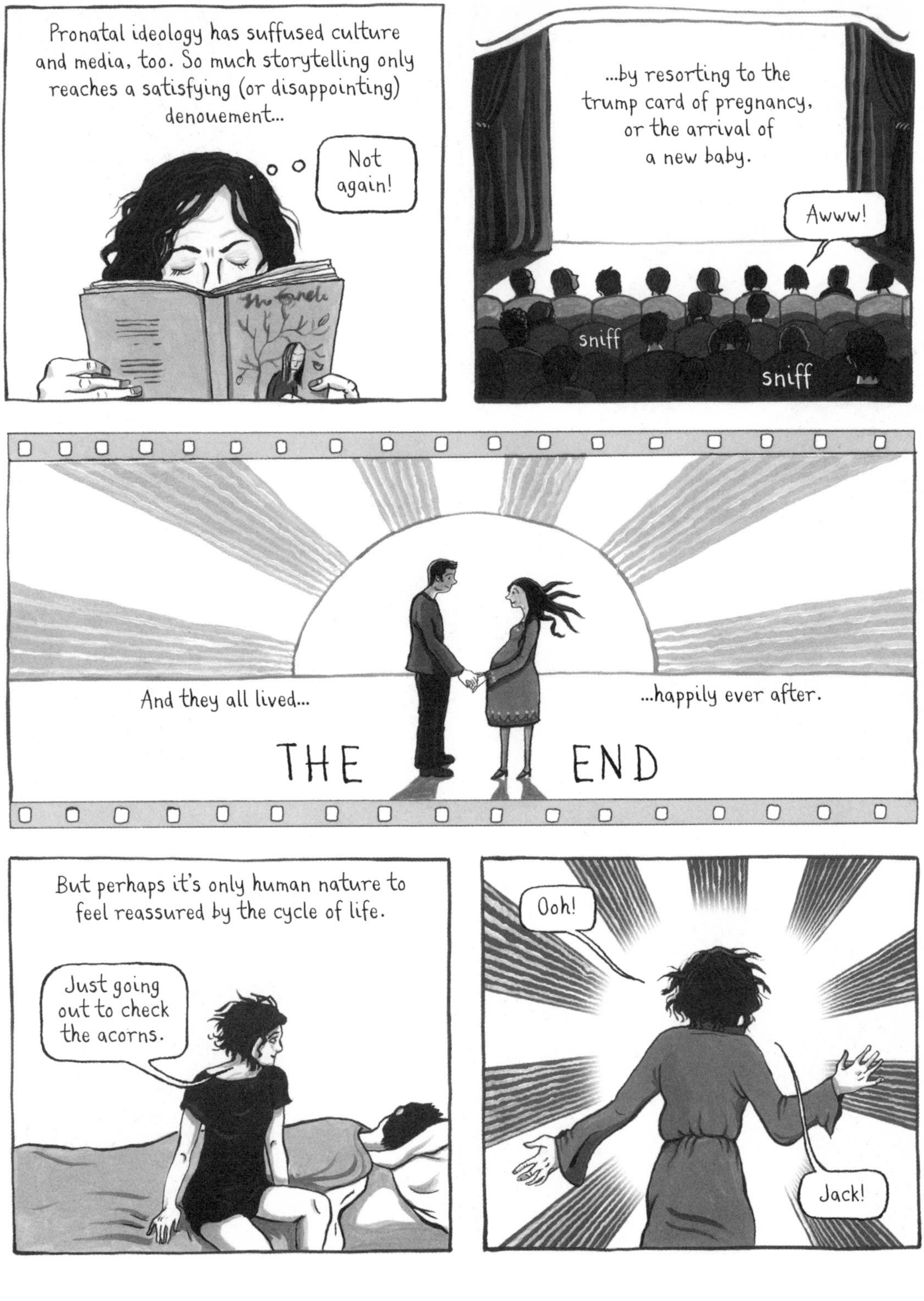
Pronatal ideology has suffused culture and media, too. So much storytelling only reaches a satisfying (or disappointing) denouement...
Not again!
...by resorting to the trump card of pregnancy, or the arrival of a new baby.
Awww!
sniff
sniff
And they all lived...
...happily ever after.
THE END
But perhaps it's only human nature to feel reassured by the cycle of life.
Just going out to check the acorns.
Ooh!
Jack!

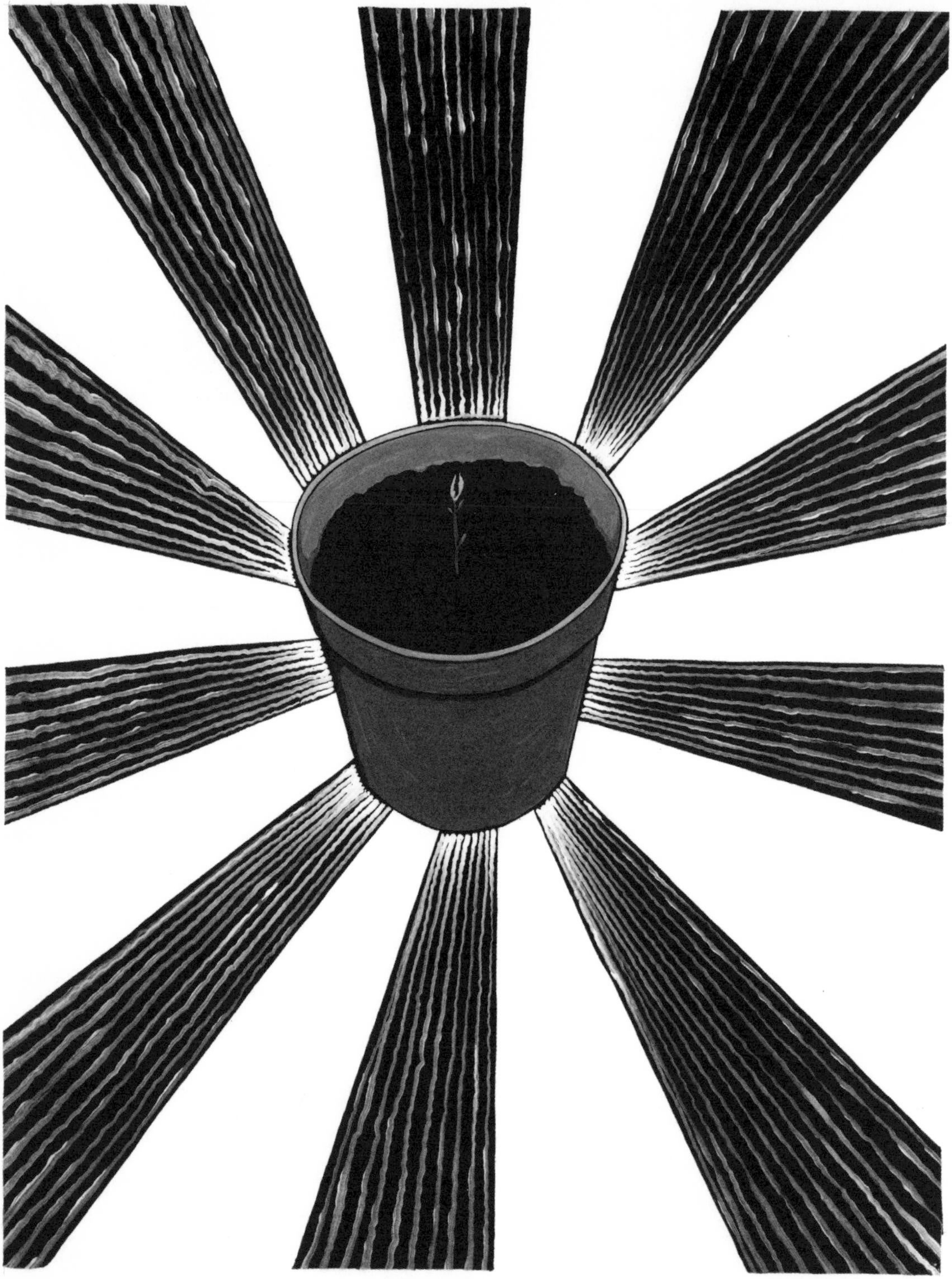

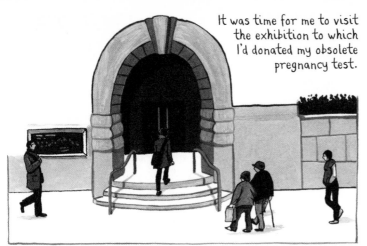

It was time for me to visit the exhibition to which I'd donated my obsolete pregnancy test.

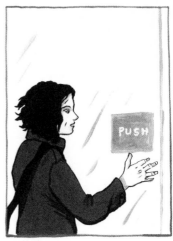

PUSH

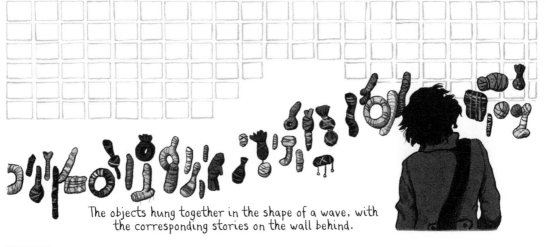

The objects hung together in the shape of a wave, with the corresponding stories on the wall behind.

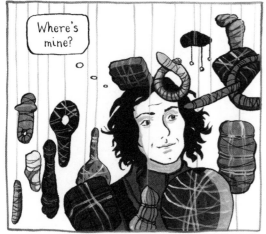

Where's mine?

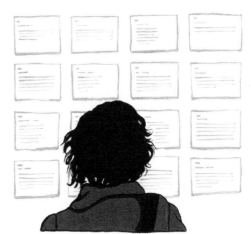

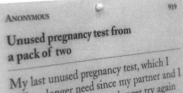

ANONYMOUS   919

**Unused pregnancy test from
a pack of two**

My last unused pregnancy test, which I
will no longer need since my partner and I
came to a decision to no longer try again
after three miscarriages. Handing it over
represents the start of my grief, which
coincided with this exhibition invitation.

Each object was wrapped and
woven with fabric, creating
the appearance of tiny
mummifications. But here
were the amulets alone, with
no dead body to weave
them around.

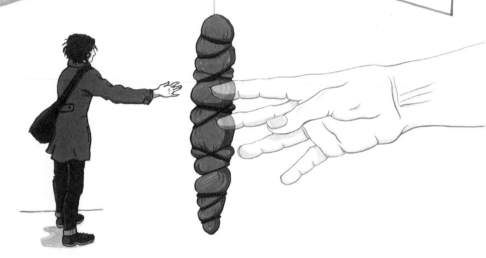

Once you give something away freely, you must relinquish all claim over it.

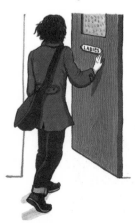
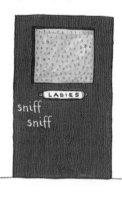

sniff
sniff

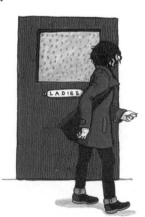

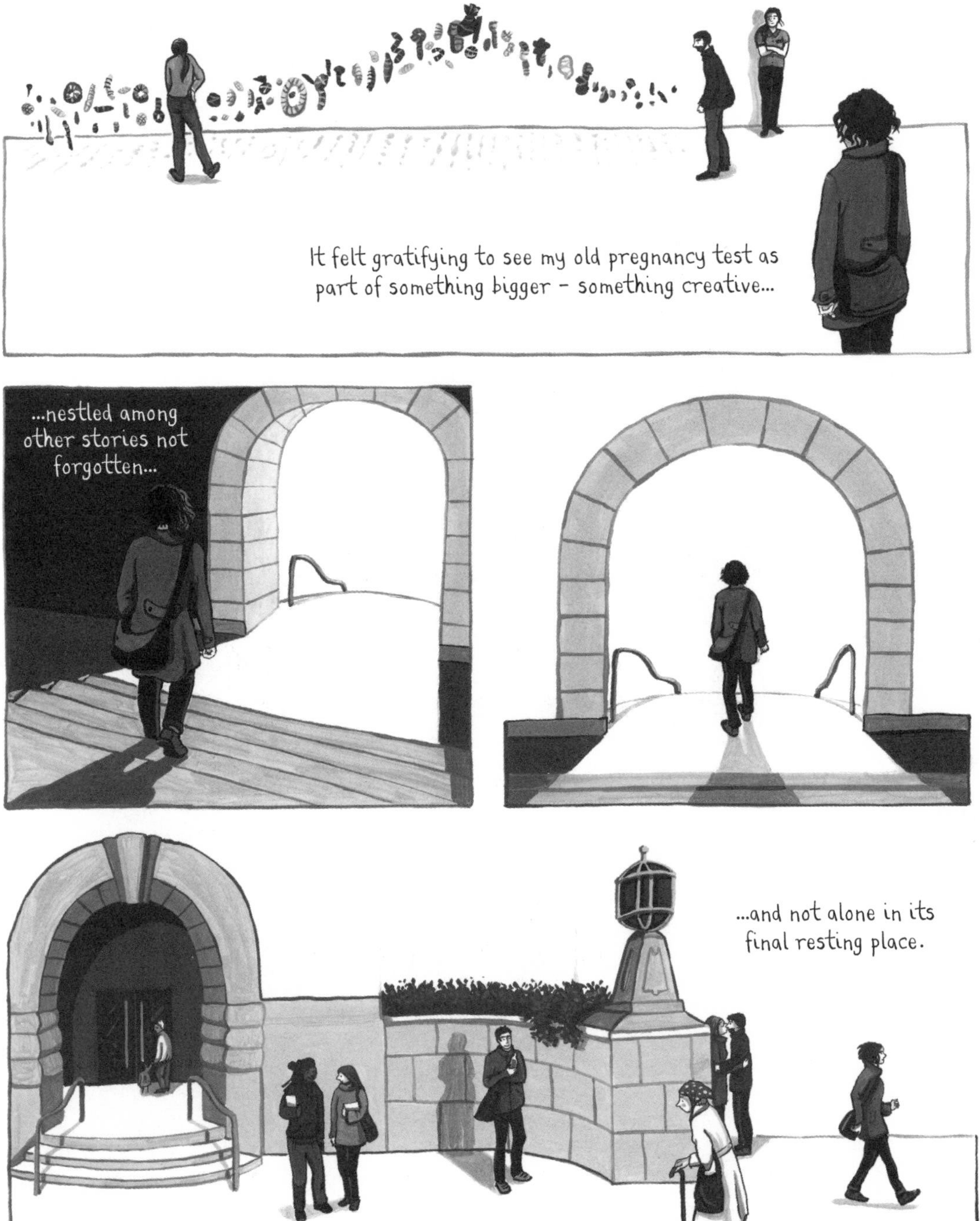
It felt gratifying to see my old pregnancy test as part of something bigger - something creative...
...nestled among other stories not forgotten...
...and not alone in its final resting place.

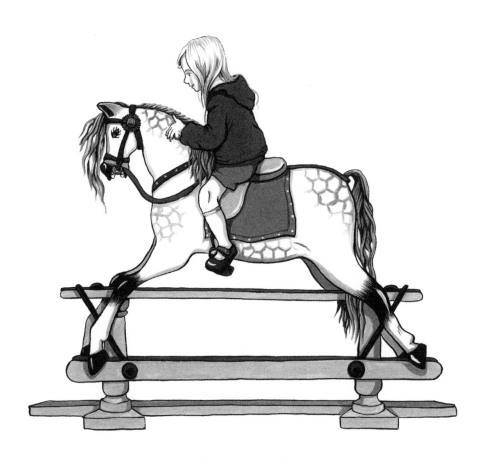

And Neddy? He eventually found a new
custodian, and is still part of my family.
I suspect he'll always find
a welcoming home.

AFTERWORD:

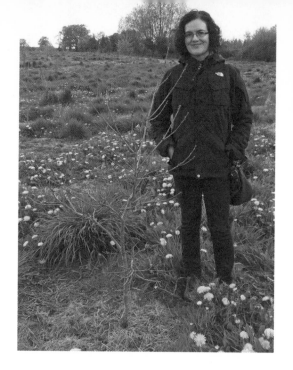

Apart from Neddy, all the names in this book have been changed, including my own. This probably seems odd given that it's a memoir, but it helped me to write more freely, and, over time, name and character became inextricably fused. Any likenesses to living people are entirely deliberate.

I've used a few photos in the book partly for means of authentication and partly to satisfy my own nostalgia. In particular, I wanted to use the photo of April and Polly on p32, because it remains the only photo in existence of me looking pregnant. In reality, that pot belly was likely a result of too much apple crumble and custard, or walking cock-eyed.

I used a very special tortoise, Rooster, as a metaphor for my illness. A tortoise is perhaps an obvious choice to illustrate fatigue, since it moves so slowly, but I also shared with Rooster a mineral deficiency which in his case led to a deformed shell. Rooster's health problem has left a visible trace whereas ME/CFS has no outward indicators — it's an invisible illness, a fact that can lead to sufferers being unfairly treated and misunderstood. Nevertheless, Rooster seemed a fitting animal to visualise what ME can feel like: however long it might have taken me to create this book, I passed the finishing line, eventually.

I collected, planted and pledged the acorns to the National Forest's 'Grow a Tree from Seed' scheme in 2009. We planted the saplings in 2012, in what is now Poppy Wood, in Derbyshire. The occasion marked the end of this story. It's a gentle, restful landscape, one I felt confident could safely harbour my oaklings, yet it was still hard to leave them to the mercy of nature. We visited them in 2015 — they grow up so fast, don't they? The National Forest's environmental project has been running for twenty-five years, reforesting areas of the Midlands that were formerly used for mining (hence the first Prologue image). After being unable to grow life in my body, it felt restorative and hopeful to make a contribution towards new ecosystems and communities — to help regenerate what used to be a damaged and barren landscape. The forest is managed, and, as such, 'my' trees might be cleared, eventually. Or they might not survive. This thought was upsetting at first, but now I've grown used to it. After all, it's only part of life's cycle of death and renewal, making way for future growth to flourish more easily. Besides, they're no longer mine: they belong to the earth, and to the creatures and people who use and inhabit that land now and in future. But it is my small connection to the future.

Paula Knight, October 2016

ACKNOWLEDGEMENTS:

Very special thanks and love to John Austin for all his hard work and support on this book. His help with scanning, digital / tidying and paint-flatting saved my arms for the artwork itself.

To Susan Hollins, for her friendship and discussions over the years about shared but contrasting memories.

Thanks to all at Myriad Editions: Candida Lacey and my editor Corinne Pearlman for taking on this story when it was but a sapling and helping it to grow stronger; to Corinne for her patience, kind reassurance and deft pruning; Vicky Blunden; Holly Ainley; and Linda McQueen.

To Kendra Boileau at Penn State University Press.

To Hannah Berry in her role as my excellent professional mentor for this project.

Thanks to Rooster, the tortoise, for not grumbling too much when rudely plucked from the undergrowth to pose for reference photos.

Other more willing models: John Austin, Deb Joffe, Kath Bridge, Bristol swans and gulls.

To the marvellous supportive communities and leaders of Graphic Medicine and Laydeez do Comics, and the opportunity to present early incarnations of this work at their events in 2011 and beyond.

Thanks to people I've met in person and online from 'childless-by-circumstance' and ME/CFS communities, who all lead valuable lives — I've benefited hugely from their collective wisdom and strength.

To the following people for their steady encouragement: MK Czerwiec, Judy Knight, Katie Green, Simon Gurr, Lucy Marcovitch, Bonnie Millard, Mita Mahato, and Ian Williams.

Experts whom I consulted from fields of health, science and education: Elizabeth Season, Lucy Marcovitch, Dr Ian Williams, Dr Brian Degger, David P. Barash (Professor of Psychology at the University of Washington), Sarah Blaffer Hardy (evolutionary anthropologist), Eva Natamba (Office for National Statistics), Arri Coomarasamy (Professor of Gynaecology, University of Birmingham).

Thanks also to: Arvon Foundation Graphic Novels Class of 2011, Tom Adams, Kay Austin, Alinah Azadeh, Eunice and John Baker, Mark Barber, Arthur Berwick, Bluelou, Gareth Brookes, Jez Butler, Darryl Cunningham, Jill Davies, Jody Day, Kate Evans, Jez Francis, David Gaffney, Andrew Godfrey, Joe Gordon, Paul Gravett, Jessica Hepburn, Richard Hollins, Polly Hulse, Sarah Lightman, Juliet Roche, Matthew Roche, Susan McLuckie, Sarah Morgan, Andy Oliver, Kenny Penman, Philippa Perry, Sam Pine, Kathryn Samson, Ben Sansum, Katie Scaife, staff of EPAC St Michael's Hospital, Nicola Streeten, Susan Squier, John Swogger, Bryan Talbot, Mary Talbot, Julie Taylor Kent, Rupert Taylor, Ravi Thornton, and my parents.

The artwork stage of this project was supported using public funding from the National Lottery through Arts Council England. This support was invaluable in allowing me time to work solely on the book.

LOTTERY FUNDED

Supported using public funding by ARTS COUNCIL ENGLAND

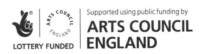

GLOSSARY

A&E: Accident and Emergency, UK

ART: Assisted Reproductive Technology

ME/CFS: Myalgic Encephalomyelitis/Chronic Fatigue Syndrome, aka PVFS (Post-Viral Fatigue Syndrome) and CFIDS (Chronic Fatigue Immune Dysfunction Syndrome), (Source: ME Association website)

Basal Body Temperature (BBT): Lowest resting body temperature, used to help chart ovulation

EPAC: Early Pregnancy Assessment Clinic

Glandular Fever: aka Infectious Mononucleosis (Mono)

GP: General Practitioner, UK

hCG: Human Chorionic Gonadotropin

IVF: In Vitro Fertilisation

NHS: National Health Service, UK

TSH: Thyroid-Stimulating Hormone

UCCA: Universities Central Council on Admissions, now known as UCAS

BIBLIOGRAPHY/SOURCES

The following books were helpful to me (see pp220–29) and are recommended to anyone who wants to read further. Those pages are a mixture of my own thoughts and things I learnt from the books:

Mother of All Myths (How Society Moulds and Constrains Mothers) by Aminatta Forna, HarperCollins Publishers, 1999

Wonder Woman (The myth of 'having it all') by Virginia Haussegger, Allen & Unwin, 2005

The Feminine Mystique by Betty Friedan, Penguin Modern Classics, 2010

Her Blood is Gold (Awakening to the Wisdom of Menstruation) by Lara Owen, Archive Publishing, 2008

The Baby Matrix (Why Freeing Our Minds From Outmoded Thinking About Parenthood & Reproduction Will Create A Better World) by Laura Carroll, LiveTrue Books, 2012

Delusions of Gender (The Real Science Behind Sex Differences) by Cordelia Fine, Icon Books, 2010

PHOTO/COLLAGE CREDITS

p32: Elizabeth Davidson; p51: Letter, kindly returned by Susan McLuckie; p105: John Austin; p112: Albert Downes, John Austin, unknown ancestor; p180: Pressed flower, Judy Knight, collected April 28, 1954; p234: *The Gifts* contributor card photo, Bristol Museum and Art Gallery

Notes on artistic works mentioned and permissions

pp25–7, 34: *How a Baby Is Made* © Per Holm Knudsen 1971, pub. Pan Books Ltd, 1975

p27: *Grease*, dir. Randal Kleiser, cinematography by Bill Butler, Paramount Pictures, 1978

pp29–30, 41: *Jackie* (magazine), pub. D.C. Thomson & Co. Ltd

p39: 'Too Much Too Young', by Jerry Dammers and Lloyd Chalmers, performed by The Specials, 1980

p47–48: 'I've Never Been to Me', by Ron Miller and Kenneth Hirsch, performed by Charlene, 1982

p49: *EastEnders*, BBC UK soap opera, 1985

pp49–50: *Threads*, BBC TV film about nuclear holocaust, 1984

p64: *Childbirth*, by Jean Dubuffet, 1944; postcard, Museum of Modern Art

p64: Postcard words by Susan Hollins, with kind permission

pp95–6, 116: 'Hoppípolla' – Sigur Rós (Birgisson/Dyrason/Holm/Sveinsson) Licensed courtesy of Universal Music Publishing Ltd

p103: *Place* by Magdalena Jetelová, Forest of Dean Sculpture Park

p108: Font, 'Pixelmix', by Andrew Tyler

pp172, 233–5: *The Gifts*, by Alinah Azadeh, Bristol Museum and Art Gallery/the shape of things, 2010

pp226-7: Font, 'Kingthings Printingkit', by Kingthings